Psychiatric Nursing Clinical Companion

DEBORAH ANTAI-OTONG,
MS, RN, CNS, PMHNP, CS, FAAN
Veterans Administration North Texas Health Care System
Dallas, Texas

THOMSON
™
DELMAR LEARNING

Australia Canada Mexico Singapore Spain United Kingdom United States

NOTICE TO THE READER

Publisher does not warrant or guarantee any of the products described herein or perform any independent analysis in connection with any of the product information contained herein. Publisher does not assume, and expressly disclaims, any obligation to obtain and include information other than that provided to it by the manufacturer.

The reader is expressly warned to consider and adopt all safety precautions that might be indicated by the activities herein and to avoid all potential hazards. By following the instructions contained herein, the reader willingly assumes all risks in connection with such instructions.

The publisher makes no representation or warranties of any kind, including but not limited to the warranties of fitness for particular purpose or merchantability, nor are any such representations implied with respect to the material set forth herein, and the publisher takes no responsibility with respect to such material. The publisher shall not be liable for any special, consequential, or exemplary damages resulting, in whole or part, from the readers' use of, or reliance upon, this material.

Delmar Learning Staff
Vice President, Health Care SBU: William Brottmiller
Editorial Director: Cathy L. Esperti
Acquisitions Editor: Matthew Kane
Developmental Editor: Marjorie A. Bruce
Editorial Assistant: Erin Silk
Marketing Director: Dawn Gerrain
Channel Manager: Jennifer McAvey
Executive Prodution Manager: Karen Leet
Project Editor: Mary Ellen Cox
Production Editor: Anne Sherman
Art/Design Coordinator: Connie Lundberg-Watkins

Printed in Canada

1 2 3 4 5 6 7 8 9 10 XXX 08 07 06 05 04 03

For more information, contact Delmar Learning, Executive Woods, 5 Maxwell Drive, P.O. Box 8007, Clifton Park, NY 12065-8007, or find us on the World Wide Web at http://www.delmarhealthcare.com

ISBN: 1-4018-1508-1

Contents

Aggressive Disorders, Suicide, and Other Self-Destructive Behaviors

1

• Key Terms

Hopelessness: A state of despondency and absolute loss of hope.

Lethality: Level of dangerousness or injury.

Self-Destructive Behavior: Behavior that tends to harm or destroy self.

Self-Mutilation: The act of self-induced pain or tissue destruction void of the intent to kill oneself.

Suicidal Ideation: Thought or idea of suicide.

Suicidal Intent: Refers to the degree to which the person intends to act on his suicidal ideations.

Suicidal Threat: Verbalization of imminent self-destructive action, which, if carried out, has a high probability of leading to death.

Suicide: The act of killing oneself.

Harm associated with suicide is a major health care concern in the United States. The need for preventive measures that target high-risk groups is great. Because mental illness is a powerful risk factor for suicide, psychiatric nurses must play key roles in its prevention.

2 CHAPTER 1 Aggressive Disorders, Suicide, and Other Self-Destructive Behaviors

SELF-DESTRUCTIVE BEHAVIORS

Causes

High-risk groups for self-mutilating are clients with mental retardation, those with pervasive developmental disorders such as autistim, those with psychosis, those who have a history of childhood abuse, or those with borderline personality disorders.

Aggression and self-injurious behaviors also have been linked to decreased serotonergic levels in clients diagnosed with borderline personality disorder.

Symptoms

Roy (1985) classified **self-destructive behaviors** as direct or indirect. *Direct patterns of self-destruction* refer to those behaviors that directly affect the client's physical and mental well-being such as suicide, anorexia, alcohol and substance abuse, and self-mutilation. *Indirect patterns of self-destruction* include high-risk behaviors that may cause harm such as promiscuity, unsafe sexual practices, prostitution, abusive relationships, dangerous sports, and compulsive gambling.

Other actions include other self-mutilation behaviors such as hair pulling, nail biting, burning, picking at wounds, and hacking or cutting. Winchel and Stanley (1992) defined **self-mutilation** behaviors as those that cause deliberate harm to one's body without the conscious intent of suicide. Self-injurious behaviors also include destruction of nails, cuticles, injurious masturbation, head banging, or rocking.

TREATMENT

Serotonin reuptake inhibitors have consequently been effective in the treatment of self-injurious behaviors, and depression suggests a biological component to these disorders. Self-injurious behaviors, such as nail-biting and hair-pulling symptoms, have been relieved by fluoxetine (Prozac) and clomipramine (Anafranil) (Primeau & Fontaine, 1987).

SUICIDE

The term **suicide** stems from the Latin word *sui*, of oneself, and *cidus* from *caedre*, "to kill." Shneidman (1985) described suicide as "the conscious act of self-induced annihilation," and he emphasized the importance of psychosocial stressors and the inability to resolve intolerable pain by stopping "consciousness."

Suicidal ideations are thoughts of injury or demise of self but not necessarily a plan, intent, or means. **Suicidal intent** refers to the degree to which the person intends to act on his suicidal ideations. A **suicidal threat** is verbalization of an imminent self-destructive action, which, if carried out, has a high probability of leading to death (Shneidman, 1985).

Causes

Illnesses such as depression, bipolar disorder, alcoholism, personality disorders, and schizophrenia increase the risk of suicide (Beck, Brown, Berchick, Stewart, & Steer, 1990; Goldberg, Garno, Leon, Kocsis, & Portera, 1998; Mann, Waternaux, Haas, & Malone, 1999; Radomsky, Haas, Mann, & Sweeney, 1999). Other risk factors include male gender, previous attempts, psychotic disorders, European American ethnicity, genetic or familial influences, panic disorder, social isolation, and aging. Over 90 percent of clients who commit suicide have a mental illness at the time of their death (Harris & Barraclough, 1998; Mann et al., 1999; Strakowski, McElroy, Keck, & West, 1996). Developmental and biological factors also place individuals at risk for suicide. See Table 1–1, Clinical Factors of High Suicide Risk.

Socioeconomic, ethnic, and cultural factors influence suicide rates. Cultural causes that buffer individuals from suicide (Gibbs, 1988; Shaffer, 1988) include:

- Negative perceptions of suicide
- Strong social support systems
- Networking generated by families who experience discrimination or extreme stress. Conversely, cultures that condone substance abuse, neglect, social isolation, and violence increase the risk of suicide (Gibbs, 1988).

Table 1–1 • Clinical Factors of High Suicide Risk

Psychological

Hopelessness
Helplessness
Depression
Cognitive Impairment

Behavioral

History of suicide attempts
Poor impulse control
Alchoholism
Substance abuse

Sociocultural

Family history of suicide or attempts
Previous attempts
Recent significant loss
Poor support systems
Chaotic or disorganized family systems

Neurobiological

Neurochemical dysregulation
Genetic
Hormonal imbalances (e.g., as detected by dexamethasone suppression and thyroid-stimulating hormone tests)
Physical illness (e.g., HIV positive, terminal, debilitating)

Major Demographic

Unmarried (separated, divorced, widowed)
Male older than 65 years of age
White (European American)
Protestant
Mental illness (e.g., depression, schizophrenia)
Alcoholism or substance abuse

HIV, human immunodeficiency virus.

Recent advances in neuroscience and neurobiology suggest a relationship between suicide and altered neurological factors such as genetics, neuroendocrine, and neurochemical functioning in the brain.

Genetic factors have also been linked to the prevalence of major depression and suicidal behavior.

Social problems such as chaotic family systems, child-parent conflict, divorce, violence, or child abuse increase the likelihood of adolescent suicide.

Stress plays a major role in adaptation, and an inability to resolve stress results in crisis. Crisis often generates disorganization and feelings of helplessness and hopelessness.

A previous suicide attempt is often the best predictor of death by suicide (Cheng, Chen, Chen, & Jenkins, 2000).

Clients with histories of poor impulse control, such as those with personality disorders, psychosis, and alcoholism, are at risk for suicide.

Suicide generally occurs within chaotic and stressful environments or relationships (Helig & Klugman, 1970).

People who are actively drinking are particularly vulnerable to suicide when they have comorbid depression and have experienced a recent loss.

Adolescence is a time of intense emotional and biological changes. Puberty increases vulnerability to stress and impaired self-concept as youths search for identity within society.

Several factors such as significant losses, feelings of isolation, and poor physical health have been found to be consistent predictors of suicidal behaviors in the older adult.

Symptoms

Major depression is represented by a constellation of core neurovegetative behaviors such as altered mood, abnormal sleeping patterns, diminished libido, abnormal eating patterns, and impaired cognitive function.

Clients with depression often feel hopeless, worthless, inadequate, and guilty. These clients have already given up and feel they do not deserve happiness.

Hopelessness is a fundamental suicide predictor.

Depressed clients may willfully distort their experiences and isolate themselves from loved ones to resolve their perception of being a burden or to be remorseful of their present illness.

Children as young as 2 or 3 years of age have been found to have suicidal behaviors, such as attempting to jump from high places, verbalizing wishes to kill oneself, and attempting to hang oneself or inject poison (Rosenthal & Rosenthal, 1984).

Depressed adolescents, like depressed adults, usually experience impaired cognitive function and coping skills. They also tend to view themselves and the world as negative or hopeless.

Key Facts

It is a common fallacy that people who threaten to kill themselves are not likely to commit suicide. The opposite is true: an estimated 20 to 30 percent of clients who commit suicide have made previous threats or attempts to do so (Leon, Friedman, Sweeney, Brown, & Mann, 1990).

Estimates of the lifetime risk of death by suicide among clients with borderline personality disorder range from 8 to 10 percent, which is similar to the prevalence among those diagnosed with major depression (Gunderson, 2001). A review of published studies by Duberstein and Conwell (1997) estimated that 30 to 40 percent of clients who commit suicide have an Axis II diagnosis, of which the most frequent was borderline personality disorder.

Suicide in older people is a major national health problem, and reducing its occurrence is a national priority. People 65 years old and older have the highest rate of completed suicides in the United States (19 deaths per 100,000 persons), and these rates are six times higher than the national average (McIntosh, 1995; National Center for Health Statistics, 1991).

TREATMENT

The nursing assessment is a vital part of identifying populations at risk for suicide. The client needs a comprehensive physical and psychosocial assessment to determine reasons for seeking treatment, level of dangerousness to self and others, present and past coping patterns, and the quality of current support systems.

Past suicide attempts must be explored along with reasons for their failure and whether the client was under the influence of alcohol or other intoxicants. Nurses can explore the meaning of past suicide attempts by asking clients the following questions:

- How many suicide attempts have you made?
- How have you tried to kill yourself (actual behavior)? Did you want to die? When was the last time?
- What are your feelings about the uncompleted attempt(s) (clues about the client's attitude regarding the attempt)?
- What were the circumstances of each (i.e., What types of stressors [changes] were you experiencing at the time?)?
- What happened before the attempt that made you believe killing yourself was an option?
- Did you plan the attempt or did you do it on the spur of the moment (impulsivity)?
- Were you drinking or abusing substances at the time or shortly before the attempt?
- What type of treatment did you receive after the attempt(s)?

Questions about past suicide attempts serve as the basis for developing nursing interventions to prevent or reduce the incidence of present or future suicides. Assessing the meaning of present and past coping patterns needs to include verbal and nonverbal cues.

Approaching the client in a calm, nonjudgmental manner is the basis of a therapeutic alliance. The primary intervention of working with the suicidal client is prevention. Effective communication is fundamental to helping the client understand his behavior. Assessing suicide risk involves recognizing risk factors and understanding the effect of psychosocial stressors on biological processes and cognitive functioning. Several considerations

(continues)

TREATMENT *(continued)*

can assist in evaluating suicide risk. They include:

- Determining whether the client has a suicidal plan. The client may express thoughts of dying, such as " I want to kill myself" or "I wish I could go to sleep and not wake up." Suicidal plans need to be taken seriously because they indicate that thorough planning and working through have already taken place. A suicide note suggests that the client is resolved to kill himself, and the ambivalence of wanting to live or die has been worked through. Assessing for suicidal plans includes asking "Are you having thoughts of killing yourself?" Nurses need to make sure that they are speaking the same language as the client, because he may not know what the word *suicide* means.
- Determining the dangerousness of the suicide attempt. It is essential to assess the level of lethality. The term **lethality** refers to the potential degree of injury caused by suicidal gestures or attempts. Direct questions need to be asked about the suicide to assess the suicidal potential. Degrees of lethality range from high risk (e.g., shooting, hanging, stabbing, or using carbon monoxide) to lower risk (e.g., overdosing on 5 acetaminophen [regular-strength] tablets). The client's perception of the incident determines the seriousness of the attempt, except in cases when the attempt is minimized.

When the client is assessed to have a definite suicidal plan, the next question involves assessing lethality. The second concern is providing safety and preventing suicide. This is generally done by offering the client referral for evaluation for acute inpatient psychiatric or other means of treatment, such as the crisis mobile team or day hospital, to provide crisis intervention and further evaluation of suicidality and the treatment of underlying mental illness.

Preoccupation with suicide or dying is a symptom of distress and ineffective coping reactions. Suicidal thoughts and plans must be thoroughly assessed to determine their duration and how they have been responded to in the past. It is also important to assess the client's reasons for not acting on the thoughts. Information needs to be documented, and the client needs to be assessed for level of dangerousness to self and others at the present time. The client also needs to be asked about specific circumstances that would make him act on the thoughts.

Most suicidal clients tend to be ambivalent about dying. That is, a part of them usually wants to die and another part wants to live. The part that wants to live usually communicates despair and pain though verbal and nonverbal cues. These cues must be taken seriously and their meaning must be thoroughly assessed. The client who has a specific plan, means, and intent is at serious risk for suicide. Questions such as, "What has stopped you from acting on these thoughts or plans in the past?" elicit information about the imminence of suicide. Some clients may respond with "I don't want to hurt my family" or "I know this is a silly idea." Inquiring about ways they have handled similar thoughts is useful in assessing impulse control and coping patterns.

Assess the clients' present and past substance abuse history, particularly when comorbid psychiatric and physical conditions exist.

Clients with chronic and debilitating illnesses need to be assessed for depression and suicide potential.

Understanding coping patterns throughout the life span helps the nurse recognize the significance of prevention and health promotion. Table 1–2 summarizes the prevalence and causative factors of suicide across the life span.

Childhood suicidal behaviors often represent a family problem. Ideally, assessing the children should take place in an emotionally and physically safe environment. For older children, a quiet room is adequate. Younger children require a room with ample space for toys and art materials. Assessing the child's role within the

(continues)

Table 1–2 • **Prevalence and Causative Factors of Suicide across the Life Span**

	Prevalence	Causative Factors
Childhood	Unknown (some accidents may be suicide); predicted to increase 13% for ages 10–14 years by 2000	Affective disorder (depression), family and developmental factors
Adolescence	6–13% have attempted suicide; predicted to increase 94% for ages 15–19 years by 2000	Affective disorders, conduct and antisocial disorders, substance abuse, family disorganization
Early and Middle Adulthood	15% of those with major ` depression commit suicide; 15% of those with schizophrenia commit suicide; 80% of those who commit suicide have made previous attempts; 15% of alcoholics commit suicide	Depression, schizophrenia, previous attempts, lack of psychosocial resources, alcoholism and substance abuse, major psychiatric and physical health problems
Older Adulthood	17% have attempted suicide	Loss, feelings of isolation, poor physical health status
Total Population	12% have attempted suicide	Mental illness, alcoholism

Note. Data from *Vital Statistics of the United States: Vol. 2, Mortality—part A (for the years 1966–1988)*, by the National Center for Health Statistics, 1991, Washington, DC: U.S. Government Printing Office. Adapted with permission.

TREATMENT *(continued)*

family context is important to evaluating the meaning of suicidal behavior (Antai-Otong, 2001; Rauch & Rappaport, 1994). Children's understanding about death is crucial in determining the lethality of any ideation. Asking about previous experiences with death, such as the death of a pet or family member, provides some understanding about the child's grasp of death.

Assessing the adolescent requires establishing an alliance. Forming an alliance with an adolescent requires a nonthreatening approach. The nurse can begin the process with inquiries about neutral topics such as school and interests before asking about reasons for seeking treatment or family problems. This process must start as soon as possible and include taking dynamic efforts to assess the client's mental and physical status. These early nurse-client interactions foster trust and provide immediate emotional support to the adolescent and family in crisis.

All suicidal gestures are significant in children and adolescents. The youth with a history of previous attempts must be protected and probably hospitalized to evaluate the risk for harm when presenting behaviors that are dangerous to the youth or others or when outpatient treatment has failed. Outpatient treatment is appropriate when the youth does not pose an imminent danger to self or others and the family is motivated to participate in treatment. Treatment strategies are usually multimodal, consisting of crisis intervention and psychodynamic, psychopharmacologic, cognitive, behavioral, and family therapy.

Suicidal behaviors in older adults, as in other age groups, must be assessed early, and measures to prevent it are major nursing goals. Establishing therapeutic relationships are critical to this process because nurses can identify client resources and develop effective interventions that increase self-esteem and adaptive coping skills.

RESOURCES

Please note that because Internet resources are of a time-sensitive nature and URL addresses may change or be deleted, searches should also be conducted by association or topic.

Internet Resources

http://www.healthfinder.gov
Department of Health and Human Services

http://www.nami.org   National Alliance for the Mentally Ill National Web Page

http://www.cf.nlm.nih.gov   National Institute of Health

http://www.nimh.nih.gov   National Institute of Mental Health

http://www.reidpsychiatry.com
Psychiatry and the Law

2 Altered Sensory Perception Disorders and Schizophrenia

• Key Terms

Alogia: Inability to speak owing to a mental condition or a symptom of dementia.

Altered Sensory Perception: Refers to the physical and psychological changes that affect brain functioning, behavior patterns, and the five senses.

Anhedonia: Refers to an inability to experience pleasure in activities and life.

Autism: Denotes the presence of abnormal and impaired development in social and communication skills and severely restricted activity and interests.

Avolition: Decreased motivation.

Delusion: A fixed, false belief unchanged by logic.

Negative Symptoms: Denote schizophrenic symptoms associated with structural brain abnormalities. Most negative symptoms include blunted affect, inability to experience pleasure, apathy, a lack of feeling, and impaired attention.

Positive Symptoms: Refer to schizophrenic symptoms with good premorbid functioning, acute onset, and positive response to typical and atypical antipsychotics. Common positive symptoms include hallucinations, delusions, disorganized thinking and speech, and gross behavioral disturbances.

Current research indicates that the global burden of mental illness is second only to cardiovascular disease throughout the world (U.S. Public Health Service, Department of Health and Human

Services [DHHS, 1999]). In the United States, one out of five Americans incurs a mental disorder throughout any year (DHHS, 1999). Statistics for children ages 9 to 17 years are even higher, with 25 percent of them receiving mental health treatment within a year's time (DHHS, 1999). Direct costs for mental illness is estimated at more than $69 billion. Indirect costs to the individuals affected by mental disorders can be catastrophic when appropriate treatment is not accessed or available (Buckley, 2000). Persons from diverse racial and ethnic groups often have more severe outcomes from mental illness because of societal economic problems and the lack of culturally competent mental health providers. The most prevalent mental disorders involve the altered sensory brain disorders of schizophrenia and mood disorders (DHHS, 1999).

DELUSIONAL DISORDER

Delusional disorder involves a fixed false belief. Subtypes include grandiosity, jealousy, persecutory, and somatic (APA, 2000).

Causes

The functional system is comprised of the language and memory systems located within the amygdala and the hippocampus regions (e.g., Broca and Wernicke's areas, respectively) of the brain. The functional system is responsible for the integration of learning and memory within in a person's brain. It is postulated that structural changes within these areas may lead to the development of altered sensory perception problems such as hallucinations and **delusions**.

Symptoms

Individuals who incur psychosis may experience altered sensory perceptions of their smell, taste, sight, hearing, or touch senses (i.e., hallucinations, delusions, illusions).

An affected person may think he is Napoleon or the President of the United States or some other important person. Affected persons may also have *somatic* (injury or illness regarding their body), *nihilistic* (world is ending or they are dying), *persecutory* (being threatened, spied on), *religious* (having special religious powers), or *sexual* (others know about their sexual activity and that the activity causes illness) (APA, 2000).

TREATMENT

Psychiatric-based hallucinations, delusions, and illusions are best treated through the use of antipsychotic medications.

SCHIZOAFFECTIVE DISORDER

Symptoms

Schizoaffective disorder is a disturbance that has at least one month of symptoms that include two or more of the following:

hallucinations, delusions, disorganized speech, inappropriate behaviors, catatonia, and negative symptoms. Additional symptoms include mood disturbance (e.g., depressed, manic, or mixed). Schizoaffective disorder is of a shorter duration and intensity than schizophrenia.

There are a number of other disorders that may exhibit symptoms of altered sensory perception or psychosis. Among these are schizoaffective, delusional, and mood disorders.

TREATMENT

Psychiatric assessment of children is similar to that for adults. However, differential diagnosis for children is challenging because of the varied developmental stages that they undergo. The following guidelines have been suggested regarding psychiatric diagnosis in children (Perry & Antai-Otong, 1995):

- Delineation between the normal and abnormal developmental behaviors
- Length and occurrence of symptomatology
- Presenting symptomatology
- Social interaction and adaptation
- Length of abnormal or inappropriate behaviors

As with adults, a complete workup needs to be accomplished. See Table 2–1 for the diagnostic tests.

SCHIZOPHRENIA

Altered sensory perception refers to the physical and psychological changes that affect brain functioning, behavior patterns, and the five senses. Schizophrenia, one of the primary altered sensory brain disorders, has been widely researched.

Causes

The current etiology on schizophrenia delineates five primary explanations of the disorder: genetic, psychodynamic, neurobiological, substance abuse, and the diathesis stress theories (Crespo-Facorro et al., 2001; Gottesman & Moldin, 1997). All but the substance abuse theory are discussed next.

The *genetic theory* is connected to the structural changes that have been seen on computer tomography (CT) within the brains of persons diagnosed with schizophrenia. It is postulated that these structural changes lead to the development of neurological and developmental alterations. These alterations then increase a person's risk to develop schizophrenia (Gottesman & Moldin, 1997; Owen, 2000).

In addition, there seems to be a genetic pattern for development of schizophrenia within family systems (APA, 2000; Perry & Antai-Otong, 1995; Wuerker, Fu, Haas, & Bellack, 2002).

There have been some studies regarding the effect of influenza on fetal development. This research indicates that there is an increased risk for the development of schizophrenia when mothers incur influenza during their second trimester. This risk is based on structural cell proliferation changes within the hippocampus (Perry & Antai-Otong, 1995).

The *psychodynamic theory* evolved from the work of Bleuler (1950) and Freud (1959). Their works indicate that schizophrenia developed because of the psychic alterations that occurred within a person. In addition, these alterations are contingent on the poor caregiving that is provided within the child's environment. However, both of these scholars believed that the psychic alterations are somehow tied to the genetic or physiological changes that develop within the growing child's environment.

The *neurobiological theory* involves the changes that occur within the brains of persons diagnosed with schizophrenia. These changes occur within five system areas: three anatomic systems—prefrontal, limbic, and basal ganglia—and two functional systems—language and memory.

Overall, normal anatomic brain tissue and capacity are reduced in persons who

Table 2–1 • Diagnostic Tests: Children and Adolescents with a Suspected Psychotic Disorder

	Tests and Examinations	Rationale
Physical	Configuration and size of head Circumference of head Facial signs, e.g., nose, mouth, brows Handprinting or dermatoglyphics	To assess for microcephaly, hydrocephalus, Down syndrome
Neurological	Skull radiographs CT scan, MRI Electroencephalogram	Disturbances in motor areas, e.g., spasticity or hypotonia Sensory impairments, e.g., hearing, visual cranial defects, central nervous system abnormalities, and seizure disorders, to assess for Down syndrome
Laboratory	Urinalysis and serum Hearing and speech evaluations	Metabolic disorders Enzymatic abnormalities (chromosomal disorders, such as Down syndrome) Hearing and speech development, to assess for mental retardation
Psychological	Screening tests such as Gesell, Catell, Bayley (for infants) Stanford-Binet, Wechsler Intelligence Scale for Children— Revised (WISC-R), Bender-Gestalt, Benton Visual Retention tests	Developmental assessment Detection of brain damage

CT, computed tomography; MRI, magnetic resonance imaging

have schizophrenia. For example, scans of these persons' brains illustrate an enlarged third ventricle, decreased tangles, and less electrical activity. The cortex of the brain is the last section of the human brain to develop. It is responsible for the coordination of information into the rest of the brain, controls arousal and emotions, focuses attention, and assists in the formation of abstract thinking (Guyton & Hall, 2000).

The limbic system regulates an individual's emotions and memory. Someone with the diagnosis of schizophrenia has a structural change within the limbic system that often creates impulsivity, aggression, and sexually inappropriate behavior. In addition, these individuals often have problems with learning new information owing to the damage within the hippocampus area (Guyton & Hall, 2000).

Groupings of neurons are involved in the release of the neurotransmitters of dopamine (Dz), norepinephrine (NE), serotonin (5-HT), acetylcholine (M), and gamma-aminobutyric acid (GABA) within the cell body. There is a compatibility with a neurotransmitter (e.g., the key) and receptor (e.g., lock) that causes the activation mechanism of the process. It is postulated that persons with schizophrenia may have too much or too little of the neurotransmitters available. This imbalance creates the development of the positive and negative symptoms that are associated with the disorder (Fox & Kane, 1996; Wykes, Reeder, Corner, Williams, & Everitt, 1999).

One of the most popular theories regarding development of schizophrenia is the *diathesis stress*, or combination, *theory.* According to this theory, individuals develop schizophrenia based on the interaction of a number of factors. These factors include genetics, environmental (e.g., both physical and psychological), anatomic and functional systems, and the contribution of stressors (e.g., neurological dysfunction, psychobiological and environmental factors, use of alcohol and other substances, and interpersonal relationships) (Lutz & Warren, 2001). The predisposition to develop schizophrenia is created by changes within a person's physical, psychological, spiritual, or cultural environments in conjunction with the presence of stressors. This combination approach to development of schizophrenia is supported by research regarding the interaction variables (O'Connor, 1994).

The development of schizophrenia in persons is contingent on changes that occur in the anatomic, functional, and neurochemical systems of the brain. Anatomic or structural alterations may lead to functional changes in language and memory sections of the brain. In addition, alterations in the neurotransmitter system, at the release, receptor, activation, or reuptake locations, may alter the anatomic or functional systems. The consequence of these changes is the development of the positive and negative symptoms in persons incurring schizophrenia (Fox & Kane, 1996).

The diagnosis of schizophrenia is rarely made in children. However, there is some evidence indicating that some children who are diagnosed with autism may be diagnosed with schizophrenia once they become adults (Perry & Antai-Otong, 1995). **Autism** is manifested by the presence of abnormal and impaired development in social and communication skills and severely restricted activity and interests.

Symptoms

Schizophrenia is a disorder associated with a variety of a complex combination of symptoms, including hallucinations, delusions, disorganized speech, disorganization, flat affect, alogia, and avolition (APA, 2000; Bleuler, 1950). Schizophrenia generally emerges during adolescence or in the 20s or 30s. However, it may occur in later adulthood (DHHS, 1999). Women generally experience a later onset of schizophrenia and exhibit more mood symptoms than men do (APA, 2000).

Individuals diagnosed with schizophrenia often have more difficulty ascertaining their psychological and physical symptoms because of their perceptual alterations. The *DSM-IV-TR* (APA, 2000) delineates five subtypes of schizophrenia: *paranoid, disorganized, catatonic, undifferentiated,* and *residual.* The specifiers for these subtypes are defined in Table 2–2.

There are two phases for the development of schizophrenia: prodromal and active (Table 2–3). The *prodromal phase* of schizophrenia may occur acutely or has a slower onset. Symptoms within this phase include drastic alteration in the normal behavior patterns, unusual preoccupation regarding other persons, social isolation, and problems in school or work areas (APA, 2000). The *acute phase* has active overt symptoms. These include the manifestation of **positive symptoms** (e.g., hallucinations, delusions, illusions, catatonia) and **negative symptoms** (e.g., flat affect; **alogia**, which is seen as thought and speech disorganization; **anhedonia**, which is seen as lack of pleasure in activities and life; **avolition** or decreased motivation; and inattention) (APA, 2000).

A person with schizophrenia often has trouble concentrating and thinking abstractly. In addition she is often impulsive and may exhibit inappropriate behavior and actions.

Table 2–2 • Major Types of Adult Schizophrenia

Catatonic—marked by a catatonic state or stupor in which the client is unresponsive to his or her surroundings and displays a lack of spontaneous psychomotor activity (rigid posture or bizarre) or mutism

Disorganized—major symptoms include confusion or loose association, disorganized thoughts, and blunt or inappropriate affect

Paranoid—marked by one or more systematic persecutory delusions, auditory hallucinations with a single theme

Undifferentiated—manifested by pronounced delusions, hallucinations, and disorganized thought processes and behavior

Residual—generally there is an absence of pronounced delusions, hallucinations, confusion, or disorganized thoughts or behaviors

Note. Data from *Diagnostic and Statistical Manual of Mental Disorders* (4th edition Text Revision) (*DSM-IV-TR*), by American Psychiatric Association, 2000, Washington, DC: Author. Adapted with permission.

Table 2–3 • Schizophrenia: Course of the Illness

Acute (Active) Phase	Prodromal and Residual Phases
Definition Active Phase: presence of psychotic symptoms—at least one from the list of positive symptoms (*DSM-IV* Option A1)	**Definitions** Prodromal phase—clear deterioration in functioning occurring prior to active phase involving minimum of two symptoms listed below.
Symptoms Positive symptoms • Delusion • Hallucination • Disorganized speech • Bizarre or disorganized behavior Negative symptoms • Flat affect • Avolition • Alogia • Anhedonia • Attention impairment Impairment in functioning (one or more major areas) • Work • Interpersonal relations • Self-care • Failure to achieve expected levels of interpersonal, academic or occupational development	Residual phase—persistence of minimum of two symptoms following active phase. **Symptoms** • Marked social isolation and withdrawal • Marked impairment in role functioning as wage earner, student, or homemaker • Markedly peculiar behavior • Marked disturbance in speech Circumstantial Poverty of speech and content Vague Overelaborate • Odd beliefs • Unusual perceptual experiences • Marked lack of initiative, interests, energy
Minimum Duration One month	**Minimum Duration** Continuous signs persisting a minimum of 6 months Must include active-phase period lasting 1 week to 1 month

Note. Data from *DSM-IV Options Book. Work in Progress*, by American Psychiatric Association Task Force on *DSM-IV*, 1999, Washington, DC: Author. Adapted with permission.

The basal ganglia is responsible for the initiation and control of muscle activity and movements as well as postural changes. A person diagnosed with schizophrenia may have problems with her ability to determine where her body is in relationship to others. Thus, she may accidentally run into others as she walks and moves.

Persons with schizophrenia may have problems understanding language as well as communicating with other persons (DHHS, 1999).

Symptoms of schizophrenia often emerge during adolescence. However, these symptoms are more pronounced than the normal adolescent behavior. Maladaptive behaviors and symptoms may include the ones discussed in the earlier discussion in this chapter as well as the *DSM-IV-TR* (APA, 2000) criteria in Table 2–4 (e.g., extreme social withdrawal and

---

Table 2–4 • *DSM-IV-TR* Diagnostic Criteria for Schizophrenia

A. *Characteristic symptoms:* Two (or more) of the following, each present for a significant portion of time during a 1-month period (or less if successfully treated):
   (1) delusions
   (2) hallucinations
   (3) disorganized speech (e.g., frequent derailment or incoherence)
   (4) grossly disorganized or catatonic behavior
   (5) negative symptoms, i.e., affective flattening, alogia, or avolition

   Note: Only one Criterion A symptom is required if delusions are bizarre or hallucinations consist of a voice keeping up a running commentary on the person's behavior or thoughts, or two or more voices conversing with each other.

B. *Social/occupational dysfunction:* For a significant portion of the time since the onset of the disturbance, one or more major areas of functioning such as work, interpersonal relations, or self-care are markedly below the level achieved prior to the onset (or when the onset is in childhood or adolescence, failure to achieve expected level of interpersonal, academic, or occupational achievement).

C. *Duration:* Continuous signs of the disturbance persist for at least 6 months. This 6-month period must include at least 1 month of symptoms (or less if successfully treated) that meet Criterion A (i.e., active-phase symptoms) and may include periods of prodromal or residual symptoms. During these prodromal or residual periods, the signs of the disturbance may be manifested by only negative symptoms or two or more symptoms listed in Criterion A present in an attenuated form (e.g., odd beliefs, unusual perceptual experiences).

D. *Schizoaffective and Mood Disorder exclusion:* Schizoaffective Disorder and Mood Disorder With Psychotic features have been ruled out because either (1) no Major Depressive, Manic, or Mixed episodes have occurred concurrently with the active-phase symptoms; or (2) if mood episodes have occurred during active-phase symptoms, their total duration has been brief relative to the duration of the active and residual periods.

E. *Substance/general medical condition exclusion:* The disturbance is not due to the direct physiological effects of a substance (e.g., a drug of abuse, a medication) or a general medical condition.

F. *Relationship to a Pervasive Developmental Disorder:* If there is a history of Autistic Disorder or another Pervasive Developmental Disorder, the additional diagnosis of Schizophrenia is made only if prominent delusions or hallucinations are also present for at least a month (or less is successfully treated).

---

communication problems; presence of hallucinations, delusions, and illusions; bizarre thinking; and behavior patterns).

Key Facts

Schizophrenia affects approximately 1.6 percent of the population across all cultural groups (Buckley, 2000; DHHS, 1999). It is estimated that schizophrenia accounts for approximately 2.5 percent of all health care expenditures.

First-degree relatives of individuals with schizophrenia have a 10 percent greater chance of developing the disorder than do persons within the general population. There has also been an in-depth examination of the risk for both identical and fraternal twins' development of schizophrenia. Statistics indicate that there is almost a 50 percent chance of the other identical twin developing schizophrenia when one twin is diagnosed. The chance is reduced to approximately 15 percent when the twins are fraternal (Perry & Antai-Otong, 1995).

TREATMENT

When caring for the client who presents with symptoms of schizophrenia, it is important that the psychiatric-mental health nurse carefully assess the client's cultural viewpoint in order to make a differential diagnosis between a normal cultural practice and the presence of a pathologically based hallucination, delusion, or illusion.

In the past, it was thought that persons with schizophrenia became progressively more debilitated. However, the advent of the concept of recovery, new psychotropic medications, and use of psychotherapy and counseling have been instrumental in facilitating the recovery processes of persons in a different manner.

It is important for the nurse to assist clients with knowledge about the symptoms of their disorder and the treatment options for it. In addition, the use of *advance directives* has been beneficial

for clients. Advance directives are similar to those for persons with physical illnesses. Clients may make decisions regarding their level of care and use of interventions and pharmacologic treatments while they are at a maximum level of psychological health and wellness. In addition, clients will choose an *agent* or someone who is responsible for carrying out their wishes when they decompensate or are at a higher level of symptomatology that may require hospitalization and additional treatment (Srebnik & La Fond, 1999).

Traditional or typical and atypical antipsychotic medications are the ones used for treatment of schizophrenia. All of these medications in some way affect the anatomic and functional systems of the brains. Hence, they assist with ending or minimizing the presence of hallucinations, delusions, and illusions that interfere with a person's ability to recover and function appropriately on a daily basis (see Chapter 28 and Chapter 31 of the core text).

Clozapine (Clozaril) was the first atypical medication. However, additional medications have been developed, including risperidone (Risperdal), olanzapine (Zyprexa), quetiapine (Seroquel), and ziprasidone (Geodon).

Levels and dosages of the antipsychotics need to be adjusted also depending on the age and size of the client. The use of the newer antipsychotics with children is just beginning to be researched. However, current research on the use of these medications with late-in-life-onset schizophrenia indicates that lower, smaller doses of the medications work better for older adults (Goldberg, 2001).

Counseling and psychotherapy are extremely important adjuncts to the use of pharmacologic agents because persons with schizophrenia need a clear understanding of their disorder as well as how to interact with others and manage their symptoms. As previously mentioned, psychoeducation provides clients with an

(continues)

TREATMENT *(continued)*

understanding of schizophrenia, its management, and resource development to facilitate their recovery process (Jerrell, 1999).

Social skills development and stress and crisis management are other important interventions for clients to develop. The symptoms of schizophrenia may interfere with the developmental process that clients move through. Hence, their ability to know how to interact with others may be altered by the presence of their altered sensory perceptions. The use of medications may eliminate this latter occurrence. However, clients may still need assistance in appropriate social skill use.

Finally, *stress and crisis management* is another important skill for persons to learn in order to establish and maintain their recovery process. As with any chronic illness, exacerbation of symptoms may occur. Persons need to be able to manage the stress that is associated with this occurrence. In addition, stress and crisis situations are often part of everyday existence. Clients' development of knowledge about these techniques also contributes to their recovery progression.

There are some specific issues for the generalists and advanced-practice nurses as they provide psychiatric nursing treatment for their clients. Collaboration is the primary role for both the generalist and advanced-practice PMH nurse. In addition, advocacy for client rights is another important role for both practice roles. Finally, it is important for both practice roles of nurses to provide care in a holistic manner that addresses the cultural mind, body, spirit issues for clients.

The generalist nurse is involved in the initial development of the nursing treatment plan for the client. The generalist nurse implements and monitors the plan and the client's response to pharmacologic agents. The generalist nurse may be involved in psychoeducation, social skills, and good health habits classes. The nurse may also participate in the collection of data associated with research projects that clients may be involved in. Finally, the generalist nurse needs to be involved in the use of best practices within in mental health care as it pertains to direct nursing care.

The advanced-practice (AP) PMH nurse is often the coordinator of care for clients and extends the depth of the nursing process. She may be involved as a case manager and coordinator of care and provide medication management within community settings. In addition, she provides counseling and psychotherapy (Raingruber, 2000). The AP PMH nurse may develop and conduct research and evaluation on various aspects of mental health, wellness, and illness (Warren, 1999; 2000).

RESOURCES

Please note that because Internet resources are of a time-sensitive nature and URL addresses may change or be deleted, searches should also be conducted by association or topic.

Internet Resources

http://www.mentalhealth.com/book/p40-sc01.html Schizophrenia Handbook for Families

Anxiety Disorders

3

• Key Terms

Adaptation: Sustaining homeostasis; the ability to mobilize resources and adjust to demands of internal and external environments.

Anxiety: An affect or emotion arising from stress or change accompanied by biological arousal, behavioral responses, and elements of apprehension, impending doom, and tension.

Attachment Theory: Theory based on the classic works of Bowlby and Ainsworth that define attachment or bonding as an evolutionary and biological process of eliciting and maintaining physical closeness between a child and a parent or primary caregiver. This theory also infers that the infant's relationships with early caregivers are responsible for influencing future interactions and relationships.

Cognitive Processes: Higher cortical mental processes, including perception, memory, and reasoning, by which one acquires knowledge, solves problems, employs judgment, and makes plans.

Comorbidity: Coexistence of more than one psychiatric disorder.

Compulsion: Repetitive, ritualistic, unrealistic behaviors used to neutralize or prevent discomfort of stressful events, circumstances or recurring thoughts, images, or impulses such as obsessions.

Depersonalization: A person's subjective sense of feeling unreal, strange, unfamiliar, or emotionally numb.

Derealization: A subjective sense that one's environment is unreal or unfamiliar.

Desensitization: A cognitive-behavioral therapy technique developed by Joseph Wolpe that involves three steps: relaxation training, gradual or hierarchy exposure (using visual imagery or

(continues)

real situations) to an anxiety-provoking or fearful situation or object, and desensitization to the stimulus. This technique is useful in the treatment of phobias.

Dissociation: An unconscious defense mechanism that refers to a detachment or alteration in one's sense of reality, psychogenic amnesia, and perception of self and environment; used by a person to protect self from being overwhelmed by anxiety, usually from a traumatic experience. Memory and feeling related to an event are sealed off from the conscious awareness.

Eye Movement Desensitization and Reprocessing (EMDR): Involves asking the client to imagine an anxiety-provoking or traumatic memory. This technique is used to treat post-traumatic stress disorder by processing a traumatic experience in a non-threatening manner.

Homeostasis: Refers to a state of adaptation or ability to effectively manage internal and external environmental demands.

Neurotransmitter: A central nervous system biochemical involved in facilitating the transmission of impulses across synapses between neurons. Examples include serotonin, dopamine, and norepinephrine.

Obsession: Intrusive, recurrent, and persistent thoughts, impulses, or images.

Progressive Relaxation: A form of relaxation training that involves visualizing and sequentially relaxing specific muscle groups, starting with the scalp to the tips of the toes. This technique involves teaching the client to tense and relax various muscle groups in an effort to reduce tension and stress.

Separation Anxiety: Refers to a common childhood and adolescent anxiety disorder whose symptoms involve panic or intense fear of losing one's primary caregivers.

*The term **anxiety** stems from the Latin word anxietus, which means "to vex or trouble." Anxiety represents uneasiness, and it is an integral aspect of human nature because it plays a crucial role in **adaptation** and **homeostasis** (the ability to mobilize resources and adjust to demands of internal and external environments). It often extends beyond adaptive importance for the individual. Anxiety is a state arising from stress or change and frequently emanates from fear. However, anxiety differs from fear in that it is a diffuse, internal, and anticipatory reaction to danger that may be ambiguous or nonspecific, and the reaction may be disproportionate to the degree of danger.*

ANXIETY DISORDERS— GENERAL

Causes

Anxiety normally accompanies developmental changes and life span issues. Anticipating an examination or new clinical experience is an example of normal anxiety. By acting as a protective response to various situations, anxiety enables individuals to use behaviors such as studying or getting enough sleep before a big exam to reduce their sense of helplessness and frustration. These responses minimize the long-term sequelae of anxiety and promote a state of health. Conversely, maladaptive responses or failure to mobilize homeostatic processes often culminate and contribute to formation of anxiety disorders. Overwhelming and enduring anxiety often produces maladaptive responses that globally affect one's level of functioning.

The *DSM-IV-TR* (APA, 2000) describes anxiety disorders as one of the most common psychiatric conditions (Table 3–1). APA delineates major anxiety disorders as panic disorder with or without agoraphobia, specific phobia and social phobia, obsessive-compulsive disorder, posttraumatic stress disorder, acute stress disorder, and generalized anxiety disorder.

The severity of abnormal anxiety or anxiety disorders varies, but most arise from distinct causes, such as traumatic exposure and exaggerated fears or phobias, and require holistic interventions to reduce their potentially debilitating effects.

Cultural beliefs and practices mediate cognitive, biological, and behavioral responses to danger and fear and determine specific coping and avoidance responses. Cultural beliefs also influence parenting and socialization and are the basis of attachment, separation, sense of security, and one's perception of danger. Ultimately, these factors play key roles in anxiety disorders (Kirmayer, Young, Hayton, 1995).

The foundation of psychoanalytic theory is the premise that various factors, such as conflict, pleasure, morality, and fantasies, are the bases of symptoms and neurosis.

A lack of competency, or sense of nothingness, predictably results in inadequate coping skills and generates empty feelings that result in people viewing their lives as meaningless, aimless, and worthless and having ineffective coping skills. Consequently, maladaptive coping skills produce anxiety, which interferes with the individual's ability to preserve his existence.

Beck, Emery, & Greenberg (1985) defined anxiety from a **cognitive processes** perspective and asserted that it occurs when a threat or danger is perceived. (*Cognitive* refers to thought processes related to judgment, reasoning, comprehension, attitude, and perception of self, the world, and future.)

Behaviorists propose that intense or disabling anxiety is a learned maladaptive response to stress (Eysenck 1990; Wolpe, 1961; Wolpe & Lazarus, 1966).

Families and other psychosocial factors shape various personality traits and one's ability to cope and respond to stress effectively. Specific family qualities, such as a lack of warmth and nurturance or overprotectiveness, increase the likelihood of maladaptive responses in children (Andrews & Crino, 1991; Leon & Leon, 1990).

Bowlby's (1969) **attachment theory** asserted that anxiety initially occurs with separation from early primary caregivers. He described **separation anxiety** as a predictable process involving several stages:

1. Protest (separation anxiety): the child cries and often looks and calls for caregiver(s).
2. Despair (grief and mourning): the child fears that the caregiver will not return.
3. Detachment (coping/defense mechanism): the child emotionally separates from caregivers.

Biological theories of anxiety disorders historically focused on the role of the hypothalmic-pituitary-adrenal (HPA) axis and other neuroendocrine systems that contribute to the physiological and behavioral manifestations of anxiety disorders.

Table 3–1 • Specific Anxiety Disorders

Anxiety Disorder/Condition	DSM-IV-TR Criteria
Acute Stress Disorder	A. Person exposed to a traumatic event that posed threat to self or others' physical integrity; impact on person involves profound fear, powerlessness, or terror
	B. During exposure or after exposure to trauma event, *three* or more of the following dissociative manifestations are present: • numbness, void of emotional responsiveness • "being in a daze" • derealization • depersonalization • dissociative amnesia
	C. The traumatic event is persistently reexperienced in one of the following: recurrent vivid memories, nightmares, flashbacks, and distress (neurobiological arousal) arising from memory of the event
	D. Marked avoidance of stimuli behaviors
	E. Profound anxiety or autonomic arousal
	F. Interference with optimal level of function
	G. Duration of symptoms persists for at least 2 days and no longer than a month and occurs within a month of traumatic exposure
	H. Not due to a substance or medical condition • Differs from post-traumatic stress disorder because manifestations of this disorder must evolve within 1 month and resolve within this 1-month period
Anxiety due to a General Medical Condition	A. Pronounced anxiety, specific anxiety disorder (e.g., panic attacks) is chief complaint
	B. Physiological symptoms directly parallel a general medical condition (e.g., hypoglycemia, hyperthyroidism)
	C. Symptoms are not associated with another mental disorder
	D. Symptoms are not part of the course of delirium
	E. Symptoms interfere with optimal level of functioning
Substance-Induced Anxiety Disorder	A. Pronounced anxiety, specific anxiety disorder (e.g., panic attacks) is chief complaint
	B. Anxiety symptoms evolved during or within the past month of substance intoxication or withdrawal; medication use is directly associated with presenting symptoms
	C. Symptoms are not directly caused by a specific anxiety disorder
	D. Manifestations are not part of the course of delirium
	E. Symptoms interfere with optimal level of function

Note. From *Diagnostic and Statistical Manual of Mental Disorders* (4th edition Text Revision) (*DSM-IV-TR*), by American Psychiatric Association, 2000, Washington, DC: Author. Adapted with permission.

Many of the biological theories of anxiety disorders have come from examination of behavior and adaptation to internal and external stimuli that may result in a positive or negative response (Cannon, 1914; Cloninger, 1986; Eysenck, 1981; Gray, 1988; Pavlov, 1927). A combination of neurochemicals and neuroendocrine systems affects the network of brain regions whenever a person experiences anxiety. Data from animal studies and drug trials posit that dysregulation of three major **neurotransmitters**, specifically, norepinephrine (NE), serotonin (5-HT), and gamma-aminobutyric acid (GABA), contribute to the genesis of diverse anxiety disorders. Refer to Table 3–2 for a compilation of biological theories of anxiety.

Other biological factors that contribute to the genesis of anxiety disorders include the postulation by Gray (1988), which suggests that the affective and motivational systems modulate the sensation and experience of anxiety, and genetic predisposition and personality traits that contribute to neurotransmitter release and function during anxiety states.

The primary theory of anxiety disorders involves dysregulation of benzodiazepine receptors in the central nervous system (CNS). Benzodiazepine receptors have primary binding sites with GABA receptors, which sensitize them to GABA, an inhibitory neurotransmitter. GABA is the principal inhibitory neurotransmitter in the CNS and appears to play a role in modulation and reduction of NE. Presumably, the primary anxiolytic or anxiety-reducing effects of benzodiazepines result from regulating GABA receptors. The inhibitory action of GABA receptors decreases the cells' electrical excitability, hence an anxiolytic effect.

Neuroanatomical theories, like previous biological theories, support the premise that complex factors contribute to the clinical manifestations of various anxiety disorders. Neuroanatomical studies using positron emission tomography (PET) and computed tomography reveal abnormalities in glucose metabolism in the frontal and prefrontal cortex and the basal ganglia of the brain in clients with major anxiety disorders, such as panic disorder and obsessive-compulsive disorder (OCD).

Additional data from other neuroimaging studies suggest that the abnormalities in the basal ganglia and ventral prefrontal cortex are most frequently found in OCD.

Other neuroanatomical studies suggest that individuals with PD are vulnerable to precipitation of acute anxiety symptoms or physiological arousal by intravenous lactate infusion (Dager, Richards, Strauss, & Artru, 1997; Dager et al., 1999). These data support the premise regarding metabolic dysregulation in individuals with PDs. These researchers, like other scientists, hail these findings as another biological marker of anxiety disorders, specifically PD. Although these findings are not definitive, they support the premise that panic attacks and other anxiety disorders arise from specific brain regions and structures. Figure 3–1 shows specific regions of the brain with a relationship to anxiety disorders.

Genetic studies provide strong evidence of familial patterns of anxiety disorders such as generalized anxiety disorder and phobias (Kendler, Neale, Kessker, Heath & Eaves, 1992a; Kendler, Neale, Kessler, Heath & Eaves, 1992b).

Anxiety sensitivity refers to the fear of anxiety-related physiological sensations (i.e., palpitations, diaphoresis), which clients believe are life threatening. Taylor (1995), an anxiety sensitivity theorist, stated that some people are more vulnerable to this condition than others and they are likely to perceive these symptoms as dangerous and life threatening.

Researchers believe that anxiety sensitivity is a risk factor for the development of PD and predict the onset of panic attacks (McNally & Eke, 1996; Schmidt, Lerew, & Jackson, 1999; Schmidt, Lerew, & Joiner, 2000). They also believe that these findings are consistent with social learning theories that suggest a link between information-processing abnormalities in anxiety disorders and their role in anxiety disorders and sensitivity (McNally, 2001; Taylor & Cox, 1998).

Table 3-2 • Compilation of Research Data of Common Biological Theories of Major Anxiety Disorders

Anxiety Disorder	Neurotransmitter(s) Involved	Neuroendocrine System	Neuroanatomical Structures	Biological Response	Behavioral Manifestations
Panic disorder	NE or adrenergic system hyperactivity--> stimulates the limbic system and HPA axis	Activation of the HPA* and HPS† axes--> increase release of CRF, ACTH, GH	Cortical atrophy in the right temporal lobe and decreased volume in the hippocampus (brain region involved in learning and memory)	Tachycardia Tachypnea Palpitations Diaphoresis Sighing Dry mouth Difficulty swallowing Headache	Feelings of doom and fear Avoidant behaviors Hypervigilance Deficits in visual integration, reasoning, memory, and motor coordination performance
	Dysregulation or decrease of 5-HT Decreased GABA levels Overactivity of serotonin	Activation of the LC (Activation of the ANS)	Abnormalities in glucose metabolism in the frontal, prefrontal, and basal ganglia		
Post-traumatic stress disorder	NE hyperactivity	Activation of the HPA and HPS axes--> increase release of CRF, ACTH, GH Activation of the LC	Decreased blood flow to the middle temporal lobe, which plays a role in the extinction of fear through inhibition of amygdala function	Tachycardia Tachypnea Palpitations Diaphoresis Sighing Dry mouth Difficulty swallowing Headache	Feelings of doom and fear Avoidant behaviors Hypervigilance

(continues)

Table 3–2 *(continued)*

Anxiety Disorder	Neurotransmitter(s) Involved	Neuroendocrine System	Neuroanatomical Structures	Biological Response	Behavioral Manifestations
Obsessive-compulsive disorder	Dysregulation of 5-HT 1A		Abnormalities in the basal ganglia and ventral prefrontal cortex Abnormalities in glucose metabolism in the frontal, prefrontal, and basal ganglia Reduced bilateral orbital frontal and amygdala volumes and asymmetry of the hippocampus-amygdala complex	Tachycardia, increased motor activity, palpitations, diaphoresis	Deficits in visual integration, reasoning, memory, and motor coordination performance Ritualistic behaviors

Neurotransmitters: GABA, gamma-aminobutyric acid (inhibitory neurotransmitter); NE, norepinephrine (activating neurotransmitter); 5-HT, serotonin (activating neurotransmitter).

Neuroendocrine system: ACTH, adrenocorticotropic hormone; ANS, autonomic nervous system; CRF, cortisol-releasing factor; GH, growth hormone; HPA, hypothalamic-pituitary-adrenal axis; HPS, hypothalamic-pituitary-somatropin axis; LC, locus ceruleus (specialized neurons that contain the largest number of NE receptors in the ANS).

Note. Data from "Sensitization of the Hypothalamus—Pituitary—Adrenal Axis in Posttraumatic Stress Disorder," by R. Yehuda, 1997, in *Psychobiology of Posttraumatic Stress Disorder* (pp. 57–75) by R. Yehuda & A. C. McFarlane (Eds.). New York: New York Academy of Sciences; from "Psychoneuroendocrinology of Post-Traumatic Stress Disorder," by R. Yehuda, 1998, *The Psychiatric Clinics of North America, 21*, pp. 359–379. Reprinted with permission.

†*Note.* Data from "Generalized Anxiety Disorder: Neurobiological and Pharmacotherapeutic Perspectives," by K. M. Connor and J. R. T. Davidson, 1998, *Society of Biological Psychiatry, 44*, pp. 1286–1294; from "Persistence of Blunted Human Growth Hormone Response to Clonidine in Panic Disorder Following Fluoxetine Treatment," by J. D. Coplan, L. A. Papp, J. Martinez, D. S. Pine, L. A. Rosenblum, T. Cooper, et al., 1995, *American Journal of Psychiatry, 152*, pp. 619–622; from "Adrenergic Receptors: Gⁱ Protein Coupling, Effects of Imipramine, and Relationship to Treatment Outcome," by G. N. M. Gurguis, D. Antai-Otong, S. P. Vo, J. E. Blakely, P. J. Orsulak, F. Petty, et al., 1999, *Neuropsychopharmacology, 20*, pp. 162–176; from "Psychoneuroendocrinology of Anxiety Disorders," by G. M. Sullivan, J. D. Coplan, and J. M. Gorman, 1998, *The Psychiatric Clinics of North America, 21*, pp. 397–412. Adapted with permission.

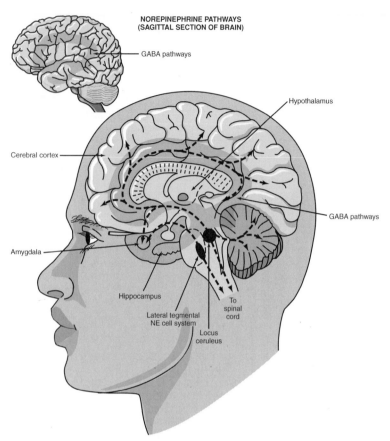

Excessive secretion of the neurotransmitter norepinephrine may be a factor in anxiety disorders. Neurons in the locus ceruleus and the lateral tegmental norepinephrine (NE) cell system receive stimuli of sensory pain or potential danger. In response, they secrete NE in excessive amounts to the cerebral cortex, limbic system (primarily the right temporal lobe), brain stem, and spinal cord to prepare for defense or escape. It has not been determined whether the extreme stress felt by a person with an anxiety disorder is caused by overstimulation of a normal NE system or by physiological differences in that person's NE system. Abnormal serotonin functioning and glucose metabolism are also believed to play a role in anxiety disorders.

Figure 3–1 Neuroanatomy illustration of specific brain regions associated with anxiety disorders. *(Illustration concept: Gail Kongable, MSN, CNRN, CCNR, Department of Neurosurgery, University of Virginia Health Sciences Center.)* **(continues)**

Puberty increases vulnerability to various anxiety disorders, particularly PD, agoraphobia, and social phobia. More interestingly, concerns about one's appearance, acceptance, interactions with peers, and self-confidence tend to replace early childhood fears (Bernstein et al., 1996; Kashani & Orvaschel, 1990).

Symptoms

Major symptoms include autonomic nervous arousal, a sense of doom, depersonalization, paresthesias, and avoidant behaviors.

Manifestations of biological responses include increased respirations and blood

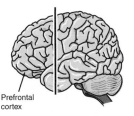

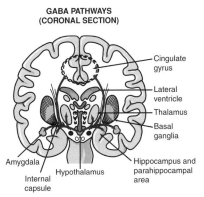

GABA PATHWAYS (CORONAL SECTION)

Prefrontal cortex

Amygdala
Internal capsule
Hypothalamus

Cingulate gyrus
Lateral ventricle
Thalamus
Basal ganglia
Hippocampus and parahippocampal area

Gamma-aminobutyric acid (GABA), an amino acid that serves as the brain's modulator, is an important inhibitory neurotransmitter. Without adequate GABA biosynthesis, release, and activity, the brain would react to the continuous bombardment of even the smallest external and internal stimuli. GABA receptors throughout the brain counteract the effects of the excitatory neurotransmitters norepinephrine and dopamine, preventing disorganized and frenzied responses to continual stimuli and dampening emotional arousal. A person with low levels of GABA or fewer GABA receptors is theoretically more susceptible to anxiety disorders.

HOW DRUGS WORK IN ANXIETY DISORDERS

Uncontrolled anxiety results from unsuccessful defense against anxiety-provoking stimuli. Sometimes anxiety may be related to chronic depression; in such cases treatment with tricyclic antidepressants or monoamine oxidase inhibitors can cause the anxiety to resolve. Drugs that enhance the action of GABA can also be effective in treating anxiety. *(See Figure 2–4 for an explanation of synaptic structures).*

1. Norepinephrine (NE) is synthesized from a dopamine and tyrosine hydroxylase reaction. GABA is synthesized from glutamate, a common amino acid.
2. NE and GABA are stored in synaptic vesicles. *Some antihypertensive drugs interfere with the uptake and storage of NE and deplete NE stores. Although they are prescribed for other reasons these drugs may have the side effect of alleviating anxiety.*
3. Vesicles migrate to the presynaptic membrane and release NE and GABA into the synaptic cleft. *Because amphetamines stimulate the release of NE and block its reuptake, they can contribute to anxiety.*
4. Stimulation of GABA receptor sites makes the target neuron less sensitive to stimulation by NE and other neurotransmitters. *Benzodiazepines such as chlordiazepoxide (Librium) and diazepam (Valium) are effective in treating anxiety because they enhance the binding of GABA to its receptor sites.*
5. The action of NE is stopped by its resorption into the presynaptic terminal. *The tricyclic drug desipramine (Norpramin), used to treat posttraumatic stress disorder, inhibits the resorption of NE, resulting in larger available amounts that may cause increased anxiety.*
6. NE present in the free state within the presynaptic terminal can be broken down by the enzyme monoamine oxidase (MAO). *MAO inhibitors (MAOIs), sometimes used to treat anxiety disorders caused by underlying depression, prevent the breakdown of NE in the presynaptic terminal.*

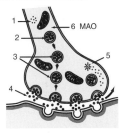

Figure 3–1 *(continued)*

pressure, tachycardia, paresthesias, headache, tightness in the chest, diaphoresis, and lightheadedness. Behavioral responses include rituals, social isolation, avoidance behaviors, help seeking, self-care deficits, and increased dependency. Motor reaction often presents as muscle tension, tremors, shakiness, stuttering, pacing, **compulsions**, and restlessness. Cognitive, or psychological, symptoms include a sense of doom or powerlessness and "going crazy or dying," help-

lessness, vigilance, rumination, preoccupations, **obsessions**, **dissociation**, distortions, and confusion. Table 3–3 lists global manifestations of anxiety responses.

Anxious persons often exaggerate the threat of danger by using faulty cognitions. Faulty or distorted cognitions are characterized by overgeneralization, "awfulizing," and "all or none" perceptions of self, others, and the world. These thoughts often generate intense anxiety and impaired social functioning (e.g.,

Table 3–3 • Global Manifestations of Anxiety Responses

Autonomic/ Biological	Motor
• Increased respirations	• Tension
• Shortness of breath	• Pacing
• Tachycardia	• Tremors
• Diaphoresis	• Stuttering
• Dizziness	• Restlessness
• Paresthesias	**Cognitive/ Psychological**
Behavioral	• Sense of doom
• Rituals	• Powerlessness
• Avoidance	• Intense fear
• Increased dependence	• Vigilance
• Clinging	• Rumination
• Following (infant)	• Helplessness
• Crying (infant or school-age child)	• Dissociation
	• Distortions
	• Confusion
	• Overgeneralization

avoidant behaviors), which cause the individual to feel powerless and helpless.

Adult clients are likely to exhibit decrements on neuropsychological testing, specifically on visual integration, reasoning, memory, and motor coordination performance (Purcell, Maruff, Kyrios, & Pantelis, 1998; Robinson, Wu, Munne, Ashtari, 1995).

Key Facts

Anxiety disorders are among the oldest, most recognizable, and prevalent mental disorders, affecting approximately 15 percent of the general population at some point during their lifetime. More significantly, anxiety is one of the most common reasons for seeking medical and psychiatric treatment (Regier, Burke, & Burke, 1990; Regier et al., 1993; Weissman et al., 1997).

Anxiety is a striking feature of most mental disorders and continues to be one of the most common mental disorders, with an estimated 15 percent of the population experiencing it at some time during their lifetime (Regier, et al., 1990). More than 25 years ago, anxiety disorders were classified as anxiety neurosis and delineated into panic and generalized anxiety disorders. The *DSM-IV-TR* (APA, 2000) defines a number of anxiety disorders, including generalized anxiety disorder (GAD); PD; phobias such as agoraphobia, social phobia, specific phobia; OCD; acute stress disorder; and PTSD. (See Table 3–1 for a list of specific anxiety disorders).

TREATMENT

Psychiatric nurses, like other health care providers, face the daily challenge of understanding the meaning of unusual symptoms and responding to various situations in a sociocultural context. An accurate interpretation of the client's experience can only occur when the nurse examines anxiety disorders within the system and sociocultural context in which they occur.

Most anxiety symptoms respond positively to both short-acting and long-acting benzodiazepine medications, which activate GABA receptors, such as lorazepam (Ativan) and diazepam (Valium), respectively (Longo, 1998).

The client must receive appropriate assessment for medical conditions that mimic anxiety disorders. Medical conditions that produce panic-like symptoms include myocardial infarction, mitral valve prolapse, endocrine disorders such as hypoglycemia, respiratory distress, and substance-related disorders. Substance-related disorders such as central nervous system stimulants, anticholinergic intoxication, or alcohol withdrawal pose a challenge to nurses assessing clients with anxiety disorders. Medical examinations are imperative and involve a complete physical examination and other diagnostic tests such as an electrocardiogram (ECG), toxicology screens, and laboratory studies such as electrolytes and cardiac enzymes. The psychobiological assessment provides pertinent information about current prescribed and

(continues)

TREATMENT *(continued)*

over-the-counter medications, past and present medical and psychiatric treatment, nutritional status, and substance-related disorders. Because of the high **comorbidity** of depressive illness, the nurse must also assess the client's risk of dangerousness toward self and others throughout treatment. This also involves assessing the client's past and present coping skills. The client's dietary habits must be a part of this assessment and include caffeine intake; beverages such as coffee, tea, soft drinks; chocolates, and over-the-counter preparations. The nurse must also ask the client and family about alternative or complementary therapies that may also contribute to anxiety such as diet preparations or other stimulants. This holistic database is critical to appropriate diagnosis and treatment of these complex disorders.

Although anxiety disorders in older adults are likely to evolve over time, distinguishing medical conditions that mimic anxiety disorders is a priority in this age group. Before treating these clients for anxiety disorders, the treatment team must make a differential diagnosis. Differential diagnoses are contingent on complete physical and psychiatric examinations.

A complete medical and psychiatric workup focuses on differential diagnoses of medical, polypharmacy, substance use, current and past coping skills, and current and past illnesses. Because polypharmacy is a major concern when caring for these clients, the nurse must ascertain information from both the client and family members regarding over-the-counter medications, herbs or other alternative therapies, treatment compliance, suicide risk, and preference. The client's nutritional status, mental status, and functional status are integral aspects of the assessment and treatment planning.

Major treatment considerations involve age-related physiological factors that affect prescribing and administering agents to older adults. Before initiating treatment, the nurse must also assess the quality of the client's support system. This is particularly significant if the client lives alone or has sensory or cognitive deficits. Because of the high rate of drug interactions, polypharmacy, and adverse drug reaction in this age group, the nurse needs to develop a plan of care that reflects age-specific issues. These clients often require lower and slower increases in drug doses. In addition, because of the high risk of suicide in this age group, they must be assessed throughout treatment for suicide risk and comorbid depressive illness.

Caring for the client with an anxiety disorder requires an understanding of complex processes, such as biological and environmental factors, that contribute to normal and abnormal anxiety.

Understanding the basis of anxiety disorders and specific interventions to treat them enables the generalist psychiatric-mental health nurse to identify the mental health needs of the client experiencing anxiety. This approach provides the basis for interventions that reduce the frequency and severity of symptoms of anxiety. Major nursing interventions include establishing rapport, enhancing present coping skills, assessing maladaptive responses, minimizing the deleterious effects of anxiety, and promoting health maintenance.

As the advanced-practice nurse assumes more responsibilities and manages more complex populations, determining differential diagnosis is a major treatment concern. For instance, performing a psychiatric evaluation also entails a review of systems. A review of systems and ordering diagnostic tests, such as ECG, laboratory studies, and drug levels, enable the nurse to gather data about the client's physical and health status and rule out conditions that have a potentially deleterious impact on certain treatment.

Psychotherapy, prescription of medications, case management, and evaluation of outcome measures are major

(continues)

TREATMENT *(continued)*

treatment foci of the advanced-practice nurse. Psychotherapy enables the nurse to assess the impact of underlying psychodynamic issues such as early childhood traumas and abuse on current symptoms and behaviors. Various theories guide the advanced-practice psychiatric mental health nurse in the decision to provide psychotherapy. Many use an eclectic brief or short-term psychotherapy approach that offers the client didactic and experiential experiences that facilitate adaptive coping skills, self-care activities, emotional support, and reinforcement of adaptive behavioral changes. During the course of treatment the nurse continuously assesses the client's educational needs; risk of dangerousness to self and others; response to treatment, both nonpharmacologic and pharmacologic; and makes appropriate referrals for physical problems.

Anxiety disorders represent a continuum of symptoms that evolve throughout the life span and affect psychosocial, biological, and occupational well-being. Their comorbidity with other medical and psychiatric disorders, such as endocrine disorders and major depressive episodes, understandably underscore the need for health care professionals to discern the complexity of the human response to internal and external demands and develop effective interventions. Effective interventions require a cultural and age-specific biopsychosocial assessment that integrate data about the client's physical and mental status.

Determining the client's current physical health status helps the psychiatric nurse to continue the holistic nursing process. Major components of this process include continuous data gathering or assessment of current symptoms and their impact on the client's current level of functioning.

Performing a mental status examination is part of the assessment process and provides vital information about the client's current mental health, judgment, insight, and strengths. The nurse must assess the client's symptoms and their chronological patterns and other assessment data in order to make accurate diagnoses according to *DSM-IV-TR* and nursing diagnoses.

Successful client outcomes result from holistic treatment planning that involves collaboration among the nurse, client, family members, other health care providers, and community resources.

Establishing a therapeutic relationship with the client and significant other is essential. A sound health teaching program begins with education about etiology, course, and treatment of an anxiety disorder. This process begins by teaching the client that symptoms of anxiety disorders arise from internal and external stimuli, which trigger an arousal of the autonomic nervous system to protect the body. Coping with anxiety is a two-part endeavor that consists of the client assessing his perception of the threat and using specific coping behaviors to reduce or eliminate distorted cognitions (Andrews & Crino, 1991). Table 3–4 lists diverse anxiety-reducing techniques that the nurse can recommend or teach the client.

The overall treatment outcomes for anxiety disorders depend on the client's ability to:

- Establish a therapeutic relationship
- Acknowledge awareness of anxiety and verbalize related feelings and thoughts
- Develop adaptive skills, such as relaxation, deep breathing techniques, and positive self-talk
- Avoid maladaptive responses
- Reduce the emotional and biological discomforts of anxiety by using anxiety-reducing techniques, including thought blocking and positive self-talk, and having the insight to take prescribed antianxiety agents when indicated
- Improve self-esteem and personal control over feelings, thoughts, and behaviors

(continues)

Table 3–4 • **Anxiety-Reducing Techniques and Interventions**

COGNITIVE-BEHAVIORAL TECHNIQUES

Cognitive Therapy

Therapy is based on principle of internal dialogue or self-talk and its impact on thoughts and feelings or emotions and behaviors. Major goals are to

- Assess the client's belief systems and cognitive distortions
- Challenge and alter the client's distorted/negative thoughts and self-defeating behaviors
- Enhance the client's coping skills

Homework assignments are used to test cognitions (e.g., stimulus $\rightarrow$ thoughts $\rightarrow$ feelings). Various behavioral techniques can be used.

Behavioral Role Rehearsal

The client role-plays anticipated stressful situations. The therapist assesses the client's reactions and provides feedback to the client as a teaching modality. The client can use modeling to shape behavior.

SYSTEMATIC DESENSITIZATION

The client is taught to maintain relaxation while imaging various stages of ranked anxiety-evoking situations. For example, for a client with agoraphobia, situations that evoke an anxiety reaction are ranked from least to most:

1. Going outside
2. Being alone
3. Driving
4. Going to a shopping mall

The client neutralizes anxiety by using deep-muscle relaxation techniques and visual imagery, while the nurse assesses the client's subjective response.

PROGRESSIVE RELAXATION

Visual imagery is the basis of this technique. Directions to the client are as follows:

- Choose a dark, quiet area.
- Close your eyes.
- Focus on all muscle groups from scalp to tips of toes.
- Tense each group of muscles and maintain tension for 4 to 8 seconds.
- Tell yourself to relax and immediately release tension.
- Progress until you have tensed and relaxed all muscles.

Progressive relaxation can also be done using deep-breathing exercises: The client lies on his or her back and inhales through the nose and exhales through the mouth.

Note. Data from *Anxiety Disorders and Phobias: A Cognitive Perspective*, by A. T. Beck, G. Emery, and R. Greenberg, 1985, New York: Basic Books; and *The Practice of Behavioral Therapy*, by J. Wolpe, 1973, New York: Pergamon Press. Adapted with permission.

TREATMENT *(continued)*

- Perform at an optimal level of functioning
- Mobilize support systems and other resources

Nursing implications in the treatment of anxiety disorders include assessing the effectiveness of psychotropics. Prescribing and administering these agents

(continues)

TREATMENT *(continued)*

is contingent on the cause and course of specific anxiety disorders, severity of symptoms, the client's preference, the presence of comorbid conditions such as major depressive episode and substance-related disorders, previous treatment response, and the client's motivation for treatment. Table 3–5 lists antianxiety or anxiolytic agents.

Traditional treatment of anxiety disorders involves prescribing pharmacologic agents, such as anxiolytic and nonanxiolytic agents, and nonpharmacologic interventions, such as cognitive-behavioral therapies. In today's world, one is likely to find other treatments, including complementary therapies. Presumably, more than 60 million Americans are using daily treatments in the form of herbs. These include a bright yellow flower called St. John's wort; dietary supplements; chamomile tea; and kava and aloe for depression, sleep, and their vitalizing or calming effects. Most concerns about herbs and other complementary therapies include potential drug interactions with prescription medications, such as St. John's Wort and SSRIs.

Clients presenting with anxiety disorders can benefit from several complementary therapies that extend beyond over-the-counter herbs, minerals, and vitamins. Individuals prescribing or using complementary therapies require special training and knowledge regarding adverse and desired effects. Major alternative or complementary therapies include aromatherapy, meditation, massage therapy, and yoga.

Evaluating the effectiveness of nursing interventions is an integral part of the nursing process that begins during the initial assessment phase and continues throughout treatment. It provides invaluable data regarding the client's response to treatment, formation of adaptive coping skills, and potential risk of recurrence of symptoms. Criteria for effectiveness parallel outcome identification, the client and family member's feedback, and observations by the nurse and other mental health professionals regarding the client's response to diverse interventions.

Table 3–5 • Major Psychopharmacologic Anxiolytic Agents

Benzodiazepines (Diazepam, Alprazolam, Lorazepam, and Clonazepam)

Generalized anxiety disorder

Panic disorder

Dopamine-Norepinephrine Reuptake Inhibitors (Bupropion, sustained release)

Post-traumatic stress disorder

Nonbenzodiazepines (Buspirone)

Generalized anxiety disorder

Serotonin-Norepinephrine Reuptake Inhibitors (Venlafaxine, extended release)

Generalized anxiety disorder

Serotonin Reuptake Inhibitors/ Antidepressants (Fluoxetine)

Obsessive–compulsive disorder

Post-traumatic stress disorder

Panic disorder

Tricyclic Antidepressants (Clomipramine)

Panic disorders

Post-traumatic stress disorder

Phobic disorders

Monoamine Oxidase Inhibitors (Phenelzine)

Panic disorders

Post-traumatic stress disorder

Phobic disorders

Beta-Blockers (Propranolol)

Panic disorder

Generalized anxiety disorder

Note. Data from "Pharmacology of Antidepressants: Focus on Nefazodone," by C. L. DeVane, D. R. Grothe, & S. L. Smith, 2002, *Journal of Clinical Psychiatry, 63*(Suppl. I), pp. 10–17; and "Overview of Antidepressants Currently Being Used to Treat Anxiety Disorders," by J. P. Feighner, 1999, *Journal of Clinical Psychiatry, 60*(Suppl. 22), pp. 18–22. Adapted with permission.

ACUTE STRESS DISORDER

Causes

The diagnosis of acute stress disorder was introduced in the *DSM-IV*. Similar to PTSD, this anxiety disorder results from exposure to a traumatic and overwhelming event involving actual or threatened death, physical injury, or other threats to one's or another's integrity.

Examples of events that produce acute stress disorder include rape, witnessing a murder or other violent event, violent attacks, combat and other war experience, and surviving natural and man-made disasters.

Symptoms

A *stressor* or event (criterion A) represents the client's response and has to comprise intense fear, a sense of helplessness, or horror. Whereas PTSD represents disturbance that endures for more than 1 month, acute stress disorder must last a minimum of 2 days, and a diagnosis can only be made up to 1 month after exposure to the stressor (APA, 2000).

Another clinical difference between acute stress disorder and PTSD is the presence of a dissociative response to the trauma in the former. Hence, the diagnosis of acute stress disorder requires at least three dissociative symptoms (criterion B), such as "being in a daze," **derealization**, and depersonalization, but only one symptom from each of the reexperiencing or intrusive thoughts (cognitive) (criterion C), avoidance (criterion D), and arousal (biological) (criterion E) categories. Derealization describes a subjective sense that the environment is unreal or strange. Impairment (criterion F) is also necessary to make this diagnosis (APA, 2000).

TREATMENT

Because of the potential deleterious and long-term effects (i.e., PTSD) of acute stress disorder, early identification is crucial. Psychiatric nurses need to identify high-risk groups and initiate early interventions to promote adaptive resolution of traumatic and stressful events. The constellation and intensity of symptoms direct treatment planning. Crisis Intervention Stress Debriefing (CISD) is a crisis model developed by Mitchell (Mitchell & Dyregov, 1993; Robinson & Mitchell, 1993) for disaster workers exposed to traumatic events who are experiencing acute and chronic symptoms of intense anxiety. The basis of this intervention is the provision of immediate emotional support to individuals suffering from abnormal situations. It offers them a supportive environment that encourages and validates their experience and provides education about current and potential behavioral, psychological, biological, and cognitive responses.

Although some clients may benefit from this intervention, others may require professional help, such as psychotherapy or pharmacologic intervention, to manage acute and chronic symptoms such as frightening nightmares, depression, intense and enduring arousal or activation of previous traumatic memories, and PTSD symptoms.

GENERALIZED ANXIETY DISORDER

Causes

Presently, there is a paucity of research that conceptualizes this anxiety disorder, hence, a distinct definition remains obscure. A lack of clarity also makes it difficult to distinguish from *normal worrying or apprehension*. The *DSM-IV-TR* (APA, 2000) describes the cardinal feature of GAD as apprehensive worrying. It further describes it as a pervasive, frequently *uncontrollable* worrying that extends to concerns about daily living and minor life stressors.

Symptoms

Primary symptoms of GAD include nervousness, irritability, apprehension, agitation, tension, tachycardia, diaphoresis, shortness of breath, difficulty falling and staying asleep, and edginess (APA, 2000). Symptoms of GAD tend to overlap those of panic and depressive disorders. GAD differs from PD in that it rarely remits and its onset occurs during earlier developmental stages, with an absence of autonomic nervous system arousal. Table 3–6 presents the prevalence and primary symptoms of anxiety disorders. See also Table 3–4 for anxiety-reducing techniques and interventions and Table 3–5 for major psychopharmacologic anxiolytic agents for major anxiety disorders.

OBSESSIVE-COMPULSIVE DISORDER

Causes

A more recent comprehensive study of childhood-onset OCD and tic disorder in 50 children (Swedo et al., 1998) adds another dimension to the biological basis of this complex anxiety disorder. Data from this study show that some disorders may reflect a pediatric autoimmune neuropsychiatric disorder (PANDAS) arising from group A beta-hemolytic streptococcal [GABHS].

Symptoms

The emergence of OCD symptoms during childhood generally presents as repetitive, ritualistic behaviors and thoughts (Hanna, 1995). Epidemiological studies of children with OCD show a pattern of the following symptoms:

- Obsessive thoughts with common themes of fears of contamination, sexual, or religious
- Rituals, such as washing, checking, arranging, and cognitive rituals
- Repeatedly rewriting a letter or number until it was perfect

Examples of compulsions are repetitive hand washing, counting, checking, touching, cleaning, or hoarding. The client with OCD often attempts to alleviate the anxiety that arises from his obsessions by performing various rituals, or compulsions.

The complexity of OCD challenges nurses to make differential diagnoses, including those with similar clinical presentations, such as obsessive-compulsive personality disorder (OCPD).

Conversely, clinical features of OCPD disorder involve "perfectionism" and emotional constriction, orderliness, rigidity, and indecisiveness. The most obvious impact of these features involves social functioning. Many of these clients have impaired social skills, seem "serious" most of the time, and are inflexible and rigid about their ideas. Moreover, their indecisiveness stems from their need to be perfect and obsessions about routines and orderliness.

Key Fact

Obsessive-compulsive disorder (OCD) affects children and adolescents along with adults. One third to one half of adults with OCD report a childhood or adolescent onset, again suggesting the continuum of anxiety disorders across the life span (Mataix-Cols et al., 2002; Price, Rasmussen, & Eisen, 1999).

TREATMENT

Major treatment modalities for the child with OCD are consistent with adult treatment and include cognitive therapy and psychopharmacology. The developmental stage, severity of symptoms, and parental involvement determine interventions. Cognitive-behavioral therapy is useful for stopping ruminating thoughts. This approach attempts to modify negative perceptions of self and improves the child's self-observation concerning obsessions. It also fosters independence and adaptive behavioral change.

(continues)

Table 3–6 • Primary Symptoms and Prevalence of Anxiety Disorders

	DSM-IV-TR Criteria	Prevalence
Panic Disorder (with or without agoraphobia)	• Shortness of breath • Dizziness • Diaphoresis • Palpitations • Depersonalization • Chest pain • Feelings of doom • Concern of having another attack • Avoidance behaviors • Fear of being in open places	• Isolated recurrent attacks: 10% of adult population • Full criteria for panic attacks: 3.6% of adult population • Full-blown attack: 1.6% of population (Weissman & Merikangas, 1986) • Thirty percent to 50% of population with panic attacks have agorophobia (APA, 2000)
Specific Phobia (formerly called Simple Phobia)	• Arousal of anxiety in and avoidance of specific circumstances; natural, environmental type (e.g., snake or spider phobia) or situational (e.g., fear of heights or flying)	• Lifetime prevalence: 10–11.3% (APA, 2000)
Social Phobia	• Persistent fear and avoidance of circumstances that expose one to embarrassment or humiliation (e.g., public speaking or eating in restaurants)	• Lifetime prevalence in men: 1.7% • Lifetime prevalence in women: 2.8% (Regier et al., 1990a)
Obsessive-Compulsive Disorder	• Thoughts or images of excessive worries regarding life situations (obsessions) • Ritualistic behaviors such as handwashing, counting, or hoarding (compulsions)	• Lifetime prevalence in U.S.: 1.2–2.4% (Karno et al., 1988)
Post-traumatic Stress Disorder	• Recurrent nightmares • Hypervigilant behavior • Intrusive thoughts of traumatic event • Autonomic arousal generated by nightmares, thoughts, or images • Acute or delayed symptoms	• Lifetime prevalence in men: 0.5% • Lifetime prevalence in women: 1.2% (Epstein, 1989)
Generalized Anxiety Disorder	• Restlessness • Tension • Arousal of autonomic nervous system • Agitation/irritability • Free-floating anxiety	• Lifetime prevalence of general population: 3–5%

Note. Data from *Diagnostic and Statistical Manual of Mental Disorders* (4th edition Text Revision) (*DSM-IV-TR*), by American Psychiatric Association, 2000, Washington, DC: Author. Adapted with permission.

TREATMENT *(continued)*

One such approach consists of a 16-session cognitive-behavioral therapy incorporating exposure response prevention (ERP) in conjunction with anxiety management training (AMT). AMT encompasses relaxation, coping skills, breathing exercises, and coping statements (March, Mulle, & Herbel, 1994). **Desensitization**, or exposure to biological cues, helps the child and parents recognize fear or anxiety-evoking incidents.

Parents also play active roles in the child's treatment program during various stages. Psychoeducation provides a forum for family support and reinforcement techniques that reduce compulsive rituals. Similarly, family therapy is vital to decreasing the family's involvement in the child's rituals and dealing with dysfunctional family dynamics. Group therapy is effective in reducing anxiety, improving social skills, and assessing the meaning of symptoms or behaviors (Kendall, 1993; Lenane, 1991).

Psychopharmacologic interventions have been used successfully to treat OCD in children. Major psychotropics, such as those used in adults (SSRIs and tricyclic agents, such as clomipramine) have been among these agents (American Academy of Child and Adolescent Psychiatry, 1998). Despite diverse treatment and the advent of SSRIs and other antiobsessional agents, OCD symptoms persist and have a chronic course for a significant number of clients.

Major pharmacologic interventions for OCD include SSRIs such as fluvoxamine (Luvox), paroxetine (Paxil), and sertraline (Zoloft), and clomipramine (Anafranil)—a tricyclic with serotonergic properties.

Nonpharmacologic interventions for OCD include cognitive-behavioral therapies (Beck et al., 1985). See Tables 3–4 and 3–5 for the pharmacologic and non-pharmacologic interventions used to treat anxiety disorders.

PANIC DISORDER

Causes

The term *panic* originates from the Greek work *panikos*, meaning "fear." Clinical features of PD vary, and symptoms persist for at least 1 month. Panic attacks have a sudden onset of unanticipated intense anxiety generated by arousal of the sympathetic nervous system such as tachycardia, lightheadedness, diaphoresis, paresthesias, and a sense of doom.

Symptoms

Profound fear or sense of imminent danger and an urge to escape may also accompany PD and underlie symptoms of agoraphobia. Normally, panic attacks peak within 10 minutes (APA, 2000). They also vary in their occurrence and intensity, ranging from experiencing multiple episodes for several months at a time to daily attacks for a brief period, with months separating the next episode (APA, 1998).

Key Facts

PD is rarely found before the peripubertal period; however, retrospective studies of adults show that this disorder probably begins by adolescence or young adulthood. These studies also support a continuum of various anxiety disorders across the life span. Approximately 20 to 40 percent of clients with PD experience their initial panic attack before age 20. Women are two to three times more likely to suffer from a PD than men (Weissman et al., 1997).

TREATMENT

Because of the intensity of panic attacks, management of *acute symptoms* of PD involves the use of benzodiazepines such as clonazepam (Klonopin). Long-acting agents are less addictive than shorter-acting, high-potency agents such as alprazolam (Xanax). Major benefits of

(continues)

TREATMENT *(continued)*

clonazepam include its rapid effectiveness and that it is well tolerated. Its long-acting property makes it highly effective in the acute management of PD. These agents should not be used in clients with a history of a substance-related disorder owing to their addictive properties and risk for relapse. In the event of a substance-related disorder or history of substance use, clients can benefit from nonpharmacologic interventions such as deep breathing and relaxation exercises. Maintenance treatment for PD often consists of antidepressant agents such as SSRIs. Antidepressant agents are especially useful in the treatment of PD and comorbid depressive illnesses.

Historically, the treatment focus of PD was to stop or reduce the frequency of panic attacks. Contemporary treatment extends beyond this approach and centers on treating anticipatory anxiety, phobic avoidance, concomitant depression, and level of functioning. Medications from various classes are proving to be effective in managing major symptoms of panic disorder. These classes comprise SSRIs (Ballenger, Wheadon, Steiner, Bushnell, & Gergel, 1998) and tricyclic antidepressants (Mavissakalian, Perel, Talbott-Green, & Sloan, 1998). Other agents include monamine oxidase inhibitors, and calcium channel blockers. Nonpharmacologic interventions such as behavioral and cognitive therapies have also been reported to enhance antipanic agents. **Progressive relaxation**, guided imagery, and deep muscle relaxation are examples of these therapies (Barlow, 1997; Beck, Skodol, Clark, Berchick, & Wright, 1992; Loerch et al., 1999). Progressive relaxation is a form of relaxation training that involves visualization and progressive relaxation of specific muscle groups. The goal of this technique is tension and stress reduction. In addition, the client with PD must be continuously assessed for suicide risk and other maladaptive coping behaviors.

POST-TRAUMATIC STRESS DISORDER

Causes

In the past century, PTSD has appeared in the literature under several names: hysteria, war neurosis, shell shock, and battle fatigue. Regardless of the terminology used, this disorder comprises a complex constellation of symptoms that evolve in survivors of traumatic or overwhelming stressful events.

Symptoms

The emergence of PTSD symptoms may occur immediately after the event or later. Acute PTSD symptoms may occur within 6 months; after this time, symptoms are referred to as delayed. The major symptoms of PTSD in adults fall into three major groups:

1. Persistent recurrent and intrusive thoughts; flashbacks (a sense of reliving the event); dreams of the trauma; intense psychological distress at exposure to internal or external cues such as smells, sounds, or visual event)
2. Avoidance behaviors or **depersonalization**; inability to recall certain aspects of trauma; lack of interest in things that were formerly pleasurable, feeling of detachment, or isolation; restriction in range of feelings (unable to feel happy)
3. Biological responses such as emotional numbing, hypervigilance, and autonomic nervous system arousal (APA, 2000; Morgan, Hill, Fox, Kingham, & Southwick, 1999; Wang, Wilson, & Mason, 1996). PTSD, like other anxiety disorders, is likely to have other comorbid conditions such as depression, other anxiety disorders, and substance-related disorders.

TREATMENT

Youth interventions must focus on strengthening the youth's individual and family repertoire of coping skills.
(continues)

TREATMENT *(continued)*

Adaptive responses to trauma are likely to occur when interventions provide an atmosphere of acceptance and empathy. This process involves fostering enduring adaptation of the child's resilience and facilitating healthy resolution of the traumatic incident. Similarly, it involves facilitating grief resolution in both the child and parents. Finally, treatment must center on preventing the traumatic event to interfere with normal growth and development and minimizing maladaptive responses in the child and family.

The following are suggestions for helping the child experiencing severe trauma to express feelings:

- Establish a trusting relationship by assessing the child alone, speaking in a nonthreatening voice tone, affording proper space between the child and the nurse. This process also involves introducing and explaining the purpose of the visit, reassuring confidence and safety, and considering the child's individual attributes and developmental stage.
- Engage the child by asking him to draw a picture, or invite the child to play with puppets and other toys.
- Tell a story using metaphors that are similar to the youth's traumatic experience, pointing out the character's possible reactions to the incident.
- Engage the youth in clinical debriefing, which involves reviewing and processing the traumatic event and assessing the emotional meaning of the experience, or personal impact. The nurse must be prepared to hear the entire experience, including the horrific details, sadness, and crying that may emerge during this process. This process is enhanced through play therapy, drawing, puppets and other toys, as well as telling a story.

The treatment of childhood PTSD, like other childhood anxiety disorders, is multimodal and includes cognitive-behavioral approaches, individual and family therapy, psychoeducation, and pharmacologic interventions. Ideally, treatment occurs during the acute phase or within the first 3 months after the trauma. The cognitive-behavioral model comprises a rapid exposure approach. Currently, there is a lack of empirical data regarding the use of pharmacologic agents in childhood PTSD.

Similarly to other anxiety disorders, clients with PTSD often benefit from a holistic treatment approach that integrates pharmacologic and nonpharmacologic interventions such as cognitive-behavioral therapy, desensitization, and progressive relaxation exercises. This program must tailor the client's ability to tolerate intense feelings and biological arousal and motivation for treatment.

A relatively new method of treating PTSD is **eye-movement desensitization and reprocessing (EMDR)**. EMDR involves asking the client to imagine an anxiety-provoking or traumatic memory. The primary goal of this technique is to move information and facilitate processing a traumatic experience in a nonthreatening manner when the client's nature processes are blocked (Barron, Curtis, & Grainger, 1998; Rosenbaum, 1997; Shapiro, 1995). Special training is necessary to perform EMDR.

Health education is an integral part of the client's treatment planning and must include signs and symptoms of PTSD, current treatment options, and the role of family members as a team member.

SEPARATION ANXIETY DISORDER

Separation anxiety disorder is associated with psychosocial, learning, and genetic factors. It is one of the most common diagnoses in children, affecting girls more than boys (Black, 1995).

Symptoms

Children with separation anxiety experience panic or excessive worrying about losing their primary caregiver. They are reluctant to go to school or depart from the caregiver because of the fear of separation. These symptoms exist for at least 4 weeks and produce significant or subjective distress (APA, 2000). A number of children may even ruminate or have morbid fears about losing their parents, getting lost, or having accidents.

Other behavioral responses include the fear of being harmed, frequent crying when primary caregivers leave the room, and refusal to attend school. These children are often reluctant or refuse to go to sleep, fear the dark, and experience nightmares. Some children may even complain of somatic problems such as nausea, palpitations, faintness, headaches, stomach pain (butterflies in stomach), fretfulness, and whining (APA, 2000).

TREATMENT

Cognitive-behavioral interventions that involve exposure-based or desensitization approaches show promise in the treatment of separation anxiety disorder. This approach uses stepwise exposure that assists the child in confronting fearful situations and focusing on the maladaptiveness of cognitive distortions. Family psychoeducation must focus on teaching parents how to support the child and maintain parent-child boundaries without reinforcing maladaptive behaviors.

Psychopharmacologic interventions enhance cognitive-behavioral techniques and other therapies as well as reduce the distress of biological responses to fearful circumstances. Pharmacologic interventions include antidepressant agents such as SSRIs, (e.g., fluoxetine), tricyclic agents (e.g., imipramine), beta-receptor antagonists (e.g., propranolol), and buspirone in the treatment of separation anxiety disorder (Bernstein, et. al., 1996).

- Assess the parents' understanding about separation anxiety.
- Encourage parents to express their feelings about the child's symptoms.
- Provide health education about separation anxiety and teach cognitive-behavioral approaches to their child's care.
- Make referrals to various community support groups for parents of children with anxiety disorders.

SOCIAL PHOBIA

Social phobia, also known as social anxiety disorder, refers to a fear of performance situations and subsequent avoidance behaviors, particularly when the child fears humiliation or embarrassment when under the scrutiny of others.

Causes

Factors that increase the risk of social phobia in children and adolescents include modeling of shy, aloof behaviors by the primary caregivers, child abuse, early traumatic childhood losses, chronic medical problems, and impaired social skills (Andrews & Crino, 1991; Leon & Leon, 1990).

Symptoms

Social phobia in children and adolescents involves distress in a broad range of interpersonal encounters such as formal speaking, eating in front of others, using public restrooms, and speaking to authority figures (Biederman et al., 2001).

Avoidant behaviors in children and adolescents are manifested as persistent or extremely constricted social interaction with unfamiliar people to the point of intense social impairment of interaction with peers. These behaviors may occur as early as 2½ years of age and endure for at least 6 months for diagnosis. Behaviors of children tend to be associated with a desire to be involved with others. If this disorder continues into adulthood, it is linked with avoidant personality disorder (APA, 2000).

Adult symptoms of social phobia are comparable to the childhood type and include a fear of performance situations such as public speaking, eating in front of others, or writing in public, ensuing avoidance behaviors.

TREATMENT

A multimodal approach that consists of psychosocial and family interventions provides the most effective treatment outcomes for the child with social phobia. Treatment consists of cognitive-behavioral interventions that involve gradual exposure, cognitive reconstructing, coping skills, assertiveness training for shyness, and anxiety self-monitoring. The focus of cognitive reconstructing is modifying maladaptive negative self-statements that interfere with problem-solving behaviors (Albano & Chorpita, 1995).

The diverse clinical symptoms of clients experiencing social phobia are perplexing and require accurate assessment, differential diagnoses, and interventions that reduce its debilitating form and restore quality of life. Interventions for this disorder are similar to other anxiety disorders and include both pharmacologic and nonpharmacologic approaches. Pharmacologic approaches include a broad spectrum of antidepressants such as SSRIs (Baldwin, Bobes, Stein, Scharwachter, & Faure, 1999; Stein, Fyer, Davidson, Pollack, & Wiita, 1999; Stein et al., 1998), MAOIs (Schneier et al., 1998), beta-adrenergic blockers, and long-acting benzodiazepines.

Nonpharmacologic interventions include various psychotherapies such as individual, cognitive-behavioral therapy, desensitization, rehearsal, an array of homework assignments, progressive muscle relaxation, and abdominal deep breathing exercises (Beck et al., 1985; Wolpe, 1961; 1973).

RESOURCES

Please note that because Internet resources are of a time-sensitive nature and URL addresses may change or be deleted, searches should also be conducted by association or topic.

Internet Resources

http://www.apna.org American Psychiatric Nurses Association

http://www.nami.org National Alliance for the Mentally Ill

http://www.nimh.nih.gov/anxiety/anxietymenu.cfm National Institute of Mental Health (website on anxiety disorders)

http://www.adaa.org Anxiety Disorders Association of America

Attention Deficit Disorder

4

• Key Terms

Cognitive: The mental process involved in obtaining knowledge, including the aspects of perceiving, thinking, reasoning, and remembering.

Comorbidity: A psychiatric or physical disorder that occurs with a primary psychiatric disorder.

Hyperactivity: Extra active; having too much energy to handle. An activity level that is out of proportion for the situation, setting, and person's developmental level.

Impulsivity: A tendency to act suddenly and without thought. An inability to delay gratification, which reflects a lack of personal control and inability to manage feelings and emotions.

Inattention: A failure to focus attention on those elements of the environment that are most relevant to the task at hand.

Learning Disability: A condition that makes it difficult for a person to learn information in a usual manner.

Overarousal: To be excessively excited or stimulated.

Personal Boundaries: A mental idea of how one experiences and maintains a line of separation between oneself and the world.

*Attention-deficit hyperactivity disorder (ADHD) is the most common neurobehavioral disorder among school-age children. The main characteristics of the disorder are **inattention**, **impulsivity**, and **hyperactivity**.*

ATTENTION DEFICIT HYPERACTIVITY DISORDER

Causes

Alcohol and other drugs ingested by the mother are transferred through the placenta to the fetus. Steinhaus, Williams, & Spohr (1993) studied children suffering from fetal alcohol syndrome. They found attention deficits and behavioral problems similar to those of ADHD children; however, they also found that the children who were affected by alcohol were more impaired intellectually. These findings were further supported by studies conducted by Naison and Hiscock (1990).

Studies of children with significant lead ingestion demonstrate deficits in global IQ function, visual and fine motor coordination, and in behavior. School failure resulting from learning and behavior problems was also more frequent in the group exposed to lead.

These findings suggest that there may be a group of children with ADHD symptoms that are at least in part a result of lead exposure. The studies provided no evidence that treatment for lead poisoning would improve the cognitive or behavioral functioning of these children (Wyngarden, 1988).

The majority of children with ADHD are found to have a positive family history of ADHD. For many, it is a close family member such as a parent. Studies of parental psychopathology demonstrate that attention-deficit symptoms are more common in the fathers and uncles of ADHD children than in the relatives of non-ADHD children (Stewart, DuBlois, & Cummings, 1980).

The attention system consists of a brainstem center composed of dopamine, serotonin, and noradrenaline neurons that project to many areas of the brain, basal ganglia, and frontal lobes. Limbic, frontal, and right hemispheric cells also are part of this system. This network, which projects to all areas of the brain, is important for a regulating system whose purpose is to modulate whole brain activity. Within the cerebral hemispheres, information from the senses is converted into electrical impulses that are sent to specific areas of the cerebral cortex. Certain areas of the cerebral hemispheres are involved in translating sensory input to prepare a response. Several areas of the brain responsible for this task have been identified to function differently in children with ADHD.

One area identified is the frontal lobes. The frontal lobes are the area of the brain responsible for the executive functions. These functions consist of initiating and sustaining activities, prioritizing, strategizing, and inhibiting impulses until the brain can weigh the possible consequences of the activity rationally. The basal ganglia are also an affected area. The basal ganglia assist the frontal lobes by helping to prioritize input and by organizing and executing actions decided on by the frontal lobes. The third area is the cerebellum. The cerebellum was once thought to be involved primarily in muscular coordination, balance, and movement. It is now recognized to play a role in emotion and higher level cognitive functions.

The attention system may regulate the processing of information and concentration through coordination of several groups of nerve cells, primarily serotonin, dopamine, and norepinephrine. This system adjusts the sensitivity of the brain to stimuli and regulates the degree of activity, attention, concentration, as well as impulsivity. For example, the attention system regulates a person's ability to concentrate on reading and the cerebral cortical centers determine comprehension.

Children with ADHD likely have varying degrees of differences within the attention system. They are unable to change their degree of attention appropriately as required by tasks or situations. The high degree of variability of ADHD symptoms could be seen as variability in effectiveness of the attention system.

Children with language, socialization, **cognitive**, and other behavioral difficulties that are the result of life experiences because of abnormal development or illness also exhibit attention-related problems (Goldstein & Goldstein, 1999).

Symptoms

ADHD is characterized by attention skills that are developmentally inappropriate for the clients' age and may include the symptoms of hyperactivity and impulsivity.

The child with attention difficulties, impulsive behaviors, and increased motor activity presents a challenge to parents, teachers, peers, and health care providers. These symptoms create problems for the child and family in many settings, with the demands of the setting influencing the severity of the symptoms. At some point in the child's life the impact of these symptoms on his academic, social, or leisure functioning causes the child to be brought to the attention of mental health providers.

Symptoms of ADHD are usually first noticed in early childhood. The symptoms of excess motor activity are frequently detected when the child is a toddler, although children this age are normally active and curious. The child with ADHD, however, will be more active and impulsive than his peers. Symptoms of inattention in toddlers or preschool age children are not easily observable because young children rarely experience demands for sustained attention. As children mature the symptoms become more conspicuous. By late childhood or early adolescence, the symptoms of excess motor activity are less common and have been replaced by restlessness or fidgeting (APA, 2000). In most individuals symptoms attenuate during late adolescence and adulthood, although a minority will experience the full complement of symptoms into adulthood.

Comorbidity is a common occurrence with ADHD. Comorbid disorders often include **learning disabilities**, oppositional defiant disorder, conduct disorder, depression, and anxiety disorders (Wilens et al., 2002). Recognition of comorbid disorders is important because these conditions may influence the outcomes of medical and treatment interventions.

The *DSM-IV-TR* defines ADHD as a persistent pattern of inattention or hyperactivity-impulsivity, or both, that is more frequent and severe than is typically observed in individuals at a comparable level of development (APA, 2000).

Some hyperactive-impulsive or inattentive symptoms that cause impairment must have been present before age 7 years. Some impairment from the symptoms must be present in at least two settings (e.g., home and school or work). There must be clear evidence of interference with developmentally appropriate social, academic, or occupational functioning. Lastly, the symptoms do not occur exclusively during the course of another disorder, such as Pervasive Developmental Disorder, a psychotic disorder, mood, or other mental disorder. The *DSM-IV-TR* criteria are displayed in Table 4–1.

The *DSM-IV-TR* criteria are further broken down into symptoms of inattention and hyperactivity-impulsivity. These symptoms are behavioral and can be measured through direct observation of

Table 4–1 • *DSM-IV-TR* Diagnostic Criteria for Attention-Deficit/Hyperactivity Disorder

A. Either (1) or (2)

  (1) Six (or more) of the following symptoms of inattention have persisted for at least 6 months to a degree that is maladaptive and inconsistent with developmental level:

    (a) often fails to give close attention to details or makes careless mistakes in schoolwork, work, or other activities

    (b) often has difficulty sustaining attention in tasks or play activities

    (c) often does not seem to listen when spoken to directly

    (d) often does not follow through on instruction and fails to finish schoolwork, chores, or duties in the workplace (not due to oppositional behavior or failure to understand instructions)

    (e) often has difficulty organizing tasks and activities

(continues)

Table 4–1 *(continued)*

- (f) often avoids, dislikes, or is reluctant to engage in tasks that require sustained mental effort (such as schoolwork or homework)
- (g) often loses things necessary for tasks or activities (e.g., toys, school assignments, pencils, books, or tools)
- (h) is often easily distracted by extraneous stimuli
- (i) is often forgetful in daily activities

(2) Six (or more) of the following symptoms of hyperactivity-impulsivity have persisted for at least 6 months to a degree that is maladaptive and inconsistent with developmental level:
Hyperactivity
- (a) often fidgets with hands or feet or squirms in seat
- (b) often leaves seat in classroom or in other situations in which remaining seated is expected
- (c) often runs about or climbs excessively in situations in which it is inappropriate (in adolescents or adults, may be limited to subjective feelings of restlessness)
- (d) often has difficulty playing or engaging in leisure activities quietly
- (e) if often "on the go" or often acts as if "driven by a motor"
- (f) often talks excessively
Impulsivity
- (a) often blurts out answers before questions have been completed
- (b) often has difficulty awaiting turn
- (c) often interrupts or intrudes on others (e.g., butts into conversations or games)

B. Some hyperactive-impulsive or inattentive symptoms that caused impairment were present before age 7 years.

C. Some impairment from the symptoms is present in two or more settings (e.g., at school [or work] and at home).

D. There must be clear evidence of clinically significant impairment in social, academic, or occupational functioning.

E. The symptoms do not occur exclusively during the course of a Pervasive Developmental Disorder, Schizophrenia, or other Psychotic Disorder and are not better accounted for by another mental disorder (e.g., Mood Disorder, Anxiety Disorder, Dissociative Disorder, or Personality Disorder).

Code based on type:

314.01   ADHD, Combined Type:
Both Criteria A1 and A2 are met for the past 6 months

314.00   ADHD, Predominantly Inattentive Type:
Criterion A1 is met, but Criterion A2 is not met for the past 6 months

314.01   ADHD, Predominantly Hyperactive-Impulsive Type:
Criterion A2 is met but Criterion A1 is not met for the past 6 months

Coding note:

For individuals (especially adolescents and adults) who currently have symptoms that no longer meet full criteria, "In Partial Remission" should be specified

314.9   ADHD, Not Otherwise Specified:
There are prominent symptoms of inattention or hyperactivity-impulsivity that do not meet criteria for ADHD

Note. From *Diagnostic and Statistical Manual of Mental Disorders* (4th edition Text Revision) (*DSM-IV-TR*), by American Psychiatric Association, 2000, Washington, DC: Author. Reprinted with permission.

the client in the home, school, or work environment. A variety of observation rating scales have been developed that help identify and measure the severity of the core symptoms of inattention, impulsivity, and hyperactivity. Many of these include ratings of social relationships. Some of the more well-known scales are the Conners' Parent-Teacher Rating Scale, the Vanderbilt Rating Scale, and the Achenbach Child Behavior checklist. These scales are well established and have high degrees of interrater reliability. See the sample Behavior Rating Scale and instructions for use.

In 1998, Goldstein and Goldstein proposed a practical definition of ADHD to provide a logical framework from which to understand the patterns of behavior that constitute ADHD. They are outlined as follows:

1. Impulsivity: Children with ADHD have difficulty thinking before they act. They know what to do but they do not do what they know.

2. Inattention: Children with ADHD have difficulty remaining on-task and focusing attention compared with children without ADHD (APA, 2000). Children with ADHD have an inability to invest and sustain attention to task, especially repetitive, effortful, uninteresting, or unchosen tasks.

3. Hyperactivity and **overarousal**: Children with ADHD tend to be restless, overactive, and easily overaroused emotionally. They have difficulty controlling bodily movements in situations where they are required to sit still or stay in place for an extended period of time.

4. Difficulties with gratification: As a result of impulsivity children with ADHD require immediate, frequent, predictable, and meaningful rewards. They experience greater difficulty working toward a long-term goal. They do not appear to respond to rewards in a manner similar to other children without ADHD (Haenlin & Caul, 1987).

It also appears that children with ADHD tend to receive more negative reinforcement and feedback than children without ADHD. Because of the child's impulsivity and inconsistency, adults may place great pressure on them or the child perceives it this way. The child responds to this by completing tasks to the best of their ability but to gain relief from the adults' negative attention.

5. Emotions and locus of control: Children with ADHD are often on a roller coaster of emotions owing to their impulsiveness and emotional overarousal.

The symptoms of ADHD appear to arise on average between the ages of 3 to 7. This is true primarily for the symptoms of hyperactivity and impulsivity. Hyperactivity is often seen as restlessness, excessive running, inability to sit still for an age-appropriate length of time, fidgeting, or excessive talking. Impulsivity is exhibited as acting before thinking, not being able to take turns, poor **personal boundaries**, intrusive behavior, and frequently interrupting others. Many of these symptoms are behaviors often seen in young children who have not learned the skills of delayed gratification or impulse control. Refer to Table 4–2 for symptoms of ADHD across the life span.

It is estimated that 50 to 80 percent of children with ADHD will continue to experience symptoms in adolescence. Adolescents with ADHD of the hyperactive-impulsive subtype will exhibit increasing difficulty with authority and an increase in high-risk-taking behaviors. They continue to have academic difficulties primarily in the area of assignment completion and organization of schoolwork. If the children have been able to channel their energy into sports, they may exhibit difficulty showing up on time for practices or following the coach's instruction. Refer to Table 4–2.

Historically, ADHD was considered to be a disorder of childhood. There has been limited research done into the persistence of symptoms of ADHD into adulthood. Estimates are that from 20 to 35 percent of clients with ADHD eventually outgrow the symptoms or develop

Quick Guide to Using the Abbreviated ADHD Symptom Checklist-4

The Abbreviated ADHD Symptom Checklist-4 (ADHD-SC4) is a behavior rating scale whose items are based on the 18 behavioral symptoms of attention-deficit hyperactivity disorder (ADHD) as defined by the American Psychiatric Association's *Diagnostic and Statistical Manual of Mental Disorders* (DSM-IV). Individual items are worded to be easily understood by caregivers. Physicians can use the Abbreviated ADHD-SC4 as a brief screening device with parents and teachers who are concerned about child behavior at home and in school. The findings from a number of studies indicate that the Abbreviated ADHD-SC4 is a reliable and valid screening instrument for ADHD in children 3 to 18 years old, and it is a reliable and valid measure for assessing response to treatment. The checklist can be completed in less than 2 minutes, and it is quick and easy to score.

Scoring procedures. There are two different ways to score the Abbreviated ADHD-SC4: Symptom Count scores and Symptom Severity scores. The weights assigned to the response choices are as follows:

SYMPTOM COUNT: Never = 0,
   Sometimes = 0, Often = 1,
   Very Often = 1
SYMPTOM SEVERITY: Never = 0,
   Sometimes = 1, Often = 2,
   Very Often = 3

Symptom Count scores are used to screen for specific disorders. The *DSM-IV* identifies three types of ADHD: the predominantly inattentive type (Items 1–9), the predominantly hyperactive-impulsive type (Items 10–18), and the combined types (Items 1–18). The *DSM-IV* also specifies the number of symptoms necessary for a diagnosis. The minimum number of symptoms for each of the three types of ADHD is as follows: the predominantly inattentive type (six symptoms), the predominantly hyperactive-impulsive type (six symptoms), and the combined type (six symptoms of each the inattentive and hyperactive-impulsive types). Items that are checked as "Often" and "Very Often" are considered to be clinically significant.

Symptom Severity scores are used to assess the overall severity of child symptoms after a diagnosis has been established. This method of scoring is most useful when evaluating response to treatment.

Parent and teacher ratings. The accuracy of the Abbreviated ADHD-SC4 is enhanced when information is obtained from both parents and teacher(s). However, parent and teacher ratings do not always agree. Discrepancies between parent and teacher scores may indicate that either the child's behavior is different in the two settings or one of these care providers is a more accurate informant about certain child behaviors. Because this is a screening instrument, parent or teacher indications of ADHD behavior should be investigated further when the child's behavior is considered to be a serious problem by either informant.

Interpreting Symptom Count scores. The Abbreviated ADHD-SC4 does not provide diagnoses; it is simply a screening instrument. Furthermore, Symptom Count scores cannot be interpreted as verifying the presence or absence of specific disorders. If a child's Symptom Count score meets the minimum number of symptoms required for a diagnosis of ADHD, then a comprehensive clinical evaluation is necessary to determine if (a) the child really had ADHD, (b) some other variable (e.g., environmental stressor) can explain the symptom, or (c) another disorder can account for the ADHD symptoms. In addition to the behavioral symptoms, a diagnosis of ADHD requires information about the age of onset and duration of symptoms, extent of impairment in functioning, and the exclusionary conditions and disorders. According to the *DSM-IV*, onset must be by age 7 years, symptoms must have been present for a minimum of 6 months, symptoms must cause difficulties in at least two settings, symptoms must cause clinically significant distress or impairment in functioning, and symptoms are not caused by other disorders (e.g., pervasive developmental disorder, schizophrenia, mood and anxiety disorders).

User qualifications. Users of the Abbreviated ADHD-SC4 should have an understanding of the basic principles and limitations of psychological and psychiatric screening and diagnostic procedures. Only qualified professionals can render diagnoses after a thorough evaluation.

Abbreviated ADHD Symptom Checklist-4

Child's Name————————————————— Date——————————

Name of Person Completing Form ——————————————————

Relationship to Child ————————————

Directions: Indicate the degree to which each item below is a problem. Please respond to all items. Consider the child's behavior on the following days:

	Never	Sometimes	Often	Very Often
1. Doesn't pay attention to details; makes careless mistakes	0	1	2	3
2. Difficulty paying attention	0	1	2	3
3. Does not seem to listen	0	1	2	3
4. Difficulty following instructions; does not finish things	0	1	2	3
5. Difficulty getting organized	0	1	2	3
6. Avoids doing things that require a lot of mental effort	0	1	2	3
7. Loses things	0	1	2	3
8. Easily distracted	0	1	2	3
9. Forgetful	0	1	2	3
10. Fidgets with hands or feet; squirms in seat	0	1	2	3
11. Difficulty remaining seated	0	1	2	3
12. Runs about or climbs on things	0	1	2	3
13. Difficulty playing quietly	0	1	2	3
14. "On the go"; acts as if "driven by a motor"	0	1	2	3
15. Talks excessively	0	1	2	3
16. Blurts out answers to questions	0	1	2	3
17. Difficulty awaiting turn	0	1	2	3
18. Interrupts others or butts into their activities	0	1	2	3

Note. Data from *ADHD Symptom Checklist-4 Manual,* by K. D. Gadow & J. Spafkin, 1997, Stony Brook, NY: Checkmate Plus. Adapted with permission; and from *Child Symptom Inventory-4 Norms Manual,* by K. D. Gadow & J. Spafkin, 1997, Stony Brook, NY: Checkmate Plus. Reprinted with permission.

Table 4–2 • **Symptoms across the Life Span**

PRESCHOOL (3–5 years old)	SCHOOL AGE (6–12 years old)	ADOLESCENT (13–18 years old)	ADULT
• Increased motor activity	• Easily distracted	• Decreased/poor self-esteem	• Disorganized, poor planning skills
• Aggressive to others	• Homework poorly organized, frequent errors, careless mistakes, not complete	• School work is disorganized	• Forgetful, frequently loses things
• High curiosity level		• Difficulty completing long-term assignments	• Difficulty in initiation and completion of tasks, projects, assignments
• Spills, breaks things	• Blurts out answers before question is completed	• Fails to work independently	
• Rough play (often breaks, damages toys, frequent accidental injuries)	• Frequently interrupts, disrupts class	• High-risk-taking behaviors	• Poor time management skills—misjudges available time
• Demanding, argumentative	• Fails to wait turn in games	• Poor peer relations	
• Noisy, frequently interrupts others	• Often out of seat	• Difficulty with rules, laws, and authority figures	• Frequent job changes
• Excessive temper tantrums (severe and frequent)	• Perceived as being immature by adults		• Marital difficulties
• Low level of compliance with adult's requests	• Unwilling or unable to complete chores at home		• Continued inattention/ concentration problems
	• Often interrupts or intrudes on peers		• Poor frustration tolerance
	• Poor peer relations/ few friends		
	• Difficulty playing games, unable to follow directions		

Note. Adapted from *Attention Deficit Disorder (In Adults and Children): The Latest Assessment and Treatment Strategies,* by C. K. Conners & J. L. Jett, 1999, Kansas City, MO: Compact Clinicals.

the skills to effectively manage the symptoms. Refer to Table 4–2.

Key Fact

The estimated prevalence of ADHD is between 3 and 8 percent, which makes it one of the most frequently encountered chronic health disorders in mental health clinics that treat children (Barkley, 1996).

It is estimated that 3 to 5 percent of all school-age children have ADHD. This translates into a probability of 1 to 2 students in a typical classroom. Estimations of the number of affected adults vary widely, from 30 to 70 percent of those diagnosed in childhood experiencing ongoing symptoms. The incidence of occurrence in males exceeds females by a 4 to 1 ratio.

TREATMENT

Symptoms of ADHD are a good start to differential diagnosing, but it is important to gather data from a number of sources; otherwise, children with a wide variety of

(continues)

TREATMENT *(continued)*

behavioral, emotional, and developmental problems may be diagnosed inappropriately with ADHD.

The current *DSM-IV-TR* criteria are well defined and comprehensive. Before establishing a diagnosis it is important to collect data, history, and observations from a variety of sources to determine that the child meets symptom criteria in more than one setting.

Nursing responsibilities for management of the client's plan of care may include administering medications. Health teaching about the indications for use, effects, and potential side effects of medication is a major nursing responsibility. Clients and families will require education and nutritional counseling because many of the pharmacologic agents can affect the appetite, and certain food additives have been shown to exacerbate symptoms (Feingold, 1974, Kutcher, 1997).

Other nonpharmacologic interventions may include the use of psychoeducational groups such as social skills or anger management. Individual or family therapy may be added to address issues related to communication, relationships, or symptoms from other comorbid conditions. The type of therapy should be individualized and specific to the needs of the client and family, severity of symptoms, personal preference, and past response to treatment.

Providing care for the client with ADHD requires an understanding of the complexity of the disorder, symptom variations, and the influence of environmental and biological factors. The role of the nurse will vary according to educational preparation, use of nursing theoretical frameworks, clinical experience, personal interest, and the clinical care setting. Nursing roles and responsibilities vary, from administering medications to developing and implementing holistic treatment plans.

The nurse in a generalist role may work with clients with ADHD in a variety of settings. Nurses working in mental health clinics, pediatricians' offices, and schools have the most contact with these clients. Understanding the disorder, its etiology, symptoms, and types of treatment enables the nurse to work with the client and family and identify their specific mental health needs. The nurse may choose a specific theoretical framework to guide his practice, or he may follow clinical guidelines developed at the work setting. The initial goal of the nurse is to identify problems and establish a plan of intervention to reduce the frequency and severity of symptoms. Interventions include establishing the nurse-client relationship, enhancing the coping skills of the client and family, identifying maladaptive responses, and decreasing the negative impact of the symptoms of hyperactivity, impulsivity, and inattention. Another important nursing intervention is medication administration, patient education, and monitoring patient response.

The advanced-practice nurse (APN) is a nurse with a master's degree, who has the ability to apply knowledge, skills, and experience autonomously to complex mental health problems (ANA, 2000). The APN may function in the role of clinical specialist, or nurse practitioner. The APN can perform all the role functions of the generalist nurse but additionally may use psychobiological interventions to diagnose and treat mental health disorders. These interventions can include ordering diagnostic tests, evaluating symptoms and making differential diagnoses, prescribing pharmacologic agents, or providing psychotherapy.

ADHD is composed of a range of symptoms that evolve and change throughout the client's life span. The incidence of comorbidity of other psychiatric disorders (anxiety, major depression, conduct, and oppositional defiant disorders) reinforces the need for nurses to understand the complexity of human responses to actual or potential mental health problems. This understanding provides the basis for development of effective interventions. The nursing process provides a guide for nurses to address these problems systematically.

The assessment process begins with ruling out other potential illnesses or
(continues)

TREATMENT *(continued)*

factors yielding symptoms that mimic ADHD. A complete medical examination, including hearing and vision evaluations, is the initial step. Data collection should also include a review of currently used prescribed and over-the-counter medications, dietary habits, and an assessment of the client's living environment. Dietary habits are important to assess because many food additives can exacerbate symptoms. Data about the client's living environment should be carefully gathered to identify potential contributing factors such as exposure to lead, inadequate living or sleeping space, or exposure to community violence (Ferguson, Horwood, & Lynskey, 1994).

Nursing diagnoses should be based on an analysis of assessment data. The nurse working with the client with ADHD should consider the following diagnoses in developing the plan of care (NANDA, 2001):

- Alteration in Attention Process: Etiology Unknown*
- Alteration in Motor Activity, Overactive: Etiology Unknown*
- Risk for Injury: Related to Impulsivity
- Imbalanced Nutrition: Less than Body Requirements Related to Excessive Motor Activity
- Disturbed Sleep Pattern: Related to Medication Side Effects
- Impaired Social Interaction: Related to Ineffective Social Skills
- Situational Low Self-Esteem: Possibly related to rejection by Family, Peers, and Adults
- Deficient Knowledge: Related to a Lack of Understanding of ADHD, etiology, Course and Treatment
- Impaired Parenting: Related to Knowledge Deficit about ADHD

* Not in NANDA (2001)

Nursing diagnoses guide the nurse in developing an individualized, client-centered treatment plan. It identifies patterns of human response to actual or potential health problems. Nursing care is holistic in nature and focuses not only on the client but also on the family or others

affected by the client's symptoms. The goal of treatment is to return the client to optimum level of functioning and restore equilibrium within the family system and other affected environments.

Outcome identification involves establishing individualized outcome measures. Common outcome measures for clients with ADHD include:

- Adequate management of symptoms
- Adequate nutrition
- Normal sleep and rest patterns
- Understanding and insight about the nature of ADHD, its symptoms, causes, and treatments
- Effective individual coping
- Healthy family, peer, and adult interactions

Achieving successful outcomes are the result of effective treatment planning, which should be holistic and collaborative. Collaboration needs to occur between the nurse, client, family, teachers, other health care providers, and community resources.

Behavioral interventions focus on positive learning experiences that reduce symptom impact, enhance coping skills, and provide opportunities for success for the client with ADHD. Active participation of family and teachers in helping the client adapt and develop coping skills is vital to the success of treatment. The overall treatment outcomes for the family and client with ADHD are:

- Identify and implement interventions to reduce target symptoms.
- Develop an understanding of triggers that exacerbate symptoms.
- Develop adaptive skills that enhance relationships and personal functioning in school or work and the community.
- Avoid maladaptive responses.
- Use community resources and support systems effectively.

Treatment must consider a combination of pharmacologic and behavioral interventions. Simultaneous use of this combination of interventions provides superior outcomes rather than the use of either intervention alone. *(continues)*

TREATMENT *(continued)*

Evaluation of the effectiveness of the established behavioral management plan should be ongoing. The nurse, family, and child should meet on a regularly established timetable to review agreed-upon outcomes, academic and social progress, and whether or not problematic behaviors have improved. To achieve objectivity and consistency, the nurse may use a rating scale administered by teachers and parents, report cards, and reports from leaders of community-based activities.

Pharmacologic treatment of ADHD is the most studied and best understood of all pyschopharmacologic treatments in children and adolescents. Nursing implications in the treatment of ADHD vary with the nursing role but at either level includes assessing efficacy of psychotropics and patient and family education.

The APN will be involved in prescribing or recommending medications to treat the symptoms of the disorder. Diagnosis and symptom identification are key in determining the choice of pharmacologic agent. The core symptoms of ADHD—inattention, impulsivity, distractibility, and hyperactivity—have been shown to respond favorably to pharmacotherapy. Psychostimulant medication has clearly been demonstrated to be the treatment of choice in those clients who are able to tolerate them.

Before prescribing a medication, the APN will need to identify any existing comorbid conditions. ADHD often presents with comorbid conditions of depression, anxiety, conduct disorder, oppositional defiant disorder, tic disorder, or Tourette's syndrome. Clients with ADHD and either conduct or oppositional defiant disorder often do fine with psychostimulant medication (Bukstein & Kolko, 1998). Clients with ADHD and the comorbid conditions of depression, anxiety, bipolar disorder, Tourette's syndrome, or schizophrenia are less likely to respond favorably to these medications and will require further assessment (DuPaul, Barkley, & McMurray, 1994).

Medication Assessment

Baseline assessment data to be collected before initiation of medication include:

1. CBC (if pemoline is to be used, liver function tests should be obtained). ECG if TCA is used (baseline and periodic monitoring).
2. Height, weight, heart rate, and blood pressure.
3. Behavioral rating scales from a variety of adults who observe the child in different settings such as parents, extended family members, teachers, coaches, or adult mentors. Some common rating scales are Conners' Parent-Teacher Rating Scale, ADHD Rating Scale, or the Vanderbilt ADHD Rating Scale. Refer to the ADHD checklist for an example of a behavior rating scale and instructions for use.
4. A complete physical examination, including hearing and vision evaluation.

The choice of medication will be contingent on assessment data, patient symptoms, previous response to medications, patient or family preference, and social or environmental factors.

Psychostimulants are the most widely prescribed and best-researched medication used to treat ADHD. They increase the availability of certain neurotransmitters and have been found to improve focus and concentration. Common psychostimulant medications used in the treatment of ADHD include methylphenidate (Ritalin), mixed salts of a single-entity amphetamine product (Adderall), and dextroamphetamine (Dexedrine). Pemoline (Cylert) was once used first line, but because of the risk of development of serious side effects (liver failure), it is now reserved for use when first-line medications have not been successful. The majority of these medications are short acting, with effect lasting from 4 to 6 hours. There are a few psychostimulants with longer duration of action such as dextroamphetamine spansules, methylphenidate SR (a single dose of which can last for up to 8 hours), Metadate CD, and Adderall XR. Currently, both Adderall and methylphenidate have been

(continues)

TREATMENT *(continued)*

produced with a different delivery system providing efficacy up to 12 hours.

The specific dose of medicine must be determined for each individual. There are ranges based on dose per unit of body weight that are recommended and that provide guidelines for initiation of treatment. However, there are no consistent relationships among the height, weight, and age of the child and response to medication. A medication trial is often used to determine the most beneficial dosage. Medication is started at a low dose and gradually increased in frequency of administration and dosage until optimal effect is achieved. This also provides the opportunity for identification of side effects early in treatment.

Psychostimulants have been used successfully for over 50 years to treat ADHD. Although they have been found to be safe and effective, side effects may occur. The most common side effects are reduced appetite, headache, and difficulty sleeping. A relatively uncommon side effect may be the unmasking of latent tics such as eye blinking, shrugging, and clearing of the throat. Side effects are usually managed by an adjustment in dosage and scheduling of the medication.

Although psychostimulants are first-line agents in the treatment of ADHD, there are individuals who are not responsive to or cannot tolerate these medications. However, there are a variety of nonstimulating agents that have demonstrated efficacy. Table 4–3 provides an overview

(continues)

Table 4–3 • Medications Used in the Treatment of ADHD

Name	Type	How It Works	Target Symptoms
Tofranil (imipramine) Pamelor (nortryptyline)	Tricyclic antidepressants (TCAs)	Inhibits reuptake of norepinephrine and serotonin	Helps with impulsivity and hyperactivity; not effective with inattention
Ritalin, Concerta, Metadate CD (methylphenidate) Dexedrine Adderall, Adderall XR Cylert (pemoline)	Stimulants	Acts as a mild cortical stimulant with CNS action	Helps with focusing, concentration, and overactivity
Catapres (clonidine) Tenex (guanfacine)	Antihypertensives	Stimulates alpha-adrenergic receptors to inhibit sympathetic nervous system	Helps with tic disorders, aggressive behaviors, and impulsivity. Does not help with inattention
Wellbutrin (bupropion)	Antidepressant	Inhibits reuptake of dopamine and norepinephrine	Improves mood and possibly inattention; some decrease in overactivity noted in adolescents and adults
Remeron (mirtazapine)	Antidepressant	Inhibits reuptake of norepinephrine and dopamine	Helps improve mood and sleep disturbance in children with comorbid mood and sleep disorders

TREATMENT *(continued)*

of medications used to treat ADHD and their mechanism of action.

The nurse's role in medication administration will be two-fold: assessing the effects of medication and assessing the child's response to the process. Table 4–4 provides medication education guidelines for the client on a stimulant medication.

Behavior management plans are very effective in decreasing unwanted behaviors and promoting desired behaviors.

Table 4–4 • Patient Education Guide for the Client on a Stimulant Medication

• Take the medication as prescribed. If you miss a dose, do not "make it up." Just resume the medication at the next scheduled time.

• Avoid taking other medications, including over-the-counter medications, without discussing it with your health care provider or checking with your pharmacist to be sure there are no drug interactions.

• Take the medication after eating to avoid appetite problems or stomach upset.

• Avoid taking the medication late in the evening because it may disturb sleep.

• Some common side effects of this medication are:

1. Stomach upset, appetite loss, vomiting
2. Insomnia
3. Rapid heartbeat, chest pain
4. Headache
5. Irritability, nervousness, or confusion

• Keep all regularly scheduled appointments with your health care provider so that medication effects can be monitored. This may include laboratory tests, blood pressure or pulse checks, height and weight checks, or other tests like ECGs.

The plan should be developed by the adults involved with the children and incorporate behaviors across different environments such as the home, the school, public places (stores, restaurants), day care, and church. The behaviors should be clearly and simply stated and written to provide the child with visual cues.

Time-out procedures are quite effective in the management of the child with ADHD and should be incorporated into an overall behavior management plan. Time-out can be as simple as having the child sit in an isolated portion of the room, placing his head down on his desk, or sitting quietly for a few minutes.

Training parents to more effectively manage the behavior of children with ADHD is one component of parent training. Parents must also be taught to identify and modify causative or aggravating factors in the environment and advocate for their children within the educational and social environments. Nurses can be instrumental in implementing and facilitating parent education classes. It is important to help parents understand that parenting classes offer a means to obtain new skills, develop problem-solving strategies, enhance communication, and develop conflict resolution skills.

RESOURCES

Please note that because Internet resources are of a time-sensitive nature and URL addresses may change or be deleted, searches should also be conducted by association or topic.

http://www.chadd.org/ Children and Adults with Attention Deficit Disorder
http://www.add.org/ The National Attention Deficit Disorder Association

5 Bipolar Disorder

• Key Terms

Bipolar: The two extreme mood states of mania and depression illustrated in bipolar disorder.

Cyclothymia: A condition in which numerous periods of abnormally elevated, expansive, or irritable moods are experienced interspersed with periods of depressed mood. Neither mood state reaches the height nor depth to qualify as bipolar disorder.

Distractibility: The inability to maintain attention, shifting from one area or topic to another with minimal provocation, or attention being drawn too frequently to unimportant or irrelevant external stimuli.

Dysphoria: A mood of general dissatisfaction, unpleasantness, restlessness, anxiety, discomfort, and unhappiness observed in depressive states.

Euphoria: An exaggerated feeling of well-being, or elation.

Grandiosity: An inflated appraisal of one's worth, power, knowledge, importance, or identity and may include delusional thinking.

Hypomania: A clinical syndrome that indicates an elated mood state similar but less severe than that described by the term *mania* or manic episode; it generally does not cause social or occupational impairment and has a duration of more than 4 days.

Kindling: Refers to a neurological based theory, which postulates that bipolar disorder develops gradually in a progression from less severe episodes of mood disturbance and escalates over time.

Mixed State: A behavioral condition displayed for a period of at least 1 week in which manic and major depressive mood states are

(continues)

exhibited every day. Symptoms are sufficiently severe to cause impairment in social and occupational functioning.

Mood: A consistent emotional state experienced by an individual over time that influences her perception of the world. Examples may be dysphoric, elevated, expansive, euphoric, or irritable.

Racing Thoughts: A rapid series of ideas that occur during manic episodes.

*Human beings experience a variety of **moods**, from happiness to sadness to anger. Usually these can be experienced on a daily basis and can be linked to a specific precipitating event. However, in people with mood disorders, mood changes are often extreme and disproportionate to the event or not linked to any causative event at all. Often these severe changes in mood affect the individual's family, social, or work life. If these mood changes are severe enough, they can handicap the individual's ability to function and care for herself on a daily basis.*

BIPOLAR DISORDER

Bipolar I disorder is a common mood disorder whose primary symptoms include acute affective episodes with full or partial remission. This debilitating disorder has a lifetime prevalence of 1 percent (ADA, 2000).

Causes

Bipolar II disorder, as currently defined in the *DSM-IV-TR* (APA, 2000), shows diagnostic stability, a greater risk of the same disorder among relatives, a high frequency of episodes, increased risk of suicidality (usually during the depressed phase; 10 to 15 percent of those with bipolar II), and comorbidity. The diagnosis remains underused because hypomania is frequently not recognized, especially when occurring in the context of atypical depression.

Mood disorders are sometimes caused by general medical conditions or medications. These can be classified as bipolar IV. Classic examples include the depressive syndromes associated with dominant hemispheric strokes, hypothyroidism,

Cushing's disease, and pancreatic cancer (APA, 2000). Antihypertensives and oral contraceptives are the most frequent examples of medications that may cause depression.

Figure 5–1 describes one risk factor for bipolar disorder.

There are few cross-cultural studies of bipolar disorder. However, the Cross-National Collaborative Group study found

> Epidemiological risk factors for bipolar may include "when" a person is born. Torrey, Rawlings, Ennis, Merrill, and Flores (1996) report that 6 percent more people diagnosed with bipolar disorder were born during the months of December through March.

Figure 5–1 Epidemiological risk factor. Note. From: "Birth Seasonality in Bipolar Disorder, Schizophrenia, Schizoaffective Disorder and Stillbirths," by E. F. Torrey, R. R. Rawlings, J. M. Ennis, D. D. Merrill, and D. S. Flores, 1996, Schizophrenia Research, 21, pp. 141–149. Adapted with permission.

a lifetime prevalence of bipolar disorder that varied from 3 per 1,000 in Taiwan, 4 per 1,000 in Korea, 5 per 1,000 in Germany, and 6 per 1,000 in Canada and Puerto Rico, to 9 per 1,000 in the United States Epidemiologic Catchment Area (ECA data) and 15 per 1,000 in New Zealand (Weissman et al., 1996). Data are still limited about comparative rates of psychiatric disorders in minority populations in the United States. However, Robins and Regier (1991), in their National Institute of Mental Health Epidemiologic Catchment Area (ECA) study, found little variation in rates of disorders by race or ethnicity.

Descriptions of bipolar disorder and its etiology can be traced back to the early second century, when Aretaeus of Cappadocia recognized the association between melancholia and mania. It was not until the end of the 1800s that another major contribution to our understanding of this mood disorder was developed. In 1896, Kraepelin separated the functional psychosis into two groups, dementia praecox and manic-depressive psychosis. There have been many schools of thought about the classification and origins of bipolar disorder as well as other mood disorders. Psychodynamic, existential, cognitive-behavioral, and developmental theories have all been postulated as the underlying cause of the illness. Parenting, grief, or dysfunctional defense mechanisms were once seen as underlying causes for the onset of bipolar disorder. However, current research indicates that biological and genetic factors may be the most significant etiological factors. Bipolar disorder is seen as a complex disorder that has many contributors to onset. The above-mentioned theories all play an important role in understanding the interplay of etiological and precipitating or contributing factors, and the development of nonpharmacologic treatment modalities.

Because individuals with bipolar disorders may exhibit two extremely divergent sets of moods and behaviors, the neurochemical theories underlying each must be understood to successfully treat the illness. Neurochemical processes underlying depression have been identified as the biogenic amine theory. The biogenic amine theory of depression essentially implies that an imbalance or relative deficiency exists in relation to certain neurotransmitters or biogenic amines such as norepinephrine and serotonin. Deficiencies of these substances result in neurochemical imbalance.

The mechanisms that underlie the development of mania are much less understood. Limited data are available regarding specific neurochemical processes as they relate to alterations experienced with mania. It has been suggested that the symptoms of bipolar disorder result from an inability to modulate neuronal excitation. For example, it is postulated that the drug lithium acts on the inositol phosphate second messenger system inhibiting neurons to release, activate, or respond to neurotransmitters. It is also suggested that divalproex sodium (Depakote) increases gamma-aminobutyric acid (GABA)-ergic inhibitory activity (among other actions), thereby dampening aberrant neuronal excitation through a different physiological mechanism. Research is ongoing to support these hypotheses and to develop a more complete understanding of the neurochemical processes involved in mania (Ganong, 1999).

Scientific knowledge about the neuroanatomical component of bipolar disorder is just beginning and will act as a foundation for further neurochemical discovery. Findings indicate that individuals with bipolar disorder exhibit the following variations in brain structure and impaired functioning. See Table 5–1.

A number of studies have found that among people with bipolar disorder, women are more likely than men to have a thyroid disorder. Anecdotal evidence indicates that there may be some therapeutic benefit from the understanding of the relationship between the two disorders.

There is compelling evidence that links dysregulation of biological and genetic factors and alterations of specific brain regions with bipolar disorder. Research also links these factors with behaviors associated with mental health and mental illness. See Figure 5–2 for a glimpse at various brain structures associated with mental health.

Table 5–1 • Variations in Brain Structure and Impaired Functioning in Clients with Bipolar Disorder

Structural Variation/Abnormality*	Functional Impairment (All decreased)
Diencephalon (thalamus, mamillothalamic tract, and internal medullary lamina)	Memory performance
Prefrontal cortex	Verbal memory (recall of a story or single word)
Frontal subcortical	Attention dysfunction
Brain lesions	Verbal learning
Midsagittal areas reduction	Verbal fluency
Abnormal white brain matter (increase with age)	Psychomotor speed
Medial temporal lobe (hippocampus, parahippocampal and perirhinal cortices— episodes of depression and mania may result in hypercortisolemia, producing damage)	Declarative memory (conscious recollection of facts and events
Basal ganglia	

*The functional impairments do not necessarily correspond with the identified structural variation.

For a brief three-dimensional review of brain structure and functioning at the macro- and microstructural levels and a basic discussion of the effects of these functions on mental health, visit the National Institute of Mental Health (NIMH) site. To access, locate http://www.nimh.nih.gov, highlight "for the public" on the menu, and select the "science education" subheading. Use QuickTime Player or RealPlayer software to view (both can be downloaded for free). For a copy of the CD, send a request by e-mail at nimhinfo@nih.gov.

Figure 5–2 The brain's inner workings

Findings from more than 40 family, twin and adoption studies spanning six decades consistently show that the risk to relatives of those individuals with bipolar disorder is significantly greater than the risk for those individuals without bipolar disorder in the family history (see Figure 5–3). The risk of developing bipolar disorder is greatest when the disorder is present in first-degree family members

A genetic study conducted by Pauls, Bailey, Carter, Allen, and Egeland (1995) with 42 old order Amish families, which included 689 relatives, identified that an autosomal dominant inheritance model was found to be consistent with the transmission of bipolar I disorder within close relatives. This strongly supports the genetic transmission theory of bipolar disorder.

Figure 5–3 Cultural considerations. Note. *From Complex Segregation Analyses of Old Order Amish Families Ascertained Through Bipolar I Individuals, by D. L. Pauls, J. N. Bailey, A. S. Carter, C. R. Allen, & J. A. Egeland, 1995,* American Journal of Medical Genetics, 60*(4), 290–297. Reprinted with permission*

(i.e., mother, father, or siblings). One or more genes that could contribute to as many as one in four cases of bipolar disorder may be located on a region of chromosome 18. Of the genes identified, one codes for a protein that plays a specific part in chemical signal reception; the other is involved in stress hormone production, a physiological function that has been shown to be hyperexcitable in both depression and bipolar disorder. Other genetic findings include identification of region 22.3 of chromosome 21 and chromosome 11 and a possible relation with bipolar illness.

New research has indicated that another important factor plays a significant role in the development of bipolar disorder. This factor is related to an area of study called chronobiology and focuses on the circadian rhythm or sleep-wake cycle of the body. Several studies support the hypothesis that chronobiologic mechanisms are involved in the pathogenesis of bipolar disorder (Callahan & Bauer, 1999).

One theory of how bipolar disorder begins and is maintained is called the **kindling** theory. Bipolar disorder develops as a result of biologic and genetic predisposition in addition to environmental factors. This process often results in less severe episodes of mood disturbances that initially occur infrequently and escalate over time. As this repetitive cycle occurs, the mood disturbance becomes more severe at more frequent intervals, finally resulting in a full-blown bipolar disorder. This pattern is analogous to the use of kindling to build a fire.

Symptoms

According to the *Diagnostic and Statistical Manual of Mental Disorders*, 4th edition Text Revision (*DSM-IV-TR*), **bipolar** disorder is a recurrent mood disorder featuring one or more episodes of mania or mixed episodes of mania and depression (American Psychiatric Association [APA], 2000; Goodwin & Jamison, 1990). Bipolar disorder differs from major depressive disorder in that there is a history of manic or **hypomanic** (milder and not psychotic) episodes.

In bipolar disorder, the mood disturbance ranges from pure **euphoria**, or elation, to irritability to a labile admixture that also includes **dysphoria** (unpleasant mood). There are basically four different kinds of mood episodes that occur in bipolar disorder. These include episodes of *mania, hypomania, depression,* and *mixed episodes* (symptoms of both mania and depression at the same time or alternating frequently during the day).

In the manic phase of bipolar disorder thought content is often grandiose but can also be paranoid. **Grandiosity** usually takes the form both of overvalued ideas (e.g., "My computer program is the best one ever written") and of frank delusions (e.g., "I can control others in the room just by looking at them"). Auditory and visual hallucinations can complicate more severe episodes. Thinking speed increases (**racing thoughts**), with ideas typically racing through the manic person's consciousness. However, problems with **distractibility** and poor concentration often prohibit the implementation of new creative ideas.

Judgment is often compromised to varying degrees. This can be experienced as spending sprees, offensive or disinhibited behavior, drug or alcohol binges, promiscuity, or other objectively reckless behaviors. Individuals with bipolar disorder typically experience an increase in energy, libido, and activity. However, a perceived reduced need for sleep can deplete physical reserves and complicate the course of the disorder.

If the client with mania is delirious, paranoid, or catatonic, the behavior is difficult to distinguish from that of a client with schizophrenia. Most people with bipolar disorder have a history of remission and at least satisfactory functioning before onset of the index episode of illness.

According to the *DSM-IV-TR* (APA, 2000), bipolar depression includes type I (prior mania) and type II (prior hypomanic episodes only). About 1.1 percent of the adult population suffers from the type I form, and 0.6 percent suffers from the type II form (Goodwin & Jamison, 1990). It also includes cyclothymia and bipolar disorder not otherwise specified. Tables 5–2 through 5–10 describe the particular criteria sets used to specify the nature of the current or most recent epi-

---

Table 5–2 • Diagnostic Criteria for 296.0x Bipolar I Disorder, Single Manic Episode

A. Presence of only one Manic Episode and no last Major Depressive Episodes.

   Note: Recurrence is defined as either a change in polarity from depression or an interval of at least 2 months without manic symptoms.

B. The Manic Episode is not better accounted for by Schizoaffective Disorder and is not superimposed on Schizophrenia, Schizophreniform Disorder, Delusional Disorder, or Psychotic Disorder Not Otherwise Specified.

Specify if:

   Mixed: If symptoms meet criteria for a Mixed Episode

If the full criteria are currently met for a Manic, Mixed, or Major Depressive Episode, specify its current clinical status and/or features:

   Mild, Moderate, Severe Without Psychotic Features/Severe With Psychotic Features
   With Catatonic Features
   With Postpartum Onset

If the full criteria are not currently met for a Manic, Mixed, or Major Depressive Episode, specify the current clinical status of the Bipolar I Disorder or features of the most recent episode:

   In Partial Remission, In Full Remission
   With Catatonic Features
   With Postpartum Onset

Note. From *Diagnostic and Statistical Manual of Mental Disorders* (4th edition Text Revision) (*DSM-IV-TR*), by American Psychiatric Association, 2000, Washington, DC: Author. Reprinted with permission.

Table 5–3 • Diagnostic Criteria for 296.40 Bipolar I Disorder, Most Recent Episode Hypomanic

A. Currently (or most recently) in a Hypomanic Episode.

B. There has previously been at least one Manic Episode or Mixed Episode.

C. The mood symptoms cause clinically significant distress or impairment in social, occupational, or other important areas of functioning.

D. The mood episodes in Criteria A and B are not better accounted for by Schizoaffective Disorder and are not superimposed on Schizophrenia, Schizophreniform Disorder, Delusional Disorder, or Psychotic Disorder Not Otherwise Specified.

Specify:

   Longitudinal Course Specifiers (With and Without Interepisode Recovery)
   With Seasonal Pattern
   With Rapid Cycling

Note. From *Diagnostic and Statistical Manual of Mental Disorders* (4th edition Text Revision) (*DSM-IV-TR*), by American Psychiatric Association, 2000, Washington, DC: Author. Reprinted with permission.

---

sode in individuals who have had recurrent mood episodes. In addition to these particular variations of bipolar disorder there also are mood disorders caused by general medical conditions or by substances. The diagnostic criteria for these two conditions can be seen in Tables 5–11 and 5–12.

Table 5–4 • Diagnostic Criteria for 296.4x Bipolar I Disorder, Most Recent Episode Manic

A. Currently (or most recently) in a Manic Episode.

B. There has previously been at least one Major Depressive Episode, Manic Episode, or Mixed Episode.

C. The mood episodes in Criteria A and B are not better accounted for by Schizoaffective Disorder and are not superimposed on Schizophrenia, Schizophreniform Disorder, Delusional Disorder, or Psychotic Disorder Not Otherwise Specified.

If the full criteria are currently met for a Manic Episode, specify its current clinical status and/or features:

    Mild, Moderate, Severe Without Psychotic Features/Severe With Psychotic Features

    With Catatonic Features

    With Postpartum Onset

If the full criteria are not currently met for a Manic Episode, specify the current clinical status of the Bipolar I Disorder and/or features of the most recent Manic Episode:

    In Partial Remission, In Full Remission

    With Catatonic Features

    With Postpartum Onset

Specify:

    Longitudinal Course Specifiers (With and Without Interepisode Recovery)

    With Seasonal Pattern (applies only to the pattern of Major Depressive Episodes)

    With Rapid Cycling

Note. From *Diagnostic and Statistical Manual of Mental Disorders* (4th edition Text Revision) (*DSM-IV-TR*), by American Psychiatric Association, 2000, Washington, DC: Author. Reprinted with permission.

Table 5–5 • Diagnostic Criteria for 296.6x Bipolar I Disorder, Most Recent Episode Mixed

A. Currently (or most recently) in a Mixed Episode.

B. There has previously been at least one Major Depressive Episode, Manic Episode, or Mixed Episode.

C. The mood episodes in Criteria A and B are not better accounted for by Schizoaffective Disorder and are not superimposed on Schizophrenia, Schizophreniform Disorder, Delusional Disorder, or Psychotic Disorder Not Otherwise Specified.

If the full criteria are currently met for a Mixed Episode, specify its current clinical status and/or features:

    Mild, Moderate, Severe Without Psychotic Features/Severe With Psychotic Features

    With Catatonic Features

    With Postpartum Onset

If the full criteria are not currently met for a Mixed Episode, specify the current clinical status of the Bipolar I Disorder and/or features of the most recent Mixed Episode:

    In Partial Remission, In Full Remission

    With Catatonic Features

    With Postpartum Onset

(continues)

Table 5–5 *(continued)*

Specify:
>   Longitudinal Course Specifiers (With and Without Interepisode Recovery)
>   With Seasonal Pattern (applies only to the pattern of Major Depressive Episodes)
>   With Rapid Cycling

Note. From *Diagnostic and Statistical Manual of Mental Disorders* (4th edition Text Revision) (*DSM-IV-TR*), by American Psychiatric Association, 2000, Washington, DC: Author. Reprinted with permission.

Table 5–6 • Diagnostic Criteria for 296.5x Bipolar I Disorder, Most Recent Episode Depressed

A. Currently (or most recently) in a Major Depressive Episode.

B. There has previously been at least one Manic Episode or Mixed Episode.

C. The mood episodes in Criteria A and B are not better accounted for by Schizoaffective Disorder and are not superimposed on Schizophrenia, Schizophreniform Disorder, Delusional Disorder, or Psychotic Disorder Not Otherwise Specified.

If the full criteria are currently met for a Mixed Episode, specify its current clinical status and/or features:
>   Mild, Moderate, Severe Without Psychotic Features/Severe With Psychotic Features
>   Chronic
>   With Catatonic Features
>   With Melancholic Features
>   With Atypical Features
>   With Postpartum Onset

If the full criteria are not currently met for a Major Mixed Episode, specify the current clinical status of the Bipolar I Disorder and/or features of the most recent Major Depressive Episode:
>   In Partial Remission, In Full Remission
>   Chronic
>   With Catatonic Features
>   With Melancholic Features
>   With Atypical Features
>   With Postpartum Onset

Specify:
>   Longitudinal Course Specifiers (With and Without Interepisode Recovery)
>   With Seasonal Pattern (applies only to the pattern of Major Depressive Episodes)
>   With Rapid Cycling

Note. From *Diagnostic and Statistical Manual of Mental Disorders* (4th edition Text Revision) (*DSM-IV-TR*), by American Psychiatric Association, 2000, Washington, DC: Author. Reprinted with permission.

According to *Mental Health: A Report of the Surgeon General* (U.S. DHHS, 1999), manic episodes occur, on average, every 2 to 4 years, although accelerated mood cycles can occur annually or even more frequently. The type I form of bipolar disorder is about equally common in men and women, unlike major depressive disorder, which is more common in women.

Table 5–7 • Diagnostic Criteria for 296.89 Bipolar II Disorder

A. Presence (or history) of one or more Major Depressive Episodes.

B. Presence (or history) of at least one Hypomanic Episode.

C. There has never been a Manic Episode or a Mixed Episode.

D. The mood symptoms in Criteria A and B are not better accounted for by Schizoaffective Disorder and are not superimposed on Schizophrenia, Schizophreniform Disorder, Delusional Disorder, or Psychotic Disorder Not Otherwise Specified.

E. The symptoms cause clinically significant distress or impairment in social, occupational, or other important areas of functioning.

Specify current or most recent episode:

   Hypomanic: if currently (or most recently) in a Hypomanic Episode

   Depressed: if currently (or most recently) in a Major Depressive Episode

If the full criteria are currently met for a Major Depressive Episode, specify its current clinical status and/or features:

   Mild, Moderate, Severe Without Psychotic Features/Severe With Psychotic Features

   Chronic

   With Catatonic Features

   With Melancholic Features

   With Atypical Features

   With Postpartum Onset

If the full criteria are not currently met for a Hypomanic or Major Depressive Episode, specify the current clinical status of the Bipolar II Disorder and/or features of the most recent Major Depressive Episode (only if it is the most recent type of mood episode):

   In Partial Remission, In Full Remission

   Chronic

   With Catatonic Features

   With Melancholic Features

   With Atypical Features

   With Postpartum Onset

Specify:

   Longitudinal Course Specifiers (With and Without Interepisode Recovery)

   With Seasonal Pattern (applies only to the pattern of Major Depressive Episodes)

   With Rapid Cycling

Note. From *Diagnostic and Statistical Manual of Mental Disorders* (4th edition Text Revision) (*DSM-IV-TR*), by American Psychiatric Association, 2000, Washington, DC: Author. Reprinted with permission.

There are six separate criteria sets for bipolar I disorder: single manic episode, most recent episode hypomanic, most recent episode manic, most recent episode mixed, most recent episode depressed, and most recent episode unspecified.

According to the current *DSM-IV-TR* (APA, 2000) classification system, the diagnosis of bipolar II requires the presence of a full hypomanic and a major depressive episode. A diagnosis of bipolar II cannot be made in individuals who experience fewer than four characteristics of hypomania, do not manifest the first criterion (elevated, expansive, or irritable mood), or have symptoms apparent only to themselves, as well as individuals whose hypomania is not preceded by a major depressive episode.

Table 5–8 • Diagnostic Criteria for 296.7 Bipolar I Disorder, Most Recent Episode Unspecified

A. Criteria, except for duration, are currently (or most recently) met for a Manic, a Hypomanic, a Mixed, or a Major Depressive Episode.

B. There has previously been at least one Manic Episode or Mixed Episode.

C. The mood symptoms cause clinically significant distress or impairment in social, occupational, or other important areas of functioning.

D. The mood symptoms in Criteria A and B are not better accounted for by Schizoaffective Disorder and are not superimposed on Schizophrenia, Schizophreniform Disorder, Delusional Disorder, or Psychotic Disorder Not Otherwise Specified.

E. The mood symptoms in Criteria A and B are not due to the direct physiological effects of a substance (e.g., a drug of abuse, a medication, or other treatment) or a general medical condition (e.g., hyperthyroidism).

Specify:

Longitudinal Course Specifiers (With and Without Interepisode Recovery)

With Seasonal Pattern (applies only to the pattern of Major Depressive Episodes)

With Rapid Cycling

Note. From *Diagnostic and Statistical Manual of Mental Disorders* (4th edition Text Revision) (*DSM-IV-TR*), by American Psychiatric Association, 2000, Washington, DC: Author. Reprinted with permission.

Table 5–9 • Diagnostic Criteria for 301.13 Cyclothymic Disorder

A. For at least 2 years, the presence of numerous periods with hypomanic symptoms and numerous periods with depressive symptoms that do not meet criteria for a Major Depressive Episode.

Note: In children and adolescents, the duration must be at least 1 year.

B. During the above 2-year period (1 year in children and adolescents), the person has not been without the symptoms in Criterion A for more than 2 months at a time.

C. No Major Depressive Episode, Manic Episode, or Mixed Episode has been present during the first 2 years of the disturbance.

Note: After the initial 2 years (1 year in children and adolescents) of Cyclothymic Disorder, there may be superimposed Manic or Mixed Episodes (in which case both Bipolar I Disorder and Cyclothymic Disorder may be diagnosed) or Major Depressive Episodes (in which case both Bipolar II Disorder and Cyclothymic Disorder may be diagnosed).

D. The symptoms in Criterion A are not better accounted for by Schizoaffective Disorder and are not superimposed on Schizophrenia, Schizophreniform Disorder, Delusional Disorder, or Psychotic Disorder Not Otherwise Specified.

E. The symptoms are not due to the direct physiological effects of a substance (e.g., a drug of abuse, a medication) or a general medical condition (e.g., hyperthyroidism).

F. The symptoms cause clinically significant distress or impairment in social, occupational, or other important areas of functioning.

Note. From *Diagnostic and Statistical Manual of Mental Disorders* (4th edition Text Revision) (*DSM-IV-TR*), by American Psychiatric Association, 2000, Washington, DC: Author. Reprinted with permission.

Table 5–10 • 296.80 Bipolar Disorder Not Otherwise Specified

The Bipolar Disorder Not Otherwise Specified category includes disorders with bipolar features that do not meet criteria for any specific Bipolar Disorder. Examples include:

1. Very rapid alteration (over days) between manic symptoms and depressive symptoms that meet symptom threshold criteria but not minimal duration criteria for Manic, Hypomanic, or Major Depressive Episodes

2. Recurrent Hypomanic Episodes without intercurrent depressive symptoms

3. A Manic or Mixed Episode superimposed on Delusional Disorder, residual Schizophrenia, or Psychotic Disorder Not Otherwise Specified

---

Note. From *Diagnostic and Statistical Manual of Mental Disorders* (4th edition Text Revision) (*DSM-IV-TR*), by American Psychiatric Association, 2000, Washington, DC: Author. Reprinted with permission.

Table 5–11 • Diagnostic Criteria for 293.83 Mood Disorder Due to . . . (Indicate the General Medical Condition)

A. A prominent and persistent disturbance in mood predominates in the clinical picture and is characterized by either (or both) of the following:

   (1) depressed mood or markedly diminished interest or pleasure in all, or almost all, activities

   (2) elevated, expansive, or irritable mood

B. There is evidence from the history, physical examination, or laboratory findings that the disturbance is the direct physiological consequence of a general medical condition.

C. The disturbance is not better accounted for by another mental disorder (e.g., Adjustment Disorder With Depressed Mood in response to the stress of having a general medical condition).

D. The disturbance does not occur exclusively during the course of a delirium.

E. The symptoms cause clinically significant distress or impairment in social, occupational, or other important areas of functioning.

Specify type:

   With Depressive Features: if the predominant mood is depressed but the full criteria are not met for a Major Depressive Episode

   With Major Depressive-Like Episode: if the full criteria are met (except Criterion D) for a Major Depressive Episode)

   With Manic Features: if the predominant mood is elevated, euphoric, or irritable

   With Mixed Features: if the symptoms of both mania and depression are present but neither predominates

---

Note. From *Diagnostic and Statistical Manual of Mental Disorders* (4th edition Text Revision) (*DSM-IV-TR*), by American Psychiatric Association, 2000, Washington, DC: Author. Reprinted with permission.

Cyclothymia, sometimes categorized as bipolar III, is marked by manic and depressive states, yet neither is of sufficient intensity nor duration to merit a diagnosis of bipolar disorder or major depressive disorder. The diagnosis of cyclothymia is appropriate if there is a history of hypomania but no prior episodes of mania or major depression.

Mixed states can be described as the coexistence of depressive and manic symptoms. Mixed states have not received

Table 5–12 • Diagnostic Criteria for Substance-Induced Mood Disorder

A. A prominent and persistent disturbance in mood predominates in the clinical picture and is characterized by either (or both) of the following:

(1) depressed mood or markedly diminished interest or pleasure in all, or almost all, activities

(2) elevated, expansive, or irritable mood

B. There is evidence from the history, physical examination, or laboratory findings of either (1) or (2):

(1) the symptoms in Criterion A developed during, or within a month of, Substance Intoxication or Withdrawal

(2) medication use is etiologically related to the disturbance

C. The disturbance is not better accounted for by a Mood Disorder that is not substance induced. Evidence that the symptoms are better accounted for by a Mood Disorder that is not substance induced might include the following: the symptoms precede the onset of the substance use (or medication use); the symptoms persist for a substantial period of time (e.g., about a month) after the cessation of acute withdrawal or severe intoxication or are substantially in excess of what would be expected given the type or amount of the substance used or the duration of use; or there is other evidence that suggests the existence of an independent non-substance-induced Mood Disorder (e.g., a history of recurrent Major Depressive Episodes).

D. The disturbance does not occur exclusively during the course of a delirium.

E. The symptoms cause clinically significant distress or impairment in social, occupational, or other important areas of functioning.

Note: This diagnosis should be made instead of a diagnosis of Substance Withdrawal only when the mood symptoms are in excess of those usually associated with the intoxication or withdrawal syndrome and when the symptoms are sufficiently severe to warrant independent clinical attention.

Codes (Specific Substance-Induced Mood Disorder):

(291.89 Alcohol; 292.84 Amphetamine [or Amphetamine-Like Substance]; 292.84 Cocaine; 292.84 Hallucinogen; 292.84 Inhalant; 292.84 Opioid; 292.84 Phencyclidine [or Phencyclidine-Like Substance]; 292.84 Sedative, Hypnotic, or Anxiolytic; 292.84 Other [or Unknown] Substance)

Specify type:

With Depressive Features: if the predominant mood is depressed

With Manic Features: if the predominant mood is elevated, euphoric, or irritable

With Mixed Features: if the symptoms of both mania and depression are present but neither predominates

Specify if:

With Onset During Intoxication: if the criteria are met for Intoxication with the substance and the symptoms develop during the intoxication syndrome

With Onset During Withdrawal: if criteria are met for Withdrawal from the substance and the symptoms develop during, or shortly after, a withdrawal syndrome

---

Note. From *Diagnostic and Statistical Manual of Mental Disorders* (4th edition Text Revision) (*DSM-IV-TR*), by American Psychiatric Association, 2000, Washington, DC: Author. Reprinted with permission.

extensive research evaluation. They can be expressed on a continuum ranging from psychotic features to milder and subclinical states. Frequently, the entire episode presents with severe depression with agitated features and acceleration of thought suggestive of a depressive mixed state.

The most consistent findings to date have been the appearance of specific abnormalities, or lesions in the white matter of the brain in people with bipolar disorder. White matter consists of groups of nerve cell fibers surrounded by fatty sheaths that appear white in color. These sheaths help the transmission of electrical signals within the brain. Although the white matter abnormalities appear in many parts of the brain in individuals with bipolar disorder, they tend to be concentrated in areas that are responsible for emotional processing. These brain changes appear more often than expected in young people with bipolar disorder. This finding suggests that the white matter abnormalities seen in MRI are related to the presence of the disorder.

The indicated neuroanatomical changes and functional impairments have been identified in individuals who are euthymic and stable in their disease as well as those who are acutely ill. Cognitive dysfunction seems to be associated with severity and chronicity of the illness and with increasing age although research with adolescents has indicated similar findings (Dasari et al., 1999; Martinez-Aran et al., 2000).

Although some individuals may experience only a single episode of mania and depression in their lifetimes, over 95 percent of people with bipolar disorder have recurrent episodes of depression and mania throughout their lives. The probability of experiencing new episodes of depression or mania increases with each subsequent episode despite treatment. There is also evidence that the time between episodes decreases during the course of the illness. The marked changes in mood, personality, thinking, and behavior that are part of the disorder often have significant effects on interpersonal relationships across the life span.

Papolos and Papolos (1999) reported many parents describing their children with bipolar disorder as being different from early infancy. Frequently, parents described their infants as sleeping erratically; not sleeping long; being irritable, fussy, and difficult to settle; temperamental; and extremely anxious, often experiencing great difficulty with separation from the mother. Night terrors, rages, fear of death, and behaviors that fit into the diagnostic category of oppositional defiant disorder are often an aspect of bipolar disorder.

Bipolar disorder is frequently missed or misdiagnosed in the older adult. Depression is beginning to be more readily diagnosed both in primary care settings and in community settings. However, the mood elevation, increase in energy and activity, and other subtle manifestations of bipolar disorder are often left unrecognized. Bipolar disorder in the older adult increases the risk of suicide. Complicating the assessment and diagnosis of bipolar disorder in the geriatric population is that the client may present with various medical conditions, such as dementia.

Key Facts

Bipolar disorders are a major public health concern. Bipolar disorder I affects 1 to 1.5 percent of the general population of the United States affecting equal numbers of males and females (U.S. DHHS, 1999). Bipolar II has been identified as affecting 0.5 to 0.6 percent of the population, with females being more affected than males (U.S. DHHS, 1999). Overall economic costs of bipolar disorder in the United States is estimated at $45 billion per year.

Males have more manic episodes, are more likely to be hospitalized with a manic episode, and are likely to have a comorbidity of substance abuse and dependence. In the initial episode of mania, males display more hyperactivity, grandiosity, and risky behavior, and females more often display racing thoughts and distractibility. Of individuals hospitalized for mania, 30 percent remain unemployed for 6 months and 23 percent for 1 year.

TREATMENT

Because of the vulnerability of individuals with this disorder, it is imperative that nurses understand the course, presentation, and opportunities for intervention from a life span perspective. Some factors are unique according to age categories, whereas other issues apply regardless of age group.

Three major categories of psychotropic medications are used in the successful treatment of bipolar disorder: antidepressants, mood stabilizers, and antipsychotics. Table 5-13 lists the top-rated choices for initial medications.

There are two properties that define mood stabilizers: (1) they provide relief from acute episodes of mania or depression or prevent them from occurring, and (2) they do not worsen depression or mania or lead to increases in cycling. Pharmacologic treatment of bipolar disorder often requires a combined pharmacologic approach. This often involves an antidepressant and a mood stabilizer (Tables 5-14 and 5-15). Antidepressants are used for the depressed phase of bipolar disorder with dosages and side effects being similar to those used to treat unipolar depression. However, because mania can be a side effect of an antidepressant, clients are often concurrently maintained on therapeutic levels of a mood stabilizer (APA, 2000; Sachs et al., 2000). Before administering mood stabilizers, nurses need to check basic laboratory studies, including electrolytes, complete blood count (CBC), chemistries, electrocardiogram (ECG) and pregnancy tests in women of childbearing age. Because these agents are harmful to the developing fetus, nurses also need to ask questions about birth control methods. Health education is an integral part of caring for the client with bipolar disorder.

Lithium carbonate was the first psychotropic agent shown to prevent recurrent episodes of illness. The two major indications for use of lithium are prevention and treatment of mania.

(continues)

Table 5-13 • Top-Rated Choices for Initial Medications*

Euphoric mania or hypomania	Lithium or divalproex
Mixed or dysphoric mania	Divalproex
Mania with psychosis	Divalproex or lithium with antipsychotic (atypical or conventional)

*Assumes no contraindications; adjunctive medications added subsequently if indicated.

Note. From "The Expert Consensus Guideline Series. Medication Treatment of Bipolar Disorder 2000," by G. S. Sachs, D. J. Printz, D. A. Kahn, D. Carpenter, and J. P. Docherty, 2000, *Postgraduate Medicine*, p. 8. Reprinted with permission.

Table 5-14 • Commonly Used Mood Stabilizers, Usual Adult Doses and Therapeutic Serum Levels

Mood Stabilizer	Adult Dose Range	Therapeutic Serum Levels
Lithium (Eskalith, Lithobid, Lithonate)	600–1800 mg/d	0.6–1.2 mEq/L
Divalproex (Depakote)	750–4200 mg/d	50–100 µ/ml
Other anticonvulsants used as mood stabilizers		
Carbamazepine (Tegretol, Carbatrol)	400–1600 gm/d	4–12 µ/ml
Lamotrigine (Lamictal)	300–500 mg/d	N/A
Topiramate (Topamax)	400–1600 mg/d	N/A

Table 5–15 • Antidepressants Used in Bipolar Disorder

Bupropion (Wellbutrin)

Selective Serotonin Reuptake Inhibitors (SSRIs):

Fluoxetine (Prozac)

Fluvoxamine (Luvox)

Paroxetine (Paxil)

Sertraline (Zoloft)

Venlafaxine (Effexor)

If these are ineffective or cause undesirable side effects, other choices include:

Mirtazapine (Remeron)

Nefazodone (Serzone)

*Monoamine oxidase inhibitors:

Phenelzine (Nardil)

Tranylcypromine (Parnate)

†Trycyclic antidepressants:

Amitriptyline (Elavil)

Desipramine (Norpramine, Pertofrane)

Imipramine (Tofranil)

Nortriptyline (Pamelor)

---

*These are effective but require the client to stay on a special diet to avoid dangerous side effects.

†Tricyclics are more likely to cause side effects or set off manic episodes or rapid cycling than newer ADP agents.

TREATMENT *(continued)*

Several anticonvulsants have been found effective in the treatment of bipolar disorder. The most frequently used are valproic acid (Depakene), also known as divalproex (Depakote), and carbamazepine (Tegretol). Consensus and practice guidelines concerning the treatment of bipolar disorders indicate the efficacy of newer agents such as lamotrigine (Lamictal) and topiramate (Topamax) (APA, 2000; Sachs et al., 2000). The most common side effects of lamotrigine (Lamictal) include dizziness, headaches, somnolence, and a dangerous allergic rash. Major side effects associated with topiramate include ataxia, dizziness, and kidney stones.

Benzodiazepines are antianxiety agents that are often used in the acute phase of mania or to treat the accompanying symptoms of overwhelming anxiety and panic in the client experiencing bipolar symptoms. These medications are used for a brief time, until long-term medications can become therapeutic. Common benzodiazepines include lorazepam (Ativan), clonazepam (Klonopin), and alprazolam (Xanax).

Calcium channel blockers can be used for treatment-resistant mania as well as for clients who cannot tolerate lithium. Clients who cannot tolerate lithium include those who are pregnant or who may have sustained some degree of brain injury. Verapamil (Calan) and nifedipine (Procardia) are examples of calcium channel blockers used for treatment (APA, 2000; Blanco, Lage, Olfson, Marcus, & Pincus, 2002; Sachs et al., 2000).

Antipsychotics are often used as an adjunct to antidepressant therapy to treat psychotic symptoms of either acute mania or depression in the client with bipolar disorder (APA, 2000; Lehne, Moore, Crosby, & Hamilton, 1998; Sachs et al., 2000) until the mood stabilizer becomes effective. There are two kinds of antipsychotics used today: the "older," or "conventional," types and the "newer," or "atypical," types. Serious problems can occur with the use of older, or conventional, antipsychotics such as the potential to develop tardive dyskinesia. Today the atypical antipsychotics are usually the first choice for clinicians. See Table 5–16 for a list of atypical antipsychotics.

(continues)

Table 5–16 • Current Atypical Antipsychotics

Olanzapine (Zyprexa)

Quetiapine (Seroquel)

Risperidone (Risperdal)

Clozapine (Clozaril)

Ziprasidone (Geodon)

TREATMENT *(continued)*

Electroconvulsive therapy (ECT) is an effective and often lifesaving treatment for mania or depression if pharmacologic interventions fail or if symptom severity requires immediate relief (APA, 2000). ECT continues to be criticized by some but remains a safe and effective treatment with minimal side effects.

Milieu management is important if the client requires hospitalization in order to be stabilized. Stabilization can be viewed in terms of medications, moods, and behaviors. Clients can be hospitalized for stabilization of either mania or severe depression. Regardless of the reason for admission, environmental stimuli must be controlled and managed appropriately to meet the individual needs of the patient and others on the unit. Awareness and prevention of suicidal and homicidal intent may necessitate that the client be managed one-on-one with a psychiatric professional. It is imperative that the nurses understand that suicidal or homicidal intent can be expressed in many ways. Aggressive behaviors can quickly escalate and be directed internally or externally (toward the self or others). Once the client is stabilized, psychoeducational classes are helpful in maintaining biological and psychological equilibrium. This will be followed up in the community or outpatient setting. In summary, effective milieu management requires three essential elements: safety, limit setting, and stabilization. Table 5-17 lists some specific instructions for the client.

Appropriate identification of nursing focused problems or diagnoses must be a result of an ongoing thorough assessment. Table 5-18 includes a list of common nursing diagnoses when developing a plan of care for an individual with bipolar disorder. Areas of assessment that provide the most specific data related to bipolar disorder include mood, motor activity-energy, sexual interest, sleep, irritability, speech (rate and amount), language-thought processes, content of speech, disruptive-aggressive behavior,

(continues)

Table 5–17 • **Learning to Live with Bipolar Disorder**

- Maintain a stable sleep pattern
- Maintain a regular pattern of activity
- Do not use alcohol or other substances (includes legal and illegal)
- Ask for and use the support of family and friends
- Reduce stress at home and at work
- Be aware of your own early warning signs (often the first clue is change in sleep needs)
- Develop a repertoire of problem-solving skills
- Develop emotional tolerance/regulation skills
- Develop awareness of automatic negative thinking and approaches to combat them

Table 5–18 • **Common Nursing Diagnoses**

Risk for activity intolerance	Deficient knowledge
Impaired adjustment	Imbalanced nutrition: less than body requirements
Impaired verbal communication	Impaired parenting
Compromised family coping	Risk for powerlessness
Interrupted family processes	Self-care deficit
Dysfunctional grieving	Risk for situational low self-esteem
Ineffective health maintenance	Social isolation
Hopelessness	Disturbed thought processes
Ineffective coping	Risk for self-directed violence
Risk for injury	Risk for other-directed violence

Note. From *Nursing Diagnosis: Definitions and Classification 2001–2002*, by North American Nursing Diagnosis Association (NANDA), 2001, Philadelphia: Author. Adapted with permission.

TREATMENT *(continued)*

appearance, and insight regarding the current situation. In today's mental health care system, clients are only admitted to inpatient settings when they exhibit the most severe symptoms. Assessment (and treatment) is performed within a restricted period; therefore, the nurse must be efficient and precise in accomplishing these activities. One standardized instrument that can assist the nurse in systematic assessment in these areas is the Young Rating Scale for Mania (Young, Biggs, Ziegler, & Meyer, 1978).

The nurse caring for an individual with bipolar disorder, as with all psychiatric disorders, must identify incremental goals through which the client makes measurable, attainable (realistic) steps toward improvement. These incremental goals or outcomes in bipolar disorder are prioritized according to (1) safety and physiological functioning, (2) improved coping, and (3) return to preillness level of functioning. The nurse needs to identify outcomes directed at both the individual and the family or significant others to support the client's successful transition and growth.

Implementation and evaluation of care must be considered jointly when working collaboratively with clients and their families. Successful reintegration of the client into the family and the community is a long-term goal that hinges on successful coordination of interventions and evaluation of their effectiveness.

RESOURCES

Please note that because Internet resources are of a time-sensitive nature and URL addresses may change or be deleted, searches should also be conducted by association or topic.

Internet Resources

http://www.nami.org   National Alliance for the Mentally Ill

http://www.ndmda.org   National Depressive and Manic-Depressive Association (NMDA)

http://www.mhsource.com   National Alliance for Research on Schizophrenia and Depression (NARSAD)

http://www.ffcmh.org   Federation of Families

Cognitive
Disorders

6

• Key Terms

Alzheimer's Disease (AD): A condition characterized by progressive loss of memory, intellect, language, judgment, and impulse control. Neurofibrillary tangle and neuritic plaques are found in the cerebral cortex, particularly the hippocampus.

Aphasia: Loss of power of expression by speech, writing, or signs of loss of comprehension of spoken or written language owing to brain injury or pathology.

Apraxia: Loss of ability to carry out familiar, purposeful movements in the absence of paralysis or other motor or sensory impairments, especially the inability to make proper use of an object.

Cognitive Disorders: Those conditions in which "the predominant disturbance is a clinically significant deficit in cognition or memory that represents a significant change from a previous level of functioning" (APA, 2000).

Delirium: A medical syndrome characterized by acute onset and impairment in cognition, perception, and behavior. Also known as acute confusion.

Dementia: A condition manifested in the insidious development of memory and intellectual deficits, disorientation, and decreased cognitive functioning.

Dysarthria: Imperfect articulation of speech caused by muscular weakness resulting from damage to the central or peripheral nervous system.

Executive Function: Ability to set a goal, make decisions, and implement appropriate activities toward meeting that goal.

(continues)

• Key Terms *(continued)*

Focal Neurological Signs: Specific signs of neurological impairment such as blurred vision, aphasia, and the like.

Multi-infarct Dementia (MID): A probable irreversible dementia caused by many small strokes, or a large stroke.

Potentially Reversible Dementia: A condition characterized by an acute onset, causing neurological symptoms and changes in level of consciousness. If treated in time, the condition may be reversed. See *delirium*.

Probable Irreversible Dementia: Progressive loss of intellectual functioning caused by permanent brain damage.

Cognitive disorders are those conditions in which "the predominant disturbance is a clinically significant deficit in cognition or memory that represents a significant change from a previous level of functioning" (American Psychiatric Association [APA], 2000, p. 135). In the third revised edition of the Diagnostic and Statistical Manual of Mental Disorders (DSM-III-R), the term "organic" was applied to many cognitive disorders in which psychological and behavioral abnormalities are "associated with transient or permanent dysfunction of the brain" (APA, 1987, p. 98).

COGNITIVE DISORDERS— GENERAL

Causes

During intrauterine life the developing brain is exquisitely sensitive to changes in the biochemical environment and the supply of essential nutrients, especially glucose and oxygen. If disrupted this can result in temporary or permanent impairment. Additionally, injury and localized brain disease can result in the direct loss of nervous tissue (Figure 6–1 and see Figure 6–2). Obviously, if these disruptions or assaults occur early in fetal life, they can and often do have catastrophic results. Examples include congenital malformations and severe mental retardation. The birth process itself can be a difficult transition when the most dangerous occurrence is anoxia, which is worsened when combined with prematurity.

With age, there is an impairment in neurotransmission, especially with the serotonin, cholinergic, and dopamine systems (Strong, 1998). These changes may predispose the older person to signs of cognitive and affective disorders. Pronounced deficits may be related to severe cognitive disorders in older adults.

Psychosocial changes seem to occur with aging that affect coping and general health. Losses occurring with aging include aspects of all five physical senses and changes in body functioning that affect psychosocial activity. In addition, older adults frequently experience the loss of a spouse, friend, sibling, occupation, home, income, and possibly a child. These losses can

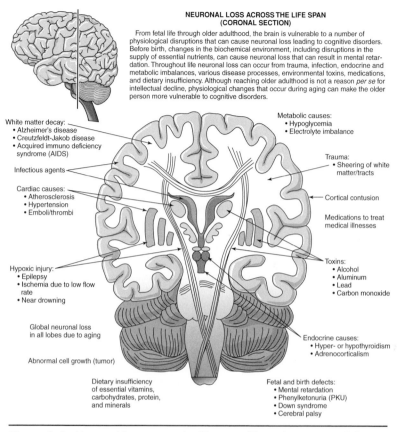

NEURONAL LOSS ACROSS THE LIFE SPAN
(CORONAL SECTION)

From fetal life through older adulthood, the brain is vulnerable to a number of physiological disruptions that can cause neuronal loss leading to cognitive disorders. Before birth, changes in the biochemical environment, including disruptions in the supply of essential nutrients, can cause neuronal loss that can result in mental retardation. Throughout life neuronal loss can occur from trauma, infection, endocrine and metabolic imbalances, various disease processes, environmental toxins, medications, and dietary insufficiency. Although reaching older adulthood is not a reason *per se* for intellectual decline, physiological changes that occur during aging can make the older person more vulnerable to cognitive disorders.

White matter decay:
• Alzheimer's disease
• Creutzfeldt-Jakob disease
• Acquired immuno deficiency syndrome (AIDS)

Infectious agents

Cardiac causes:
• Atherosclerosis
• Hypertension
• Emboli/thrombi

Hypoxic injury:
• Epilepsy
• Ischemia due to low flow rate
• Near drowning

Global neuronal loss in all lobes due to aging

Abnormal cell growth (tumor)

Dietary insufficiency of essential vitamins, carbohydrates, protein, and minerals

Metabolic causes:
• Hypoglycemia
• Electrolyte imbalance

Trauma:
• Sheering of white matter/tracts

Cortical contusion

Medications to treat medical illnesses

Toxins:
• Alcohol
• Aluminum
• Lead
• Carbon monoxide

Endocrine causes:
• Hyper- or hypothyroidism
• Adrenocorticalism

Fetal and birth defects:
• Mental retardation
• Phenylketonuria (PKU)
• Down syndrome
• Cerebral palsy

Figure 6–1 Neuronal loss across the life span. *(Illustration concept: Gail Kongable, MSN, CRN, CCRN, Department of Neurosurgery, University of Virginia Health Sciences Center.)*

present extraordinary burdens on the older person and must be kept in mind when caring for a geriatric patient. Tables 6–1 and 6–2 summarize psychosocial theories of aging and issues across the life span.

Symptoms

The different clinical presentations of organic mental disorders reflected differences in the localization, mode of onset, progression, duration, and nature of the underlying pathophysiological process. Because the term "organic mental disorder" implies that "nonorganic" mental disorders do not have a biological basis, the

term was not used in *DSM-IV-TR* (APA, 2000). The subtitle of Organic Mental Disorders versus "inorganic" mental disease in the *DSM-III-R* suggests a mind-body dualism. Therefore, in the *DSM-IV-TR*, disorders known to be caused physically are listed under the category that best describes the psychiatric features, so that a mood disorder induced by substance abuse is listed as a mood disorder. **Delirium, dementia**, and amnestic disorders are categorized as "cognitive disorders." In this way, organic disorders refer to a condition caused by something outside a mental disorder, but the mind-body dualism is softened.

Table 6–1 • Psychosocial Theories of Aging

Factor	Hypothesis
Disengagement*	Aging individuals and society gradually withdraw from each other for mutual benefit. Theory's popularity undermined by the recognition that each individual has a different aging pattern and the process often damages both society and the aged.
Activity†	Aging individuals should be expected to maintain norms of middle-aged adults: employment, activity, replacement of lost relationships. Age-related physical, mental, and socioeconomic losses may present legitimate obstacles to maintaining activity, thereby reducing universality of theory.
Development/ Continuity‡	Basic personality, attitude, and behaviors remain constant throughout the life span. Allows multiple options for aging and recognizes the individuality of the aging process.

Note. *From *Growing Old: The Process of Engagement,* by E. Cummings and W. E. Henry, 1961, New York: Basic Books. Adapted with permission.

†From *Older People,* by R. J. Havinghurst and R. Albrecht, 1953, New York: Longmans. Adapted with permission.

‡From *Middle Age and Aging,* by B. Neugarten, 1968, Chicago: University of Chicago Press. Adapted with permission.

Table 6–2 • Losses/Changes with Age

Stage	Age (yr.)	Task
Young adulthood	20–28	Development of life dream; separation from nuclear family. Erikson: Intimacy vs. isolation
Adulthood	29–39	Changing commitments; childbearing and childrearing; self-identity. Erikson: Generativity vs. stagnation
Middle adulthood	40–65 or 70	Reintegration of self-identity; launching family; accepting physical aging; redefined attitudes about money, religion, and death. Erikson: Generativity vs. stagnation
Late adulthood	65–70 and older	Capacity to feel whole in spite of diminishing health; adjusting to decreased physical strength, health; to retirement; reduced income; death of spouse. Feeling of enduring significance; adjusting and adopting social roles; maintaining maximum independence. Erikson: Ego integrity vs. despair

Note. From *Childhood and Society,* by E. Erikson, 1963, New York: W.W. Norton. Adapted with permission.

Included among cognitive disorders discussed in this chapter are those that affect younger persons, such as mental retardation and those that generally affect older persons, such as dementia and delirium. These syndromes are highly variable; they will be different from person to person and over time in the same individual.

Many physiological changes occur in the older adult that can affect memory function. There are changes in fat-to-lean body mass ratios and water balance that make medication prescription and electrolyte balances challenging. Liver and kidney dysfunction may occur and can also affect these areas. This must be kept in mind when prescribing medication or diagnosing an older adult who presents with "confusion."

Different species have different life span averages. A summary of pertinent physiological age-related changes and biological theories can be found in Tables 6–3 and 6–4.

Table 6–3 • Physiological Age-Associated Changes

System Affected	Change Noted	Age Span (yr)
Total body water		
Men	Declines from 60% to 54%	20–80
Women	Declines from 54% to 46%	20–80
Muscle mass	30% decrease	30–70
Taste buds	70% decrease	30–70
Renal perfusion	Reduced by 50%	30–70
Brain weight	Reduced by 6% to 11%	After age 50
Cardiac reserve	Decreases from 4.6 to 3.3 times resting cardiac output	25–70
Cerebral blood flow	Reduced by 20%	30–70
Reproductive system	Menopause (in women)	Around age 50
Liver	Loses mass	50 and older
Immune system	Declines	50 and older

Table 6–4 • Biological Theories of Aging

Factor	Hypothesis
Free radical structure	Altered cellular structure; thought to be caused by environmental pollutants
Cross-link of collagen	With age, collagen becomes more insoluble and rigid
Programmed cells	Biologic clock triggers events (e.g., onset of puberty, menopause, etc.)
Autoimmune reactions	The body forms antibodies against itself. Plays a role in the development of infections, cancer, diabetes mellitus, atherosclerosis, hypertension, and rheumatic heart disease
Lipofuscin	A relationship exists between age and the amount of accumulated lipofuscin
Somatic mutation	With age, defective cells multiply and lead to organ abnormalities, and system dysfunction
Stress	Wear and tear impair efficiency of cellular function, leading to physical decline
Radiation	Ultraviolet light decreases life span
Nutrition	Quality and quantity of diet is thought to influence life span

TREATMENT

The psychiatric nurse who is devoted to biological, psychological, social, and spiritual care of clients must also search for contributing factors related to cognitive disorders in an effort to identify the full array of potential nursing interventions.

An understanding of normal growth and development provides a framework for assessing the child or adolescent with a psychiatric or medical condition. Although theoretic concepts differ, theorists agree that development proceeds in a sequential manner along a prescribed continuum. Stages defined in each model are characterized by certain tasks or goals that must be mastered before a child can successfully progress to the next level.

As assessment and treatment proceed, it is important for the psychiatric nurse to remember that when using a developmental framework there is a wide variation within "normal" development. Growth and development occur fairly rapidly from birth to 3 years but is less dramatic through the latency period. During puberty and adolescence the rate of growth increases sharply and behavior is more labile again.

The nurse must recognize the importance of family, the support of significant others, the school, and the community, and include these persons in all stages of the nursing process.

When caring for a client with a cognitive disorder, some general guidelines can be followed:

- Perform a thorough assessment to ascertain the client's physical, emotional, and mental health status, focusing on strengths and weaknesses. This assessment includes results of diagnostic tests, use of medications, and the course of the disorder.
- Explore the client's previous environment and consult with caregivers to develop a care plan that is individualized and will enhance quality of life. Initiate the services of the interdisciplinary team and incorporate recommendations into a total plan of care.
- Modify the environment to promote optimal functioning. Most clients with cognitive disorders need structure and modified stimulation, and it is important to identify the client's likes and dislikes to help her feel secure.
- Monitor medications and diagnostic tests and be alert for signs and symptoms of delirium, especially in the very young and very old. Monitor the effects of medication and report any untoward effects. If delirium is suspected, implement interventions immediately.
- Include the family or primary caregivers in the plan of care. Often these primary caregivers are forgotten when the professional "takes over." Persons who have been caring for these clients can feel "left out" and frustrated if their valuable knowledge and experience is not sought after or used. Educate the family or primary caregiver on the course of the disorder, appropriate medications, signs of illness, and the need to take care of herself.
- Initiate the services of the case manager or social worker to help coordinate continuity of care and obtain the necessary support services across the continuum of health care and home settings.

The interdisciplinary team is important in designing comprehensive, holistic care for the person who is ill. This team consists of nurses, physicians, social workers, teachers and, possibly, special therapists such as physical and occupational therapists. The interdisciplinary team can develop a plan of inpatient and outpatient care that is appropriate for the person who is ill and her family on both inpatient and outpatient bases. Community resources such as partial hospitalization, special education, case management, day programs, assisted living, visiting nurses, and respite are examples. In caring for the cognitively impaired child or adult, it

(continues)

TREATMENT *(continued)*

is necessary for the psychiatric nurse to recognize the importance of caring for the caregiver as well. With a healthy caregiver, positive outcomes are possible.

In the medical examination, the physician and other health care providers look for any underlying medical disorders that might cause the symptoms associated with cognitive disorders. The neurological evaluation is not usually helpful when the psychiatric symptoms are caused by a medical condition. The neurological examination is usually normal and remains so until the disorder or disease is far advanced.

Diagnosis is based on symptoms, results of physical examination and history, and *DSM IV-TR* criteria.

AMNESTIC DISORDER

Causes

The main features of amnestic syndrome are inability to remember recent events and its relatively uncommon occurrence in children (APA, 1987; 1994; 2000). It may be found in childhood and adulthood, however, if the individual has experienced head trauma, hypoxia, lead or carbon monoxide poisoning, or herpes simplex encephalitis. It may also be related to alcohol withdrawal, sedative hypnotic, or anxiolytic intoxication in adults. The *DSM-IV-TR* classifies amnestic disorders as those caused by a general medical condition such as physical trauma or vitamin deficiency; Substance Induced Persisting Amnestic Disorder, which includes medications that are prescribed for the client; and Amnestic Disorder Not Otherwise Specified.

Symptoms

The primary feature of amnestic disorders is the loss of short-term memory that is directly caused by a physical disorder or a substance such as a medication, alcohol, or a toxin (APA, 2000).

TREATMENT

Nursing care of people with amnestic syndrome includes making sure they wear identification because they appear and sound normal. In early stages of the disease, clients may benefit from concrete memory aids such as calendars (marked off by others), schedules, and clocks. Later, careful supervision is required because clients may become lost in all but the most overlearned environments.

DELIRIUM

Causes

Causes of delirium are often a mystery. The disorder is hypothesized to be a response to cerebral oxidative system and the effects on neurotransmitters (Rasin, 1990) or a stress reaction mediated by elevated plasma cortisol and its effects on the brain (St. Pierre, 1996). Other factors that may contribute to the disorder are personal factors, such as isolation and traumatic relocation, and perceptual factors, such as the vision and hearing impairments experienced by so many older adults (Stanley, 1999). Many conditions produce symptoms of delirium. These are highlighted in Table 6–5.

Symptoms

DSM-IV-TR Diagnostic Criteria for Delirium Due to . . .
(Indicate the general medical condition.)

A. Disturbance of consciousness (i.e., reduced clarity of awareness of the environment) with reduced ability to focus, sustain, or shift attention.

B. A change in cognition (such as memory deficit, disorientation, language disturbance) or the development of a perceptual disturbance that is not better accounted for by a preexisting, established, or evolving dementia.

C. The disturbance develops over a short period of time (usually hours to days) and tends to fluctuate during the course of the day.

Table 6–5 • **Factors Associated with the Development of Delirium**

Category	Factor	Category	Factor
Body fluids and kidney function	Fluid/electrolyte disturbances Dehydration/volume depletion Hypocalcemia Hypokalemia Abnormal sodium level Low serum albumin High blood urea nitrogen (BUN) Elevated creatinine Azotemia Proteinuria Chronic renal disease	Age, gender, and living arrangement	Age 65 and older (higher incidence at age 80 or older) Male gender (suggested, nonsignificant relationship) Limited social contact (suggested, nonsignificant relationship) Admission from an institution
Sensory and neurological function	Sensory disturbances Pain (unmanaged or poorly managed) Neurological disease Cognitive impairment/brain damage/dementia (one of the most commonly identified risk factors, especially in older adults)	Infection and trauma	Symptomatic infection Urinary tract infection Respiratory infection Elevated white blood cell count at admission Emergency admission Fracture Falls Orthopedic surgery Physical illnesses (usually two or more in conjunction) Severity of illness
Circulation and oxygenation	Low blood pressures Cardiovascular disease Congestive heart disease Aortic aneurysm surgery Elevated prothrombin time (PT) Low hematocrit Abnormal arterial blood gases Respiratory insufficiency Noncardiac thoracic surgery	Effects of pharmaceuticals	Multiple medications (usually greater than four) Drugs with anticholinergic or central nervous system (CNS) effects Drug toxicity Psychoactive drug use Narcotic use Drug or alcohol abuse Drug withdrawal
Metabolism and body temperature	Metabolic disturbances Nutritional deficiencies Abnormal blood glucose Elevated aspartate aminotransferase (AST)/serum glutamic oxaloacetic transaminase (SGOT) Abnormal body temperature	Impaired physical or functional ability	Activity of daily living (ADL) impairment Urinary problems/incontinence

Note. From *Research-Based Protocol: Acute Confusion/Delirium*, by C. G. Rapp and M. G. Titler, 1998. Iowa City: The University of Iowa Gerontological Nursing Interventions Research Center. Adapted with permission.

D. There is evidence from the history, physical examination, or laboratory findings that the disturbance is caused by the direct physiological consequences of a general medical condition.

Coding Note: If delirium is superimposed on a preexisting Dementia of the Alzheimer's Type or Vascular Dementia, indicate the delirium by coding the appropriate subtype of the dementia, e.g., 294.1 Dementia of the Alzheimer's Type, With Late Onset, With Delirium.

The essential features of delirium are reduced ability to maintain attention to external stimuli and to appropriately shift attention to new external stimuli, and disorganized thinking, as manifested by rambling, irrelevant, or incoherent speech. The disorder also presents with altered or clouded consciousness with sensory misperceptions (hallucinations, delusions, or illusions); disturbances in the sleep-wake cycle and level of psychomotor activity (agitation to stupor); disorientation to person, place, or time; and memory impairment. The onset is rapid and the course typically fluctuates throughout the day and night. The duration is typically brief and death ensues if pathological processes are not resolved (APA, 2000).

Associated features of delirium include anxiety, fear, depression, irritability, anger, euphoria, and apathy. Emotional disturbances are very common and quite variable with delirium. Some persons experience rapid and unpredictable changes from one emotional state to another. Fear is commonly experienced as a response to threatening hallucinations or delusions (APA, 2000). These responses can result in the individual's attempts to escape the environment and subsequent falls; removal of medical equipment such as catheters and intravenous lines; disturbing vocalizations such as yelling and screaming; and a predilection to attack others (Rapp & Titler, 1998).

Prodromal signs and symptoms of delirium are insomnia, distractibility, excessive sensitivity to light and sound, drowsiness, anxiety, vivid dreams or nightmares, complaints of difficulty remembering, dispro-portionate fatigue, and a short attention span (Stanley, 1999). Autonomic signs (tachycardia, sweating, flushed face, dilated pupils, and elevated blood pressure) commonly occur. Chronic conditions experienced by so many older adults can contribute to confusion. These include cardiac and respiratory problems, myocardial infarctions, arrhythmias, and respiratory problems, all of which can affect the central nervous system.

Key Fact

Delirium is the most common psychiatric disorder encountered by health care personnel. Up to 50 percent of all persons admitted to acute hospitals experience acute confusion delirium (St. Pierre, 1996). Unfortunately, only 3 of 10 cases are recognized by physicians or nursing staff because of incomplete assessment or preconceived notions of aging. Delirium superimposed on dementia is even less likely to be recognized (Fick & Foreman, 2000).

TREATMENT

More than 20 terms have been used to describe delirium (i.e., organic brain syndrome, acute confusional state, acute brain failure, etc.). From a clinical standpoint it is crucial that delirium be recognized and an etiologic factor determined promptly. In older adults, delirium is often the first sign of an underlying medical problem (such as an acute infection, fecal impaction, or myocardial infarction) and if it is not diagnosed and properly treated, it may result in death (Inouye, Rushing, Foreman, Palmer, & Pompei, 1998; Lipowski, 1990; Rapp & Titler, 1998).

Refer to Table 6–6 for drugs most likely to be linked with the incidence of delirium. Because of physiological changes that occur with normal aging, the psychiatric nurse must be aware of the dictum "start low and go slow," which means that the dose of medication should be the lowest possible therapeutic dose, and

(continues)

Table 6–6 • **Commonly Used Drugs Causing Delirium**

Group	Examples
Analgesics	Opiates, salicylates
Antiarrhythmics	Lidocaine, procainamide
Antibiotics	Cephalexin, gentamicin, penicillin
Anticonvulsants	Phenytoin
Antihypertensives	Methyldopa
Anti-inflammatory	Indomethacin, steroids
Antineoplastic	5-fluorouracil, methotrexate
Antiparkinsonian	Levodopa, bromocriptine
Gastrointestinal	Cimetidine
Psychotropics	Antidepressants, barbiturates, benzodiazepines, lithium, neuroleptics
Sympathomimetics	Amphetamines, phenylephrine
Miscellaneous	Drug withdrawal (alcohol, barbiturates, benzodiazepines)
	Bromides
	Disulfiram
	Timolol eyedrops
	Theophylline

TREATMENT *(continued)*

increases in dose must be made slowly, after assessing for effects. Older adults are also likely to take many medications for multiple chronic conditions, which may be prescribed by multiple practitioners (Stoehr, 1999). Withdrawal syndromes may contribute to episodes of delirium. When a person suddenly discontinues use of sedative-hypnotics or alcohol, a withdrawal delirium can result.

Initial physiological interventions include detecting early signs, aggressively searching for the cause, and treating any underlying medical condition. Drug reactions or interactions and infection should be ruled out first (Foreman & Zane, 1996; Rapp, 1998; St. Pierre, 1996). Often, delirium can be attributed to new drugs and urinary tract and respiratory infections. Changing the medication regimen and treating infections can produce reversal of the disorder. Correction of underlying physiological problems must be initiated slowly, with frequent monitoring (Stanley, 1999). These may include correction of blood glucose levels, treating metabolic disturbances, hydration, replacing electrolytes, and balancing the acid-base systems. Delirium is prevalent after surgery and during major physical crises, such as burns, and must be treated proactively. The older adult and the very young are very susceptible to the development of delirium. If they do develop delirium, it is a grave prognostic sign, perhaps resulting in coma and death. Thus, recognition and prompt treatment are imperative.

Supportive interventions have shown promise in decreasing the degree of confusion and prompt restoration of cognitive function (Stanley, 1999). These include environmental interventions controlling noise and external stimuli, providing adequate lighting, and maintaining an uncluttered environment. Other interventions include reassuring and calming communication, gentle reality orientation, validation of feelings, and the involvement of family and significant others.

Delirium management is the provision of a safe and therapeutic environment for the individual who is experiencing an acute confusional state.

Activities include: identify etiological factors causing delirium; initiate therapies to reduce or eliminate factors causing the delirium; provide unconditional positive regard; provide the client with information about what is happening and what can be expected to occur in the future; avoid demands for abstract thinking, if the client can think only in concrete terms; limit the need for decision making,

(continues)

TREATMENT *(continued)*

if frustrating/confusing to the client; respond to the theme/feeling or tone, rather than the content, of the hallucination or delusion; remove stimuli, when possible, that create misperception in a particular client (e.g., pictures on the wall or television); maintain a well-lit environment that reduces sharp contrasts and shadows; inform client of person, place, and time, as needed; provide a consistent physical environment and daily routine; provide caregivers who are familiar to the client; use environmental cues (e.g., signs, pictures, clocks, calendars, and color coding of environment) to stimulate memory, reorient, and promote appropriate behavior; provide a low-stimulation environment for client in whom disorientation is increased by overstimulation.

At times, clients with delirium may be so agitated, assaultive, or paranoid that immediate symptomatic control is required, either to prevent these clients from harming themselves and others or to quiet them sufficiently for medical evaluation and treatment to be accomplished. Sometimes clients must be treated symptomatically even before a definite diagnosis can be made. The antipsychotics and non-benzodiazepines are the drugs most often used to help control patients in these out-of-control situations. There is little evidence that one group is more effective than another in managing delirium. Each class of medication has certain advantages and disadvantages. The choice is often made on the basis of the specific effect desired or the specific side effect to be avoided. Many of the same medications are used to manage the behaviors of the person with a probable irreversible dementia.

It is imperative that behaviors be monitored before the medication is implemented to determine possible external causes of the behavior such as stimuli, time of day, or a certain caregiver. It is then important to monitor behaviors after beginning medication management to determine the effect of the medication. In addition, the client should be monitored for possible side effects on a continual basis, particularly because the client is likely unable to voice concerns. The following is an overview of medications used for delirium and dementia.

Of the antipsychotic medications, the more potent agents such as haloperidol, olanzapine, and risperidone (Haldol, Zyprexa, and Risperdal, respectively) are most frequently chosen because they are very effective without sedation. These drugs can be administered by an injection (with the exception of Zyprexa and Risperdal), which is useful in acute psychiatric crisis. Cardiovascular function should be monitored closely in clients being treated with high doses of antipsychotics, but this may be impossible in the severely agitated client. Regardless of antipsychotics chosen, it is desirable to switch from intravenous (IV) or IM to PO administration as soon as the client begins to cooperate with treatment.

Because the incidence of extrapyramidal side effects (especially acute dystonic reactions) is high with antipsychotic agents, particularly with adolescents and young adults, it may be necessary to give benztropine mesylate (Cogentin) with the antipsychotic agent. In older adults, it may not be advisable to add a medication such as Cogentin for two reasons. First, older adults do not demonstrate the acute dystonic reactions as frequently as young persons do. Secondly, it may be desirable to avoid the use of potent anticholinergic agents unless they are essential. With chronic use of antipsychotics, the client must be monitored with the Abnormal Involuntary Movement Scale (AIMS). Older adults are at higher risk for tardive dyskinesia.

The benzodiazepines are probably as effective in controlling the severe psychiatric manifestations of delirium and dementia as are the antipsychotic agents and, in many clients, they may be the drug of choice. Their effect on cardiovascular and respiratory function is minimal, but they usually are more sedating than the more potent antipsychotic agents. The

(continues)

TREATMENT *(continued)*

benzodiazepines are powerful anticonvulsants, and this characteristic is desired when working with a client who is delirious from drug or alcohol intoxication or has the potential for seizure activity. In older adults, it is important to use shorter-acting benzodiazepine sedatives (Serax, Ativan) rather than the longer acting ones (Klonopin, Valium) because of the extended half-life, potential for accumulation with liver dysfunction, worsened cognitive deficits, and drug interactions.

Pharmacologic treatment of the symptoms of delirium and dementia is necessary when:

- The symptoms interfere seriously with medical evaluation or treatment.
- The individual's behavior is dangerous to self or others.
- The symptoms cause the client intense personal distress.

DEMENTIA

Causes

Dementia is a global impairment of cognitive functioning, memory, and personality that occurs without a disturbance in consciousness or level of alertness. Dementias are acquired, unlike mental retardation, which is usually congenital. Although dementia is found predominantly in older adults, some neuropsychiatric disorders (epilepsy, brain tumors, traumatic head injury, or AIDS) may cause dementia in childhood and adolescence.

The most common probable irreversible disorders seen in children are mental retardation (MR), attention-deficit hyperactivity disorder (ADHD), and epilepsy, although epilepsy can occur throughout the life span. **Alzheimer's disease (AD)** is the most prevalent form of dementia in adults, followed by **multi-infarct dementia (MID)**, mixed (AD and MID), and rare disorders of adults and children, some of which are discussed briefly in this section.

Table 6–7 • Causes of Mental Retardation

Genetic	Acquired
Down syndrome	Rubella and prenatal viruses
Klinefelter's syndrome	Toxins
Phenylketonuria (PKU)	Placental insufficiency
	Blood type incompatibility
Hypothyroidism	Anoxia
Tay-Sachs disease	Birth injury
	Prematurity
	Infection—meningitis, encephalitis
	Poisons—lead, medicine
	Poor nutrition
	CNS insult
	Sociocultural factors

The etiology of mental retardation is often unknown, but causes of mental retardation can be grouped into two main factors: heredity and acquired. Table 6–7 summarizes these factors.

Epilepsy is a condition characterized by sudden, recurrent, and transient disturbances of mental functioning or body movements that result from excessive discharging of groups of brain cells (Goetz, 1999). Based on this definition, the psychiatric nurse will recognize that epilepsy is not a specific disease but is comprised of a group of symptoms that have different causes in different individuals.

Four genes have been located that are associated with Alzheimer's disease (AD). Autosomal dominant genes on chromosomes 1, 14, and 21 are associated with earlier onset AD, and a gene on chromosome 19 carries a risk factor that is connected with later onset AD; 92. The early-onset (ages 30–50) familial AD is associated with the 14th chromosome discovered in 1992 (Mullan et al., 1992; Schellenberg et al., 1992; Van Broeckhoven et al., 1992). The genes on chromosomes 1 and 21 are associated with AD that has an onset from age 49 to 65 (Levy-Lahad et al., 1995; St. George-Hyslop et al., 1992).

The etiology of AD cannot totally be explained by genetics. Persons with AD who have at least one other relative affected are categorized as familial, which could include genetics or some environmental trigger. Persons with AD with no known family history are classified as sporadic.

A clear biochemical abnormality associated with AD was discovered in 1976. This chemical, choline acetyltransferase (CAT) was reduced by 90 percent in the hippocampus and cerebral cortex of AD patients. CAT is a catalyst for the neurotransmitter, acetylcholine, which is responsible for functioning of the hippocampus, paramount in the formation of memory (Figure 6–2). Other neurotransmitters such as norepinephrine, serotonin, and somatostatin have been found to be deficient in the brains of persons with AD and may contribute to behavioral impairments manifested by persons with AD (Strong, 1998).

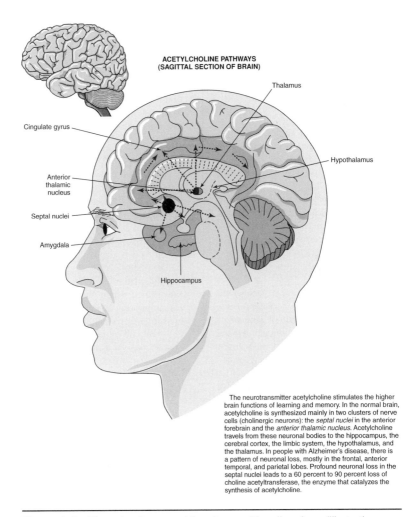

**ACETYLCHOLINE PATHWAYS
(SAGITTAL SECTION OF BRAIN)**

Thalamus

Cingulate gyrus

Hypothalamus

Anterior thalamic nucleus

Septal nuclei

Amygdala

Hippocampus

The neurotransmitter acetylcholine stimulates the higher brain functions of learning and memory. In the normal brain, acetylcholine is synthesized mainly in two clusters of nerve cells (cholinergic neurons): the *septal nuclei* in the anterior forebrain and the *anterior thalamic nucleus*. Acetylcholine travels from these neuronal bodies to the hippocampus, the cerebral cortex, the limbic system, the hypothalamus, and the thalamus. In people with Alzheimer's disease, there is a pattern of neuronal loss, mostly in the frontal, anterior temporal, and parietal lobes. Profound neuronal loss in the septal nuclei leads to a 60 percent to 90 percent loss of choline acetyltransferase, the enzyme that catalyzes the synthesis of acetylcholine.

Figure 6–2   The role of neuronal loss in cognitive disorders. *(Illustration concept: Gail Kongable, MSN, CRN, CCRN, Department of Neurosurgery, University of Virginia Health Sciences Center.)*

Vascular dementias are associated with ischemic cerebral injury. The most common vascular dementia is multi-infarct dementia (MID) resulting from vascular diseases that cause multiple small or large cerebral infarcts. These infarcts can produce dementia as a dominant symptom. The onset is generally acute, and unlike AD, the stages are clear cut or stepwise, with clear decline associated with each infarct.

The client may have a history of transient ischemic attacks (TIAs), hypertension, strokes, diabetes mellitus, vasculitis, and cardiac arrhythmias. Family history of stroke or cardiovascular disease are common (Ham, 1992; Jarvik, Lavertsky, & Neshkes, 1992).

Symptoms

Significantly subaverage intellectual functioning that originates during the developmental period and accompanied by deficits in adaptive functioning is defined as mental retardation (APA, 2000). The subaverage intellectual functioning is accompanied by significant limitations in adaptive functioning in two of the following skills: communication, self-care, home living, social or interpersonal skills, use of community resources, self-direction, functional academic skills, work, leisure, health, and safety.

Grand mal seizures are a tonic-clonic attack with a loss of consciousness. These are the most common form of generalized seizures. Many clients experiencing grand mal seizures will report vague warning symptoms of discomfort, anxiety, mood changes, or physical discomfort such as headache, upset stomach, sweating, or changes in body temperature. An aura often immediately precedes a full-blown seizure. Dizziness, fainting, and sensory phenomena (lights, dots, sounds, odors, and tastes) are the more frequent kinds of auras.

Alzheimer's disease is characterized by progressive loss of memory, especially short term; language impairments; poor impulse control; and poor judgment. The course of the disease is anywhere from 2

DSM-IV-TR Diagnostic Criteria for Mental Retardation

A. Significantly subaverage intellectual functioning: an IQ of approximately 70 or below on an individually administered IQ test (for infants, a clinical judgment of significantly subaverage intellectual functioning).

B. Concurrent deficits or impairments in present adaptive functioning (i.e., the person's effectiveness in meeting the standards expected for his or her age by his or her cultural group) in at least two of the following areas: communication, self-care, home living, social/interpersonal skills, use of community resources, self-direction, functional academic skills, work, leisure, health, and safety.

C. The onset is before age 18 years.

Code based on degree of severity reflecting level of intellectual impairment:

Mild Mental Retardation: IQ level 50–55 to approximately 70
Moderate Mental Retardation: IQ level 35–50 to 50–55
Severe Mental Retardation: IQ level 20–25 to 35–40
Profound Mental Retardation: IQ level below 20 or 25
Mental Retardation, Severity Unspecified: when there is strong presumption of Mental Retardation but the person's intelligence is untestable by standard tests.

---

to 20 years, with 10 years being the average. Experts stage the disease in three stages, four stages (Hall & Buckwalter, 1987), and seven stages (Reisburg, Ferris, Leon, & Crook, 1982). The four stages of AD and associated symptoms are listed in Table 6–8.

Persons with AD have three possible behavioral responses: baseline, anxious, and dysfunctional (Hall, 1991; Hall & Buckwalter, 1987; Hall & Titler, 1997). Baseline behaviors include a basic awareness of the environment and ability to

Table 6–8 • Stages of Alzheimer's Disease

Stage	Manifestations
1. Forgetfulness	Short-term memory losses: Misplace, forget, lose things
	Compensate with memory aides: Lists, routine, organization
	Express awareness of problem: Concern about abilities
	May become depressed: Complicates symptoms and makes worse
	Not diagnosable at this stage
2. Confusion	Progressive memory decline: interferes with all abilities; short term most impaired, long term follows later
	Disorientation: Time, place, person, thing
	Instrumental activities of daily living (IADLs): money management, legal affairs, transportation difficulties, housekeeping, cooking
	Denial is common but give clues that fear "losing their mind"
	Depression is more common; aware of deficits and frightened
	Confabulation and stereotyped word usage: Covering up for memory losses
	More problems when: stressed, fatigued, out of own environment, ill
	Day care and in-home assistance is commonly needed
3. Ambulatory dementia	Functional losses in ADLs (in approximate order of loss): willingness and ability to bathe, grooming, choosing among clothing, dressing, gait and mobility, toileting, communication, reading, and writing skills
	Loss of ability to reason, to plan for safety, and communicate verbally
	Frustration is common
	Becomes more withdrawn and self-absorbed
	Depression resolves as the person's awareness of her memory loss and disability decreases
	Becomes less "accessible" to others—unable to retain information or use past experiences to guide her behavior
	Communication becomes more and more difficult with loss of language
	Behavioral evidence of reduced stress threshold: up at night, wandering, pacing, confused, agitated, belligerent, combative, withdrawn
	Institutional care is usually needed
4. Endstage	Does not recognize family members, or even her own image in a mirror
	No longer walks; little purposeful activity
	Is often mute and may yell or scream spontaneously
	Forgets how to eat, swallow, and chew; weight loss is common and may become emaciated
	Develops problems associated with immobility: pneumonia, pressure ulcers, urinary tract infections, and contractures
	Incontinence is common; may have seizures
	Most certainly institutionalized at this point

interact and function, limited only by the amount of neurological deficits. The client remains cognitively and socially accessible—he can communicate and respond. When the client becomes anxious, he is beginning to feel stress. The client may complain of feeling uneasy. Eye contact is poor or absent and increase in psychomotor activity may appear in response to noxious stimuli. However, the client remains intact.

The client becomes dysfunctional if stress levels continue or increase. As a result, the client becomes catastrophic and cognitively and socially inaccessible. Communication is impaired and the client is unable to interpret the environment appropriately. The individual may actively avoid the noxious stimuli and become fearful and panic stricken. The result is increased confusion, purposeful wandering, night awakening, "sundowner's syndrome," agitation, fearfulness, panic, combativeness, and sudden withdrawal.

The person with MID may have more language difficulties than the person with

---

DSM-IV-TR Diagnostic Criteria for Dementia of the Alzheimer's Type

A. The development of multiple cognitive deficits manifested by both memory impairment (impaired ability to learn new information or to recall previously learned information)
  1. one (or more) of the following cognitive disturbances:
     a. **aphasia** (language disturbance)
     b. **apraxia** (impaired ability to carry out motor activities despite intact motor function)
     c. agnosia (failure to recognize or identify objects despite intact sensory function)
     d. disturbance in **executive functioning** (i.e., planning, organizing, sequencing, abstracting)

B. The cognitive deficits in criteria A1 and A2 each cause significant impairment in social or occupational functioning and represent a significant decline from a previous level of functioning.

C. The course is characterized by gradual onset and continuing cognitive decline.

D. The cognitive deficits in Criteria A1 and A2 are not due to any of the following:
  1. other central nervous system conditions that cause progressive deficits in memory and cognition (e.g., cerebrovascular disease,

Parkinson's disease, Huntington's disease, subdural hematoma, normal-pressure hydrocephalus, brain tumor)
  2. systemic conditions that are known to cause dementia (e.g., hypothyroidism, vitamin B12 or folic acid deficiency, niacin deficiency, hypercalcemia, neurosyphilis, HIV infection)
  3. substance-induced conditions

E. The deficits do not occur exclusively during the course of delirium.

F. The disturbance is not better accounted for by another Axis I disorder (e.g., Major Depressive Disorder, Schizophrenia).

Code based on type of onset and predominant features:

Without Behavioral Disturbance: if the cognitive disturbance is not accompanied by any clinically significant behavioral disturbance.

With Behavioral Disturbance: if the cognitive disturbance is accompanied by a clinically significant behavioral disturbance (e.g. wandering, agitation).

Specify Subtype:
  With Early Onset: if onset is at age 65 years or below
  With Late Onset: if onset is after age 65 years

AD, as well as **focal neurological signs** and symptoms. Emotional lability, depression, and crying spells are frequently observed. Other deficits may include **dysarthria**, hemi-neglect, movement dis- orders, or a subtle paresis. The course of the disease is fluctuating and intermittent. Delirium may occur with each infarct, clearing with time, with no return to base- line cognitive functioning.

DSM-IV-TR Diagnostic Criteria for Vascular Dementia

A. The development of multiple cognitive deficits manifested by both
1. memory impairment (impaired ability to learn new information or to recall previously learned information)
2. one (or more) of the following cognitive disturbances:
   a. aphasia (language disturbance)
   b. apraxia (impaired ability to carry out motor activities despite intact motor function)
   c. agnosia (failure to recognize or identify objects despite intact sensory function)
   d. disturbance in executive functioning (i.e., planning, organizing, sequencing, abstracting)

B. The cognitive deficits in Criteria A1 and A2 each cause significant impairment in social or occupational functioning and represent a significant decline from a previous level of functioning.

C. Focal neurological signs and symptoms (e.g., exaggeration of deep tendon reflexes, extensor plantar response, pseudobulbar palsy, gait abnormalities, weakness of an extremity), or laboratory evidence indicative of cerebrovascular disease (e.g., multiple infarctions involving cortex and underlying white matter) that are judged to be etiologically related to the disturbance.

D. The deficits do not occur exclusively during the course of a delirium.

Code based on predominant features:

With Delirium: if delirium is superimposed on the dementia

With Delusions: if delusions are the predominant feature

With Depressed Mood: if depressed mood (including presentations that meet full symptom criteria for a Major Depressive Episode) is the predominant feature. A separate diagnosis of Mood Disorder due to a general medical condition is not given.

Uncomplicated: if none of the above dominates in the current clinical presentation

Specify if:
With Behavioral Disturbance

DSM-IV-TR Diagnosis Criteria for Dementia Due to Other General Medical Conditions

A. The development of multiple cognitive deficits manifested by both
1. memory impairment (impaired ability to learn new information or to recall previously learned information)
2. one (or more) of the following cognitive disturbances:
   a. aphasia (language disturbance)
   b. apraxia (impaired ability to carry out motor activities despite intact motor function)
   c. agnosia (failure to recognize or identify objects despite intact sensory function)
   d. disturbance in executive functioning (i.e., planning, organizing, sequencing, abstracting)

(continues)

(continued)

B. The cognitive deficits in Criteria A1 and A2 each cause significant impairment in social or occupational functioning and represent a significant decline from a previous level of functioning.

C. There is evidence from the history, physical examination, or laboratory findings that the disturbance is the direct physiological consequence of one of the general medical conditions listed below.

D. The deficits do not occur exclu-

sively during the course of a delirium.

Code based on presence or absence of a clinically significant behavioral disturbance:

Without Behavioral Disturbance: if the cognitive disturbance is not accompanied by any clinically significant behavioral disturbance

With Behavioral Disturbance: if the cognitive disturbance is accompanied by a clinically significant behavioral disturbance (e.g., wandering, agitation)

TREATMENT

These assumptions are basic principles of nursing care for all clients and should be used in caring for all persons with dementia (Hall & Buckwalter, 1987):

1. All humans require some control over their person and their environment and need some degree of unconditional positive regard.
2. All behavior is rooted and has meaning; therefore, all catastrophic and stress-related behaviors have a cause.
3. The confused or agitated client is not comfortable and should be regarded as frightened. All clients have the right to be comfortable.
4. The client exists in a 24-hour continuum. Care cannot be planned or evaluated on an 8-hour shift basis. If the client has a problem during the night, some changes need to be implemented during the day.

It is important to differentially diagnose clients with dementias so that the appropriate treatment can be instituted. Similarly, the psychiatric nurse must remember that a **potentially reversible dementia** can be superimposed on a **probable irreversible dementia**, causing excess disability. Excess disability can be defined as "a reversible deficit that is more disabling than the primary disability, existing when the magnitude of the dis-

turbance in functioning is greater than might be accounted for by basic physical illness or cerebral pathology" (Dawson, Kline, Wiancko, & Wells, 1986, p. 299). When stressors causing excess disability are removed, cognitive and physical functioning may improve. If not, the patient becomes stressed, resulting in further disability and possibly death.

Cholinesterase inhibitors (CEIs) have been used and seem to slow the progression of Alzheimer's disease (Knopman, 1998). The earliest of these was tacrine (THA or Cognex), but side effects of the drug, including gastrointestinal (GI) and liver abnormalities, have reduced its popularity. The CEI Aricept (donepezil) has been used with fewer reported side effects. Exelon therapy has been effective in improving global functioning and cognition. Nausea and vomiting are most common but are decreased with slow titration and continued use. Other therapies under investigation are estrogen for postmenopausal women, anti-inflammatory agents, and antioxidants. Persons with AD and other dementias who demonstrate agitation, aggression, or psychotic features may need to be treated with psychoactive agents such as non-benzodiazepines and novel low-dose atypical antipsychotics.

Some persons with MID may benefit from anticoagulation therapy and treat-

(continues)

TREATMENT *(continued)*

ment of underlying disease, especially hypertension, which is the most important risk factor.

Once the diagnosis of an irreversible dementing illness is established, responsibility for planning and providing daily care is assumed by the family and allied health professionals.

Individualization is usually accomplished by identifying the person's culture, past interests, and preferences, and integrating them into the generic Alzheimer's care plan or with specific treatments for problematic secondary symptoms such as wandering or agitation (Hall, 1997).

Dementia management is the provision of a modified environment for the person who is experiencing a chronic confusional state.

Activities include family members in planning, providing, and evaluating care, to the extent desired; identify usual patterns of behavior for such activities as sleep, medication use, elimination, food intake, and self-care; determine physical, social, and psychological history of the client, usual habits, and routines; determine type and extent of cognitive deficit(s) using standardized assessment tool; monitor cognitive functioning using a standardized assessment tool; provide a low-stimulation environment (e.g., quiet, soothing music; nonvivid and simple, familiar patterns in décor; performance expectations that do not exceed cognitive processing ability; and dining in small groups); provide a consistent physical environment and daily routine; give one simple direction at a time; speak in a clear, low, warm, respectful tone of voice; use distraction, rather than confrontation, to manage behavior; provide unconditional positive regard; provide caregivers who are familiar to the client (e.g., avoid frequent rotations of staff assignments); avoid unfamiliar situations, when possible (e.g., room changes and appointments without familiar people); provide rest periods to prevent fatigue and reduce stress; monitor nutrition and weight; avoid frustrating the client by quizzing with orientation questions that cannot be answered; provide cues— such as current events, seasons, location, and names—to assist orientation; select television or radio activities based on cognitive processing abilities and limit the number of choices the client has to make, so as not to cause anxiety; avoid use of physical restraints; monitor carefully for physiological causes of increased confusion that may be acute and reversible.

RESOURCES

Please note that because Internet resources are of a time-sensitive nature and URL addresses may change or be deleted, searches should also be conducted by association or topic.

Internet Resources

http://www.alz.org Alzheimer's Association

http://www.thearc.org Arc of the United States (formerly the Association for Retarded Persons in the United States)

http://www.alzheimers.org/adear Alzheimer's Disease Education and Referral Center (ADEAR)

7 Depressive Disorders

• Key Terms

Anhedonia: The inability to experience pleasure from activities that usually produce pleasurable feelings.

Dysphoria: Marked feelings of sadness.

Hyperphagia: Excessive amount of eating.

Hypersomnia: Excessive amount of sleep.

Insomnia: Inability to fall asleep, difficulty staying asleep, or early morning awakening.

Mood: An emotional state.

Psychomotor Retardation: A slowing of physical and emotional reactions, including speech, affect, and movement.

Ruminations: Repetitive or continuous thinking about a particular subject that then interferes with other thought processes.

Somatic Preoccupation: Excessively focused on one's own body functioning.

Major depressive disorders (MDDs) are highly prevalent in the general population and clinical settings. Major depression is considered a mood disorder. **Mood** *refers to an emotional state such as depressed or irritable. Epidemiological studies consistently demonstrate that about 10 percent of primary care clients experience significant depressive disorders (Ustun, 2000; Wells, Sturm, Sherbourn, & Meredith, 1996). Depression is the fourth most significant cause of global disability and by the year 2020, it is projected to become the second (Murray & Lopez, 1997a, 1997b).*

DEPRESSIVE DISORDERS

Causes

Contemporary researchers suggest that the cause of depressive disorders is complex and that a combination of neurobiological, cultural, and psychosocial factors are likely to be involved in the etiology of depressive disorders. In addition, genetic or familial patterns are also indicated as causative factors of depression.

MDD is one and one-half to three times more likely to occur in a first-degree biological relative (e.g., mother, sister, or father) affected with the disorder than among the general population. Oftentimes, a psychosocial stressor, especially the death of a loved one, divorce, or childbirth may precipitate a major depressive episode (Pincus et al., 1999).

Gender factors appear to play a role in the epidemiology of MDD (APA, 2000; Fava & Davidson, 1996). Cross-cultural community surveys consistently show a female preponderance of depressive disorders (Mavreas, Beis, Mouyias, Rigoni, & Lyketsos, 1986; Piccinelli, & Gomez-Homen, 1996). The female ratio for current depression falls between 1.3 and 2.8 (McDaniel, Musselman, & Porter, 1995; Regier, Narrow, & Rae, 1990).

A number of studies also show a high prevalence of comorbid anxiety disorder and other psychiatric disorder with major depressive illness (Noyes & Hoehn-Saric, 1998; Pincus et al., 1999).

Studies of unipolar and bipolar disorders in families consistently show that these illnesses are highly familial. Data posits that female gender, family history, and past episodes are the most salient predictors of recurrent depression.

Dysregulation of either noradrenergic (norepinephrine [NE]) or serotonergic neurotransmitter systems and mechanism of action of antidepressant drugs is the most widely accepted explanation for depression. Major theories concerning the role of NE is that there is a reduction in release or production from presynaptic neurons and an increase in presynaptic alpha 2-adrenergic activities that results in reduced NE. In addition, people with depressive disorders have dysregulation

in this system (Charney, 1998; Leonard, 1997). The major neurotransmitters that have been studied in relation to mood disorders are outlined in Table 7–1.

The hypothalamic-pituitary-adrenal (HPA) axis, including the effects of corticotropin-releasing hormone (CRH) and cortisol, also play significant roles in the etiology of depressive disorders along with second and third messenger systems (Schatzberg, 1998).

Research has consistently shown that clients with major depression (especially melancholic type) secrete abnormally large amounts of cortisol. Activation of the HPA axis, ultimately leading to the secretion of cortisol, occurs when an individual experiences psychological or physiological stress. Specifically, the hypothalamus in the brain secretes CRH, which stimulates the anterior pituitary gland to release adrenocorticotropic hormone (ACTH). ACTH acts as a messenger to the adrenal glands to secrete cortisol. Normally, cortisol then shuts off the stress response by acting on the hypothalamus to stop its secretion of CRH (Schatzberg, 1998). In the depressed person this process goes awry. The body's response to stress in effect does not shut off, resulting in hypercortisolemia. Recent studies also link high cortisol level to pronounced cognitive deficits in depressed clients, especially those with psychotic features (Belanoff, Kalehzan, Sund, Ficek, & Schatzberg, 2001; Nelson, Sax, & Strakowski, 1998).

Table 7–1 • Neurotransmitters Theoretically Involved in Mood Disorders

Monoamine neurotransmitters

    Catecholamines

        Epinephrine

        Norepinephrine (noradrenergic)

        Dopamine

    Indoleamines

        Serotonin

Cholinergic neurotransmitter

    Acetylcholine

Amino acid neurotransmitter

    Gamma-aminobutyric acid

Findings that the neurohormones, which are responsive to stress, play a prominent role in the pathophysiology of depression are also consistent with clinical observations that the onset and natural history of major depression is influenced by psychological conflict, counterproductive methods of coping, and external stressors. Another neuroendocrine theory concerning depression involves the thyroid-stimulating hormone (TSH), which is dampened on thyrotropin stimulation.

Researchers submit that abnormalities of the timing of the oscillations of the circadian pacemaker may play a role in depressive disorders. The timing of the sleep-wake cycle appears to shift later as in delayed sleep phase syndrome. The client experiencing delayed sleep phases is likely to complain of having difficulty falling asleep and difficulty awakening the next morning. Seasonal affective disorder (SAD) is associated with alterations in melatonin secretion associated with winter months and reduced light (Terman, Terman, & Ross, 1998; Wehr, 2000).

Early psychoanalytic theorists sought to understand pathological depression by comparing it with grief and mourning. Karl Abraham (1911; 1924) submitted that mourning represented the grief of a lost loved one.

Freud described that the normal grieving process following a loss involves the working through of ambivalent feelings and anger toward the lost person through recalling and expressing past experiences and feelings related to this person. Instead, anger toward the lost person is turned inward, leading to dysphoria, guilt, and loss of self-esteem. **Dysphoria** refers to marked feelings of sadness. In essence, the psychoanalytic view of depression stems from disturbances in interpersonal relations in early childhood, usually involving a loss or disappointment that interfere with forming meaningful relationships across the life span.

An individual's culture colors the experience of depression; however, a core of symptoms is found to exist across cultures (Manson, 1997). The debate between culture and diagnostic parameters has to do with a tendency of various cultures to present with somatic or physical symptoms that may actually represent emotional issues such as depression and anxiety.

Some cultures that are described as stoic (Midwestern farmers, Amish, Central Europeans) often avoid reporting symptoms of depression. They resist reporting emotional symptoms and rely more on family members and religion or spiritual rituals rather than seeking professional help. Other cultures, namely, Asian, often view the mind and body holistically and often report their symptoms using somatic terms. Because they see the mind and body as unitary rather than dualistic, they tend to focus on physical distress rather than on emotional symptoms, such as depression, resulting in an overdepiction of somatic complaints (Lin & Cheung, 1999; Uba, 1994).

The extensive work of Peter M. Lewinsohn (1974) on depression and the behavioral model is well documented. He associated depression with significant losses of important sources of positive reinforcement in a person's life or a high rate of aversive experiences.

According to this theory there are two other ways in which insufficient reinforcement may occur. In addition to the loss of reinforcement, the person may (a) lack the necessary skills to obtain reinforcement even though this is potentially available, for example, poor interpersonal skills could preclude the development of satisfying social relationships, or (b) lack of ability to enjoy available reinforcers secondary to interfering anxiety.

Reinforcement theory asserts that once a depressive syndrome has occurred, it is maintained through the reinforcing concern and sympathy as well as the negative responses that depressive behaviors elicit from others (Coyne, 1976).

The learned helplessness model of depression can be summarized as follows: Individuals develop consistent attributional styles or ways of understanding the causes of events in their lives. A particular attributional style consists of habitually attributing negative outcomes to internal, stable, global causes and ascribing positive events to external, unstable, specific causes. Mild to severe depression results when this attributional style is coupled with uncontrollable, aversive events (Rehm, 1990).

Cognitive behavioral theories of depression stem from the early works of Aaron T. Beck (1963; 1964; 1967) and his colleagues (Beck, Rush, Shaw, & Emery, 1979). The basis of the cognitive-behavioral theory is that depression, in its various forms (major, melancholic, dysthymic, and bipolar), consists of a negative cognitive triad, specific schemas, and cognitive errors, or faulty information processing.

The cognitive theory of depression suggests that disturbances in thinking are the core of depression and that other symptoms associated with depression (e.g., sad mood, an inability to experience pleasure, decreased motivation) are reinforced by the cognitive disturbances. The cognitive model does not posit a cause-and-effect relationship between cognitive dysfunction and depression; rather, the cognitive distortions are viewed as but one component of the depressive syndrome (Beck et al., 1979).

Chronic physical conditions; physical abuse; homelessness; poverty; parental separation, divorce, or death; and parental psychiatric illness all increase the risk of depression during childhood (Berman, 1999; Biederman et al., 2001; Faraone & Biederman, 1997; Kendler et al., 1995; Stevenson, 1999).

Biological, psychological, and social variables appear to increase the risk for depression in older adults. Among some clients with late-onset depression, there is evidence of neurological brain disorders associated with cerebrovascular disorders, resulting in more neurovegetative states.

Psychosocial factors increasing the risk of depression in older adults include significant loss, loneliness, and debilitating medical and mental conditions.

Bereavement is an extreme stressor with physiological, psychological, and social consequences. As with other stressors, the consequences of bereavement are variable and will be influenced by the constitutional makeup and personality of the bereaved, nature of the relationship with the deceased, and the circumstances of the death.

Symptoms

The course of MDD varies, but the average onset is the late 20s, although it may occur during childhood, adolescence, or older adulthood. A prodromal period may include anxiety symptoms and mild depression several weeks before the onset of full MDD. The onset of symptoms ranges from days to months to sudden, particularly when precipitated by a psychosocial stressor. The duration of MDD also varies but when left untreated, the episode typically lasts 6 months or longer (APA, 2000). Others may develop other mood disorders, such as bipolar disorder.

Depressed clients can exhibit anorexia or **hyperphagia** (overeating), **hypersomnia** or **insomnia**, decreased libido, and disturbances in rapid eye movement sleep and body temperature rhythms (Ganong, 1999).

In addition to depressed mood, a reduction in behavior occurs. Other symptoms such as low self-esteem and hopelessness are believed to stem from the reduced level of functioning.

The *cognitive triad* is made up of (1) a negative view of self (e.g., seeing oneself as defective, inadequate, worthless, and undesirable), (2) a negative view of the world (e.g., the world is experienced as a demanding and defeating place) in which failure and punishment are to be expected, and (3) a negative view of the future (e.g., an expectation of ongoing hardship, suffering, deprivation, and failure).

Although there are certain characteristics of depression that are consistently seen across the life span, developmental stage is important in influencing how these disorders are manifested. Table 7–2 outlines characteristics that distinguish depression in various age groups.

Younger children may exhibit behavioral problems, such as aggression, apathy, sleep disturbances, and weight loss. Children may also have an irritable versus sad or depressed mood.

Depressed adolescents may express somatic complaints and have an irritable mood. Similar to children, they tend to exhibit behavioral problems such as poor

Table 7–2 • **Characteristics of Depression across the Life Span**

Childhood

Infants and Preschoolers	Prepubertal Children
Insidious onset	May report sadness, suicidal thoughts
Apathy, fatigue, withdrawal	Irritability, self-criticism, weepiness
Poor appetite, weight loss	Decreased initiative and responsiveness to stimulation, apathy
Few spontaneously describe feeling sad	Fatigue, sleep disturbance, enuresis, encopresis, weight loss, anorexia, somatic complaints
	Poor school performance
	Social withdrawal, increased aggressiveness

Adolescence

Feelings of sadness less frequent	Poor school performance
Unhappy restlessness, boredom, irritability	Argumentativeness
Affects are intense and labile	Increased conflict with peers
Low self-esteem, hopelessness, worthlessness	Acting out behavior, e.g., running away, stealing, physical violence
Feelings of loneliness and being unloved	Sexual activity (promiscuity)
Pessimism about the future	Substance abuse
Loss of interest in friends and activities, apathy	Complaints of headaches, abdominal pain
Low frustration tolerance	Hypersomnia

Early and Middle Adulthood

Depressed mood	Decreased sexual interest and activity
Anhedonia	Psychomotor retardation
Feelings of worthlessness, hopelessness, guilt	Anxiety
Reduced energy, fatigue	Decreased appetite and weight loss or increased appetite and weight gain
Sleep disturbance, especially early morning awakening and multiple nighttime awakenings	

Later Adulthood

Frequently do not complain of depressed mood or present with tearful affect	Loss of self-esteem
Feelings of helplessness	Guilt feelings
Pessimism about the future	Depressions tend to last longer and are more severe
Rumination about problems	Perceived cognitive deficits
Critical and envious of others	Somatic complaints

(continues)

Table 7–2 *(continued)*

Constipation	Loss of motivation
Social withdrawal	Change of appetite

Fixed, Core Symptoms Across Age Groups

Suicidal ideation, diminished concentration, sleep disturbance

Note. Data from "Review of Community Prevalence of Depression in Later Life," by A. T. F. Beckman, J. R. M. Copeland, and M. J. Prince, 1999, *British Journal of Psychiatry*, *174*, pp. 301–311; and from "Mood Disorders and Suicide in Children and Adolescents," by C. S. Pataki, 2000, in *Kaplan & Sadock's Comprehensive Textbook of Psychiatry* (7th ed., pp. 2740–2757), by B. J. Sadock and V. A. Sadock (Eds.), Philadelphia: Lippincott Williams & Wilkins. Reprinted with permission.

academic and social performance, suicidal ideations, apathy, social withdrawal, rebelliousness, low self-esteem, and aggressive behaviors. They also tend to engage in risky behaviors such as promiscuity and substance abuse.

The *DSM-IV-TR* (APA, 2000) criteria for major depressive disorders include: a period of 2 weeks during which there is depressed mood or loss of interest in things that were once pleasurable (**anhedonia**) and the following:

- Alterations in appetite and weight
- Sleep disturbances, usually insomnia
- **Psychomotor retardation** or agitation
- Fatigue
- Concentration disturbances—forgetfulness, memory difficulties, difficulty making decisions
- Feelings of worthlessness, inadequacy, guilt
- Recurrent thoughts of death or suicidal ideations, plans or attempts

Anhedonia, or a loss of interest or pleasure, is usually present and the client feels apathetic or has little interest in hobbies or other pleasant activities. Family members often report that the client is socially isolative and shows less interest in sexual activity or desire. All in all, the level of impairment produced by MDD varies. Some clients may experience significant impairment and have difficulty performing normal daily responsibilities, whereas others may not. Atypical depressive symptoms are more common in adults and may include increased appetite, weight gain, or increased sleep and cravings for high carbohydrate foods (APA, 2000).

Behavioral manifestations of these underlying neurological conditions include memory difficulties, forgetfulness, and complaints of dysphoria (marked feelings of sadness). Older adults are also more likely to focus on somatic preoccupation, such as an ache here or there, and ruminations. **Somatic preoccupation** involves an excessive focus on one's body function and distress. **Ruminations** manifest as repetitive or continuous thinking about a particular matter that eventually interferes with other thought processes. The client may ruminate about not going to an outing with the family for several days and have difficulty thinking about more important matters. See Table 7–3 for differentiating characteristics of depression and dementia.

A wide range of feelings and behaviors are commonly experienced after a loss. Table 7–4 outlines how these are manifested during different periods of a person's life.

Manifestations of grief normally diminish in frequency and intensity over time. It is not uncommon or abnormal, however, for the characteristic feelings and behaviors associated with mourning to recur at various points throughout a person's life. Anniversary dates of the death, birthdays of the deceased, holidays or other occasions that remind the survivor of the deceased are typical periods when this occurs.

Table 7–3 • **Differentiating Characteristics of Depression and Dementia**

Clinical Features	Depression	Dementia
Onset	Relatively rapid	Insidious
Precursors	Many have recent history of stressful event	No clear precursor
Psychiatric History	History of depression	No history of depression
Cognitive Impairment	Fluctuates	Constant
Orientation	Oriented in all spheres	Orientation impaired
Memory	Equal or no impairment of recent and remote memory	Greater impairment in recent compared with remote memory
Learning Capacity	Usually intact	Impaired
Mental Status Results	"Don't know" answers typical Emphasizes impairments	Frequent errors Minimizes or conceals impairments
Sense of Distress (Feels Depressed)	Yes	No
Affect	Irritable, constricted	Shallow and labile
Behavior	Little effort expended to perform even simple tasks	Often struggles to perform tasks
Response to Treatment	Improvement with antidepressants or ECT	Lack of response

ECT, electroconvulsive therapy.

Note. From *Diagnostic and Statistical Manual of Mental Disorders* (4th edition Text Revision) (*DSM-IV-TR*), by American Psychiatric Association, 2000, Washington, DC: Author. Adapted with permission; from *Practice Guidelines for the Treatment of Patients With Major Depressive Disorder* (Rev. ed.), by American Psychiatric Association Work Group, 2000, Washington, DC: Author; and from "Review of Community Prevalence of Depression in Later Life," by A. T. F. Beckman, J. R. M. Copeland, and M. J. Prince, 1999, *British Journal of Psychiatry, 174,* pp. 301–311. Adapted with permission.

Table 7–4 • **Manifestations of Normal Grief across the Life Span**

Children	Adolescents	Adults	Older Adults
Feelings	Physical Sensations	Behaviors	Cognitions
Sadness	Hollowness in stomach	Sleep disturbance	Disbelief
Fearfulness		Appetite disturbance	Confusion
Angry outbursts	Chest & throat tightness	Absent-minded behavior	Preoccupation
Eating disturbance	Oversensitivity to noise	Social withdrawal	
Bowel & bladder disturbance		Dreams of deceased	
Speech disturbances	Depersonalization	Searching and calling out	
Withdrawn or excessively caregiving	Breathlessness		
	Muscle weakness	Sighing	

(continues)

Table 7–4 *(continued)*

Children	Adolescents	Adults	Older Adults
Feelings	**Physical Sensations**	**Behaviors**	**Cognitions**
Deterioration of school behavior & academic achievement	Lack of energy	Restless overactivity	Sense of presence
	Dry mouth	Crying	Hallucinations
Guilt	Similar to adult except for following:		
Tendency to grieve silently	Physical sensations more pronounced & may take on pattern similar to one present in deceased		
Denial			
Sexual promiscuity			
Alcohol & drug use	Marked irritability		
Worry about future, preservation of family and new responsibilities	Negativistic thinking		

Note. Data from *Clinical Management of Bereavement: A Handbook for Healthcare Professionals*, by G. M. Burnell and A. L. Burnell, 1989, New York: Human Sciences Press; "Bereavement Reactions, Consequences, and Care," by M. Osterweis, F. Solomon, and M. Green, in *Biopsychosocial Aspects of Bereavement*, by S. Zisook (Ed.), 1987, Washington, DC: American Psychiatric Press; *Grief Counseling and Grief Therapy: A Handbook for the Mental Health Practitioner* (2nd ed.), by J. W. Worden, 1991, New York: Springer. Adapted with permission.

Key Facts

About 50 percent of people experiencing a first episode of MDD experience recurrent symptoms within 10 years. Varying degrees of severity govern the client's prognosis and treatment.

Depression is relatively uncommon in preschoolers, but estimates among children and adolescents in the community range from 2 to 6 percent, which tends to increase with age (Birmaher, Ryan, Williamson, & Brent, 1996; Costello, 1989; Lewinsohn, Rohde, & Seely, 1998).

The prevalence of depression in adolescents has been mentioned previously and suggests that it increases with age and is more common in girls than boys (Birmaher et al., 1996).

TREATMENT

The prevalence of depressive disorders in practice settings requires astute assessment skills that enable the nurse to make an accurate nursing diagnosis and initiate

interventions that shorten the course and reduce recurrence and chronicity. Nurses also face the responsibility of working with treatment team members and identifying other psychiatric and medical conditions that mimic depressive illnesses and initiating appropriate treatment to manage them. Because the risk of suicide across the life span is significant, nurses need to assess all clients for depression and suicide and facilitate adaptive resolution of causative factors to restore clients to an optimal level of functioning.

Understanding underlying dysregulation of neurotransmitter systems provides a basis for actions of various antidepressant agents. For instance, serotonin selective reuptake inhibitors (SSRIs) such as Prozac (fluoxetine) increase serotonin in the brain, thus increasing the client's mood. By having a basic understanding of these processes, the nurse can use this information to teach clients with depression the reasons for taking antidepressant medications.

(continues)

TREATMENT *(continued)*

Because families and communities play a significant role in accepting or rejecting mental illness and mental health services, it behooves the nurse to enlist them in the client treatment planning process (Antai-Otong, 2002; Lin & Cheung, 1999). It is important for the nurse to use interventions that integrate the family and other support groups and convey a prosocial approach that facilitates symptom management and return to an optimal level of functioning.

Finally, the nurse's own culture and ethnicity may affect the perception of the client's cultural expression of distress. It is imperative for the nurse to assess the client's cultural needs and preferences, recognize the role of families and communities in defining these symptoms, and gather data that determine an accurate diagnosis and plan of care. Considerations for the client as an individual living within a social context enables the nurse to accurately assess the level of distress and initiate appropriate treatment planning.

Nurses need to elicit information from the depressed child, parents or guardians, and teachers. Children, like other age groups, must be assessed for suicide. This includes gathering information about past attempts, family history, and present family stressors. In addition to assessing the child, the family's coping skills, level of stress, history of violence, substance abuse, past history of mental and physical disorders, and suicidal behaviors must also be assessed. These data assist in making decisions about disposition; referrals and the parents or guardians ability ensure the child's safety.

Nurses need to gather relevant physical data and perform a mental status examination to rule out underlying medical and psychiatric conditions such as substance-induced mood disorder. This often requires interviewing the youth alone, then the parents or guardians and, later, the entire family. Depressed adolescents may be distrustful of adults initially, but efforts to engage the youth are cru-

cial to the assessment process (Antai-Otong, 2001).

The depressed client may feel worthless and question the nurse's interest in knowing about present symptoms, preferences, and other assessment data. Nurses need to use empathy and patience to establish a therapeutic relationship. In addition, a thorough examination must be performed to rule out medical and mental conditions. Gathering information about mood changes during the woman's menstrual cycle and postpartum and menopause offer important information about hormonal influences.

Table 7–5, Table 7–6, Table 7–7, and Table 7–8 list the diagnostic criteria for some depressive disorders found in adulthood.

Examples of interventions include reminiscence groups, music and pet therapy, and other activities that increase self-esteem and value to reduce the incidence of depression.

Disequilibrium occurs following a loss, and certain tasks need to be accomplished in order to work through the loss and regain equilibrium. These four tasks of mourning are outlined as follows:

1. To accept the reality of the loss. This first task involves accepting the fact on both an intellectual and emotional level that the person is dead and will not return. Rituals, such as the funeral, are often helpful in this process.

2. To work through to the pain of grief. Physical and emotional pain is experienced with loss and it is important for the grieving person to allow himself to feel this.

3. To adjust to an environment in which the deceased is missing. The various roles filled by the deceased (e.g., household manager, child caretaker, finance handler) will influence the extent to which the bereaved needs to develop new skills and take on new roles.

4. To emotionally relocate the deceased and move on with life. This last task can be the most difficult to

(continues)

Table 7–5 • Diagnostic Criteria for Major Depressive Episode

Note: A "Major Depressive Syndrome" is defined as criterion A below.

A. At least five of the following symptoms have been present during the same two-week period and represent a change from previous functioning; at least one of the symptoms is either (1) depressed mood, or (2) loss of interest or pleasure. (Do not include symptoms that are clearly due to a physical condition, mood-incongruent delusions or hallucinations, incoherence, or marked loosening of associations.)

   (1) depressed mood (or can be irritable mood in children and adolescents) most of the day, nearly every day, as indicated either by subjective account or observation by others.

   (2) markedly diminished interest or pleasure in all, or almost all, activities most of the day, nearly every day, (as indicated either by subjective account or observation by others of apathy most of the time).

   (3) significant weight loss or weight gain when not dieting (e.g., more than 5% of body weight in a month), or decrease or increase in appetite nearly every day (in children, consider failure to make expected weight gains)

   (4) insomnia or hypersomnia nearly every day

   (5) psychomotor agitation or retardation nearly every day (observable by others, not merely subjective feelings of restlessness or being slowed down)

   (6) fatigue or loss of energy nearly every day

   (7) feelings of worthlessness or excessive or inappropriate guilt (which may be delusional) nearly every day (not merely self-reproach or guilt about being sick)

   (8) diminished ability to think or concentrate, or indecisiveness, nearly every day (either by subjective account or as observed by others)

   (9) recurrent thoughts of death (not just fear of dying), recurrent suicidal ideation without a specific plan, or a suicide attempt or a specific plan for committing suicide

B. (1) It cannot be established that an underlying medical condition (i.e., hypothyroidism) initiated and maintained the disturbance.

   (2) The disturbance is not a normal reaction to the death of a loved one (Uncomplicated Bereavement).

   Note: Morbid preoccupation with worthlessness, suicidal ideation, marked functional impairment or psychomotor retardation, or prolonged duration suggest bereavement complicated by Major Depression.

C. At no time during the disturbance have there been delusions or hallucinations for as long as two weeks in the absence of prominent mood symptoms (i.e., before the mood symptoms developed or after they have remitted).

D. Not superimposed on Schizophrenia, Schizophreniform Disorder, Delusional Disorder, or Psychotic Disorder NOS.

NOS, not otherwise specified.

Note. From *Diagnostic and Statistical Manual of Mental Disorders* (4th edition Revision) (*DSM-IV-TR*), by American Psychiatric Association, 2000, Washington, DC: Author. Reprinted with permission.

TREATMENT *(continued)*

accomplish because it involves letting go of one's attachment to the deceased and forming new ones. This does not mean giving up thoughts and memories of the lost loved one but rather relocating these in one's emotional life in a way that allows for going on with life (Worden, 1991).

(continues)

Table 7–6 • Diagnostic Criteria for Dysthymia

A. Depressed mood (or can be irritable mood in children and adolescents) for most of the day, more days than not, as indicated either by subjective account or observation by others, for at least two years (one year for children and adolescents).

B. Presence, while depressed, of at least two of the following:
   (1) poor appetite or overeating
   (2) insomnia or hypersomnia
   (3) low energy or fatigue
   (4) low self-esteem
   (5) poor concentration or difficulty making decisions
   (6) feelings of hopelessness

C. During a two-year period (one year for children and adolescents) of the disturbance, never without the symptoms in A for more than two months at a time.

D. No evidence of an unequivocal Major Depressive Episode during the first two years (one year for children and adolescents) of the disturbance.

   Note: There may have been a previous Major Depressive Episode, provided there was a full remission (no significant signs or symptoms for six months) before development of the Dysthymia. In addition, after these two years (one year in children or adolescents) of Dysthymia, there may be superimposed episodes of Major Depression, in which case both diagnoses are given.

E. Has never had a Manic Episode or an unequivocal Hypomanic Episode.

F. Not superimposed on a chronic psychotic disorder, such as Schizophrenia or Delusional Disorder.

G. It cannot be established that an organic factor initiated and maintained the disturbance, e.g., prolonged administration of an antihypertensive medication.

Specify primary or secondary type:

   Primary type: the mood disturbance is not related to a preexisting, chronic, nonmood, Axis I or Axis III disorder, e.g., Anorexia Nervosa, Somatization Disorder, a Psychoactive Substance Dependence Disorder, an Anxiety Disorder, or rheumatoid arthritis.

   Secondary type: the mood disturbance is apparently related to a preexisting chronic, non-mood Axis I or Axis III disorder.

Specify early onset or late onset:

   Early onset: onset of the disturbance before age 21.

   Late onset: onset of the disturbance at age 21 or later.

Note. From *Diagnostic and Statistical Manual of Mental Disorders* (4th edition Text Revision) (*DSM-IV-TR*), by American Psychiatric Association, 2000, Washington, DC: Author. Reprinted with permission.

TREATMENT *(continued)*

According to the American Psychiatric Association (2000) practice guidelines for the treatment of MDD, treatment involves the following phases:

1. **Acute Phase:** Treatment options are considered, including psychopharma-cology, psychotherapy, a combination of medications, and psychotherapy or electroconvulsive therapy (ECT). Potential benefits and side effects are discussed with the client and family along with treatment options and preferences. First-line antidepressants
(continues)

Table 7–7 • Diagnostic Criteria for Melancholic Type

The presence of at least five of the following:

(1) loss of interest or pleasure in all, or almost all, activities

(2) lack of reactivity to usually pleasurable stimuli (does not feel much better, even temporarily, when something good happens)

(3) depression regularly worse in the morning

(4) early morning awakening (at least two hours before usual time of awakening)

(5) psychomotor retardation or agitation (not merely subjective complaints)

(6) significant anorexia or weight loss (e.g., more than 5% of body weight in a month)

(7) no significant personality disturbance before first Major Depressive Episode

(8) one or more previous Major Depressive Episodes followed by complete, or nearly complete, recovery

(9) previous good response to specific and adequate somatic antidepressant therapy e.g., tricyclics, ECT, MAOI, lithium

ECT, electroconvulsive therapy; MAOI, monoamine oxidase inhibitor.

Note. From *Diagnostic and Statistical Manual of Mental Disorders* (4th edition Text Revision) (*DSM-IV-TR*), by American Psychiatric Association, 2000, Washington, DC: Author. Reprinted with permission.

Table 7–8 • Diagnostic Criteria for Seasonal Pattern

A. There has been a regular temporal relationship between the onset of an episode of Bipolar Disorder (including Bipolar Disorder NOS) or Recurrent Major Depression (including Depressive Disorder NOS) and a particular 60-day period of the year (e.g., regular appearance of depression between the beginning of October and the end of November).

   Note: Do not include cases in which there is an obvious effect of seasonally related psychosocial stressors, e.g., regularly being unemployed every winter.

B. Full remissions (or a change from depression to mania or hypomania) also occurred within a particular 60-day period of the year (e.g., depression disappears from mid-February to mid-April).

C. There have been at least three episodes of mood disturbance in three separate years that demonstrated the temporal seasonal relationship defined in A and B; at least two of the years were consecutive.

D. Seasonal episodes of mood disturbance, as described above, outnumbered any nonseasonal episodes of such disturbance that may have occurred by more than three to one.

NOS, not otherwise specified.

Note. From *Diagnostic and Statistical Manual of Mental Disorders* (4th edition Text Revision) (*DSM-IV-TR*), by American Psychiatric Association, 2000, Washington, DC: Author. Reprinted with permission.

TREATMENT *(continued)*

include SSRIs, tricyclic antidepressants (e.g., desipramine [Imprimine]; nortriptyline [Pamelor]), bupropion (Wellbutrin), nefazodone (Serzone), or venlafaxine (Effexor). During this phase the client's response to treatment is monitored along with assessment of side effects.

2. **Continuation Phase:** During 16 to 20 weeks following remission of symptoms.

3. **Maintenance Phase:** Because of the high risk of relapse or recurrent symptoms, this phase is suggested to prevent recurrence.

4. **Discontinuation Phase:** Discontinuation of active treatment—the precise timing of discontinuation of treatment both somatic and psychotherapeutic, varies and often parallels the client's response and preferences. Discontinuation of pharmacologic agents requires tapering the medication over several weeks to reduce recurrence and medication discontinuation syndrome. Health education during this period also focuses on early symptoms of recurrent depressions and the importance of reporting them to their health care provider.

Electroconvulsive therapy (ECT) is the electrical induction of modified grand mal seizures for the purpose of inducing therapeutic change. It is an accepted, safe, and efficacious form of treatment for major depression although the exact mechanism of action remains unclear. Generally, ECT is used only after a trial of antidepressant medication has failed to work, although in certain situations, it might be chosen as an initial treatment; for example, a history of poor antidepressant drug response or good ECT response, or a high risk of suicidal behavior (Weiner, 1994).

Of particular importance when working with the depressed client is the risk of suicide. It is imperative for the nurse to assess the client's level of danger to self and others throughout treatment and educate family members about reporting ideations, threats, gestures, and attempts regardless of how trivial they are.

Major responsibilities of the nurse concerning somatic interventions include administration, prescribing, and monitoring drug levels and adverse side effects. Documenting the client's response is crucial along with health education about various treatment options and potential risk factors.

The primary goal of psychoanalytic psychotherapy is to effect change in personality structure rather than to simply alleviate symptoms. Therapy is aimed at improving a person's capacity for interpersonal trust and intimacy, strengthening coping mechanisms, developing the ability to experience a wide range of emotions, and enhancing the capacity to grieve. Therapy often continues for many years, although in recent decades several short-term psychoanalytic approaches have been developed.

A psychodynamic treatment approach is most commonly used in depressions that are chronic and of mild severity. Because of cost constraints associated with managed care, brief and focused psychotherapies are most likely to be used.

The primary goals of interpersonal therapy are the alleviation of depressive symptoms, improvement of self-esteem, and the development of more effective skills for dealing with social and interpersonal relationships. The therapeutic focus is on current situations in the person's life, and the course of treatment is relatively short (e.g., 12 to 16 weekly sessions). This approach was specifically developed to treat MDDs.

In interpersonal therapy the client is educated about depression, with emphasis placed on the fact of its good prognosis. One or two major problem areas are then defined and become the focus of treatment. Problem areas commonly addressed include abnormal grief reactions, interpersonal role disputes (e.g., marital conflict), role transitions (e.g., divorce),

(continues)

TREATMENT *(continued)*

and interpersonal deficits (e.g., lack of social skills). Medications are often used as an adjunct in reducing depressive symptoms (Sadovy, 2000).

The behavioral theories of depression guide the treatment approach in behavioral therapy. Which behavioral theory of depression is followed guides the treatment approach used. Regardless of the interventions used, the primary goals of therapy are to increase the number of positively reinforcing interactions with the environment and to decrease the number of negative interactions in the depressed person's life. Treatment is usually short term (4 to 12 weeks) and highly structured.

Strategies used in behavioral therapy include having the client keep a daily record of his moods and activities. Based on these records the therapist encourages increased involvement in activities associated with positive moods and avoidance of situations that trigger feelings of depression. In addition, the client is taught how to better manage reactions to negative events, that is, through preparation for such events as well as substituting positive for negative thoughts in relation to them. Time management is used to increase participation in enjoyable events. Assertiveness training and role playing may be used to address social skills deficits and problematic interaction patterns. Relaxation training is used to produce a mood state incompatible with depression. Detailed manuals that outline specific behavioral treatment approaches for unipolar, nonpsychotic depression have been developed (Sadovy, 2000).

Typically, cognitive-behavioral therapy lasts from 12 to 20 sessions and its primary goals are to alleviate depression and decrease the likelihood of its recurrence by helping the individual change his way of thinking.

The following are the three overall components to cognitive-behavioral therapy:

- Didactic teaching, in which the cognitive-behavior view of depression is explained
- Cognitive techniques, involving the eliciting and testing of negative automatic thoughts and identifying and analyzing the maladaptive assumptions on which they are based
- Behavioral techniques, such as scheduling pleasurable activities, role playing, and graded task assignments

The major principle behind these techniques is that identifying and changing maladaptive cognitions and relevant behaviors will reverse the symptoms of depression (Beck, 1963; 1964; 1967; Beck et al., 1979).

The nurse considers the client's holistic needs that include spiritual, cultural, psychosocial and environmental (American Nurses Association [ANA], 2000). The nurse asks questions about current medications, treatment, past and present surgeries, and functional status. Important questions to ask include:

- Reasons for seeking treatment at this time
- Duration and frequency of mood changes and what has worked in the past
- Family history of symptoms and treatment
- Questions about appetite and weight changes
- Sleeping patterns
- Concentration difficulties
- Social support systems
- History of suicide and circumstances
- Current and present risk of suicide and homicide
- Substance abuse history and treatment (last use)
- Legal, occupational, or interpersonal problems.

Working with the depressed client also involves administering prescribed medications, family and health education groups, and initiating various health promoting activities that increase self-esteem, ensure safety, and facilitate adaptive coping skills and resolution of present stressors and depression.

(continues)

TREATMENT *(continued)*

The advanced-practice psychiatric mental health nurse (APN) performs a comprehensive mental, physical, and psychiatric evaluation, including ordering appropriate diagnostic studies to rule out medical conditions, substance misuse, and monitoring drug levels. Based on clinical findings, the APN determines a diagnosis, collaborates with the client or family, develops a holistic treatment plan, and implements various treatments, such as prescribing, monitoring, managing, and evaluating the client's response to pharmacologic interventions.

RESOURCES

Please note that because Internet resources are of a time-sensitive nature and URL addresses may change or be deleted, searches should also be conducted by association or topic.

Internet Resources

http://nimh.nih.gov   D/ART, Public Inquiries

http://www.med.jhu.org   Depression and Related Affective Disorders Association (DRADA)

http://www.cmhc.com   Mental Health Net

Dissociative Disorders

8

• Key Terms

Dissociation: The separation of thoughts, feelings, or experiences from the normal stream of consciousness and memory.

Personality: Enduring patterns of perceiving, relating to, and thinking about the world and oneself.

Switching: The process in which one alter is changed into another.

"The dissociative disorders involve a disturbance in the integrated organization of identity, memory, perception, or consciousness. Events normally experienced on a smooth continuum are isolated from the other mental processes with which they would ordinarily be associated" (Spiegel and Maldonado (1999, p. 453). Bernstein and Putnam (1986) define **dissociation** *as the separation of thoughts, feelings, or experiences from the normal stream of consciousness and memory.*

DISSOCIATIVE DISORDERS—GENERAL

Causes

Continual exposure to overwhelming experiences in the absence of an external comforter can lead to life events being managed by varying degrees of dissociation.

The core conflict in the person experiencing trauma is the wish to deny the horrible experience, while simultaneously wishing to proclaim it to everybody (Herman, 1991). The traumatic experience is usually prolonged and engenders in the victim a deep sense of being helpless to control her own survival. The repertoire of coping mechanisms available depends on the age of the victim during the traumatic event and determines the extent to which dissociation serves as the primary or persistent defense mechanism. Research has demonstrated a significant relationship between early childhood traumas, especially sexual abuse, and chronic dissociation (Chu, Frey, Ganzel, & Matthews, 1999; Draijer & Langeland, 1999; Steinberg, 2000b).

In the normal or minor process of dissociation, the sense of self or of the affect and thought belonging to the self is never lost. In pathological dissociation, the sense of self is disconnected from the experience. Affect or thought is disowned (psychogenic fugue and amnesia) or attributed to another self, or "not me" (dissociative identity disorder). When the intensity of the trauma increases, there is a greater loss of the sense of self as well as an increasing notion of personal estrangement (Meares, 1999). Repeated application of dissociation leads to its indiscriminate use in response to a variety of stressors.

Dissociation does help a person survive and escape an overwhelming reality such as child abuse. It provides relief and time for the person to gather resources to cope with the trauma. When trauma persists, as is usually the case in child abuse, the use of dissociation persists and greatly influences personality development. Estimates of the incidence of child abuse have increased dramatically in the last decade. Coons (1998) asserts that child abuse is almost always part of the history of individuals with dissociative identity disorder.

Dissociative disorders are prevalent around the world and often occur with other psychiatric disorders such as depression, post-traumatic stress disorder, substance use disorders, and borderline personality. Sexual abuse, its severity, and combination with physical abuse and neglect have been found to be strongly linked to adult dissociation measured by the Dissociative Experiences Scale or the Structured Interview for *DSM-III* Dissociative Disorders (Draijer & Langeland, 1999; Kirby, Chu, & Dill, 1993).

A significant part of **personality** development is the lifelong process of assimilating experiences (thoughts, feelings, and actions) and using the assimilated product (understanding) to observe the self and make judgments of present-day interpersonal interactions.

In Sullivan's theory of personality development, Interpersonal Theory, the personality is conceptualized as a *self-system* that consists of three mutually interacting aspects: *good me, bad me,* and *not me.* The development of each aspect is based on significant interpersonal experiences and the intensity of anxiety caused by each experience. According to Sullivan (1953), the self-system, or personality, develops around attempts to modulate anxiety internally in the context of an interaction with a significant other.

An impressive body of research has charted the neurocircuitry underpinnings of stress reactions and fear (Garcia, Vouimba, Baudry, & Thompson, 1999; Whalen et al., 1998). The amygdala, hippocampus, and prefrontal cortex play crucial roles in modulating fear responses. There is strong clinical evidence that indicates that the amygdala is a central structure in the brain neurocircuitry and plays a pivotal role in conditioned or (learned) fear responding (Garcia et al., 1999). The hippocampus and prefrontal cortex have modulatory roles in fear conditioning by processing information about the environmental context (unconditioned stimulus). Dysregulation of the amygdala or the hippocampus, or both, results in poor contextual stimulus discrimination (misinterpretation) and leads to overgeneralization of fear responding cues (Garcia et al., 1999; Whalen et al., 1998). When overgeneralization of an environmental cue occurs, the prefrontal cortex loses the capacity to extinguish fear and anxiety or discriminate between threatening situations and innocuous situations (or repeated stimuli). Alterations in these complex brain regions contribute to maladaptive stress and trauma responses.

Significant early traumatic experiences and the lack of attachment have also been demonstrated to have long-term effects on neurotransmitters, specifically serotonin, which has been identified as a primary neurotransmitter involved in the regulation of affect (Casper, 1998).

Research on stress and trauma has also demonstrated altered limbic system function in response to chronic stress, with concurrent suppression of hypothalamic activity and dysregulation of the neurocircuitry systems. It is possible that the stress hormones released (cortisol and adrenaline) precipitate dissociative episodes directly or through influence on the amygdala, hippocampus, and prefrontal cortex. Dissociation may be precipitated by physiological or emotional changes, and the nurse must thoroughly assess the client in all domains to gain understanding of contributing factors.

The role of family dynamics in the dissociative process is highly potent for the child experiencing trauma such as physical or sexual abuse.

Dissociative symptoms help a child maintain a sense of reality during exposure to trauma. In a healthy family, the child is able to develop a wide range of soothing behaviors because of effective and protective family response, whereas in an abusive family, the only soothing the child is able to take into adulthood is a well-developed dissociative disorder. Any relationship that signals danger will elicit attachment behavior that is alternated with behavior that maintains distance (e.g., self-mutilation or dissociation).

Family dynamics around the abused child leave her with a rigid perception of interpersonal roles. That is, the child perceives all people to fall into one of the following roles: abuser, victim, rescuer, or neglectful or powerless bystander (Herman, 1991).

A child with a dissociative disorder is most likely to have a history of early sexual or physical abuse and has not been able to develop attachment because of the absence of empathetic parenting.

The adolescent with dissociative identity disorder is likely to be the more vulnerable to the pressures of peer groups and use alters to respond to each demand. In a study looking at a spectrum of traumatic events and the development of dissociative symptoms in adolescents, Brunner, Parzer, Schuld, and Resch (2000) found that even less severe forms of abuse and neglect may have a significant impact on the development of dissociative symptoms in adolescents.

Even in healthy adults, the experience of a traumatic event, such as a flood, earthquake, or car crash, may result in dissociation. Dissociation allows the individual to distance oneself from the trauma (Spiegel, 1993). Dissociation of the experience is adaptive in the sense that it gives the person time to gather her defense mechanism resources. This gathering of resources will help the person assimilate the experience without being psychologically overwhelmed. The dissociative process paces the assimilation of the experience into consciousness and modulates the anxiety.

Symptoms

Dissociative phenomena exist along a continuum, from mild and common to pathological forms (Steinberg, 2000a). Minor forms of dissociation can be inconspicuous everyday occurrences of "spacing out," for example, while driving a car or sitting in class. Midpoint on the continuum would be reported out-of-body, near-death experiences, wherein the clients have an experience of viewing their body from a vantage point above or to the side of their body. Individuals who have near-death experiences describe the occurrence of dissociative phenomena during their experience (Greyson, 2000). The more pathological forms of dissociation are amnesia, fugue, and identity disorder.

They are related to traumatic, intense anxiety antecedents. Peplau (1952) operationally defined dissociation, which is presented in Table 8–1.

Dissociation is an early primitive defense mechanism available to children until they mature and gain greater psychological capacity to accommodate ambiguity and tolerate conflict. Putnam (1997) labeled this a "normative dissociation." It is normally manifested in fantasy play and other imaginary activities. It is common for children to have elaborate, imaginary companions, and the phenomenon should not be considered pathological unless it is carried into adolescence.

Children with a dissociative disorder are often difficult to differentiate from children with attention-deficit disorder. Clients with dissociative disorders can manifest mild-to-moderate inattention and sustained concentration deficits on psychological testing (Rossini, Schwartz, & Braun, 1996). The abrupt changes in behavior and short attention and memory spans seen in hyperactive children are similar to episodes of dissociation. Often, these children suffer self-hatred and appear anxious and depressed. Silberg (1998) identified the following behavioral features common in children with dissociative disorder diagnoses:

- Amnesia, or forgetting test responses
- Staring, indicative of trance states
- Unusual or odd motor behaviors
- Fearful and angry reactions to stimuli
- Expressions of internal conflict

In an effort to counteract a not-me personification of powerlessness, the adolescent may become more aggressive and act out sexually. Denial, along with dissociation, will present in an adolescent who not only does not recall trauma but also rejects any suggestion that she is the least bit troubled.

Older adults may wander away from home and, when found, be able to state their name but not have a sense of their general location or how long they have been wandering. Clients with psychological amnesia, on the other hand, have no sense of who they are, who their family members are, or what their occupation is.

Table 8–1 • Operational Definition of Dissociation

1. In early life, certain thoughts, feelings, and/or actions of the client are disapproved by significant other persons.

2. Significant people's standards are incorporated as the client's own.

3. Later in life, the client experiences one of the disapproved thoughts, feelings, or actions.

4. Anxiety increases to a severe level.

5. The feelings are barred from awareness.

6. Anxiety decreases.

7. Dissociated content continues to appear in disguised form in the client's thoughts, feelings, and actions.

Note. Adapted from *Interpersonal Relations in Nursing,* by H. Peplau, 1952. New York: G. F. Putnam. Used by permission.

TREATMENT

Clients with a dissociative disorder often present with a multitude of somatic complaints. Thus the nurse must thoroughly assess the client's physical status as the first intervention. Simultaneously, the nurse will want to keep in mind that if the client has a history of very early trauma, the somatic complaint may be representative of a memory laid down along primitive neurological pathways that is being stimulated by something in the current environment (van der Kolk & Saporta, 1991). The client often experiences the nurse's attention to her physical complaints and the nurse's education about "body memories" to be helpful and soothing.

Any sudden onset of symptoms of dissociative disorder should first be evaluated for a possible medical etiology (Table 8–2).

The nurse who is interacting with the dissociating client will be placed in one of the family member's roles as the client re-creates the family experience. The nurse needs to observe the developing *(continues)*

Table 8–2 • Medical and Other Psychiatric Diagnoses with Symptoms Similar to Those of Dissociative Disorders

Dissociative Disorder	Signs and Symptoms	Medical or Other Psychiatric Diagnosis	Signs and Symptoms
Depersonalization disorder	Parts of body feel unreal Client has sensation of body change Client is aware of perceptual distortions	Accompanies numerous other psychiatric disorders: electrolyte disturbance, seizure disorder Ganser's syndrome (seen in men with severe personality disorder) Factitious disorder: client fabricates symptoms Toxic disorders Neoplasms	Hard to differentiate Has factitious quality—symptoms are worse when client is aware of being observed Blood chemistry is abnormal Magnetic resonance imaging, computed tomography, and positron emission tomography are abnormal
Dissociative amnesia	Begins abruptly Client is aware of memory loss and is alert before and after Depression is usually associated Physical assessment is normal	Transient global amnesia Postconcussion amnesia	Client is upset about amnesia Memory loss is generalized Amnesia *gradually* subsides Central nervous system examination is abnormal
Dissociative fugue	Client travels away from home and takes on a new identity May be associated with alcohol ingestion Evidence of secondary gain is clear	Cognitive disorder	Temporal lobe epilepsy Wandering does not result in socially adaptive behavior
Dissociative identity disorder	Changes in behavior are dramatic or sudden Client experiences either co-consciousness of or amnesia for alters Physical assessment is usually normal	Cognitive disorder	Central nervous system examination is abnormal Intoxication Street drugs are used

TREATMENT *(continued)*

role pattern and assist the client in describing her perception of their interactions. Nursing interventions such as limit setting or confrontation will cause the client to perceive the nurse as an abuser. The client's threats or acts of self-destructive behavior can initiate the dynamic, whereby the nurse perceives and experiences herself as a victim or powerless bystander.

As each of these re-created family patterns is enacted, the nurse assists the client to identify her present need and to think about how to get it met. The goal is to foster a secure base for the client in the various treatment relationships so that security will eventually be internalized.

Psychiatric nurses need to familiarize themselves with behaviors that are unique to various cultures and assess the significance of the clients' symptoms to ensure an accurate diagnosis. The nursing assessment needs to include a thorough spiritual and religious assessment along with other aspects of the mental status and physical examination to make an accurate description of the clients' symptoms.

When working with the child or adolescent with a dissociative disorder, the nurse's first goal is to ensure the client's safety. The protection and soothing that were unavailable in the client's early development must be present in the nurse-client relationship and therapeutic environment. The nurse should accept the experiences of alters in children and adolescents with dissociative identity disorder. Excessive **switching** between alters is usually the result of an environmental or interpersonal trigger similar to past trauma. A therapeutic intervention occurs when the nurse, who is in the here-and-now, reassures the client. Structure in the nurse-client relationship and physical milieu helps the client experience her self in a continuous manner. In addition the continuity of the client's self may be facilitated by the use of clearly defined limits and consequences for inappropriate behavior. Emphasis should be on talking or writing about feelings, rather than on acting on them. Children can be encouraged to keep art journals.

The nurse in advanced practice may have success in using a group therapy process for adolescents. An expressive group process will help the adolescent normalize some feelings as well as provide a consistent and healthy peer group experience.

Promotion of the client's self-soothing is a major goal for the psychiatric nurse. The child client will need concrete direction in this area. Does she have a soothing stuffed toy or a favorite story or something or someone to turn to when frightened? The adolescent can be assisted to use sports or imagery that involves relaxation as a means of soothing.

As with any other age group, it is important to differentiate between a general medical condition and a psychological etiology for a dissociative process in an adult. In amnesia with an underlying medical condition, such as severe electrolyte imbalance or head injury, general information is lost before personal information.

The psychiatric nurse can make major contributions to the diagnostic process of dissociative disorder. The nurse observes patterns of apparent dissociation in terms of particular time of day and the presence or absence of possible environmental factors. The nurse correlates these observations with the objective physiological data. The advanced-practice nurse in the community will use her extensive knowledge of physiology as well as interviewing skills to identify trauma in the assessment of a client presenting with "lost time" or a sense of "not being myself."

Anxiety that is persistent and peaks before a dissociative episode is a symptom common to all types of dissociation. Thus, benzodiazepines given p.r.n. and in maintenance doses are helpful in stabilizing the client as she works to develop nondissociative coping mechanisms.

(continues)

TREATMENT *(continued)*

Depression is also a common presenting symptom of clients with dissociative disorder and may be what first brings them into the mental health system. No particular class of antidepressant is more effective than another; each needs to be evaluated on an individual basis.

Anger and severe internal disequilibrium accompany dissociation in varying degrees. Neuroleptics can be a useful adjunct to treatment to assist the client in periods of dyscontrol or rapid dissociation. Atypical antipsychotics can be effective.

Grounding, as a concept, is meant to convey the notion of "not going away," that is, dissociating. The following techniques help clients concentrate on the here and now and move toward verbalizing what is occurring in their internal world. The nurse should teach clients these techniques.

Safe Place

Finding a safe place is a concept very familiar to survivors of abuse. The dissociative person should be encouraged to find a reasonable place in the environment where she can go and guarantee the nurse and herself safety and freedom from destructive impulses. A typical place could be a particular chair or room.

Ice in Hands

Ice helps the client focus on a physical sensation that is not harmful. When the warning signs of dissociation are present, the nurse may encourage the client to hold an ice cube securely in each hand until she can report feeling calmer.

Wrapping Self in Blanket

A person who is dissociating may start to feel not real or feel that she is going to "come apart." Wrapping a blanket around herself like a long cloak helps set the external boundaries and promote a sense of protection.

Counting Forward or Backward

Counting forward or backward is a technique used mostly by clients with dissociative identity disorder. Counting is a form of hypnosis that can be used to let an alter that is overwhelmed go in and another come forward with behavior appropriate to the situation.

Providing clients with skills to cope with their dissociative disorder is an important function of the psychiatric nurse. Essential skills are relapse prevention and journaling.

Relapse Prevention

Relapse prevention is an important skill drawn from working with chemically dependent persons. The client is taught to recognize contributing factors (triggers) to dissociation. The client and nurse then develop a concrete plan to interrupt the stimulation of a dissociative episode. The plan could include activities such as listening to music, staying with people, or engaging in a task. Then the plan is shared with the family and other health care professionals involved in the client's treatment to enlist support in implementing it whenever it is needed.

Journaling

Writing in a journal helps the client achieve several outcomes: feelings are put into words, a sense of continuity of the self is developed in the journal, and the impact of triggers is diminished.

The psychiatric nurse is pivotal in the care of the client vulnerable to or diagnosed with dissociative disorder. The generalist nurse will be on the front line of identifying the undiagnosed dissociative disorder. The nurse's other important role is to help the client develop adaptive coping skills and achieve basic symptom management, including appropriate use of medications. The nurse needs to continually assess the client's level of danger to self and others throughout treatment.

The advanced-practice psychiatric nurse may often encourage the client in a psychotherapy or case management process. Psychotherapy is the arena in which the client may retrieve memories

(continues)

TREATMENT *(continued)*

in a controlled manner to consider their impact on her life. Advanced-practice nurses require specialized training to work with clients with dissociative disorders, particularly when working with alters. The nurse needs to assess client safety continually, using short hospital stays if necessary, to help clients retrieve their capacity to feel safe.

Early case finding is an important function of the nurse working with children. Recognition that a child is being abused or is experiencing early school failure can help interrupt progression toward a much more problematic dissociative disorder in adulthood.

Psychological assessment involves collecting both subjective and objective data. The client may not always be able to report sexual or emotional trauma because the event is dissociated. The nurse should watch for signs of abuse: startle reaction, erratic sleep, and fear of objects or other people. Because some clients are not aware they dissociate, the nurse should also observe for a pattern of not remembering events and a pattern of unexplained behaviors.

Possible nursing diagnoses include:

- Disturbed personal identity
- Ineffective Coping: escape through dissociation
- Anxiety severe related to acute stressor

The process of working to identify desired outcomes is empowering. Outcomes need to be very short term in nature, so that clients are able to appreciate their progress. Planning, whether in a community or hospital setting, should be reviewed frequently.

As the client works with the nurse to implement a plan of care, the client should experience a form of support that has been missing in her life. Regardless of setting, interventions should be flexible but emphasize consistency and predictability.

The accompanying Standard of Care for clients with a dissociative disorder provides the nurse with a menu of client outcomes and nursing interventions within the six domains of nursing: psychotherapeutic interventions, therapeutic milieu, health teaching, activities of daily living, somatic therapies, and discharge planning.

DEPERSONALIZATION DISORDER

Cause

The client with depersonalization disorder is overwhelmed by feelings during a current event that is similar to a traumatic event in the past (APA, 2000).

Symptoms

Depersonalization disorder is a rapid-onset, persistent dissociative process in which the client's experience of the self or perception of the reality of the self or environment is changed. The client is able to observe the process as it occurs and verbalize discomfort (APA, 2000).

DISSOCIATIVE AMNESIA

Cause

Dissociative amnesia is usually a defense mechanism that occurs in response to an emotional conflict or an external stressor, for example, the sudden loss of a significant other (Steinberg, 2000).

Symptoms

Dissociative amnesia is a dissociative process that results in a sudden identity disturbance owing to the client's inability to recall significant personal information. Underlying general medical conditions, brain injury, and substance abuse have been ruled out as possible causes (APA, 2000). Dissociative amnesia is the most common of the dissociative disorders.

Standard of Care for the Client with a Dissociative Disorder

Nursing Diagnosis: Alteration in Continuity of Self

Client Outcome: By (date), client will demonstrate or verbalize increased continuity in one or all parameters of the self: identity, memory, experience.

Defining Characteristics:

NURSING DOMAIN	CLIENT OUTCOME	NURSING INTERVENTIONS
Psychotherapeutic interventions	1. Client states what personality is interacting with nursing staff.	1a. Collaborate with client in mapping out the alters and the purpose and function of each.
		1b. Instruct client that she is responsible for letting staff know which alter is out.
		1c. Identify with client which alters are caretakers (internal self-helpers) and can be elicited in stressful situations.
		1d. Before the client goes off the unit, have her contract to have only an appropriate alter out when off the unit.
		1e. Emphasize that all alters are responsible for care and behavior of body.
		1f. Respond to client as a whole person.
		1g. Encourage host personality to engage all alters in writing in a journal.
	2. Client relates memories of self-system to present peer relationship patterns.	2a. Educate client about dysfunctional attachment/trust patterns from past abuse.
		2b. Initiate *brief* contact frequently with client during first 72 hours of hospitalization.
		2c. Problem-solve with client regarding how she may feel safe in the presence of another client or nurse who reminds client of trauma.
	3. Client maintains progressively longer experience of here-and-now reality.	3a. Teach client basic structure of journal: Work 5 to 10 minutes daily. Choose one event of day. Write about thoughts and feelings related to the event.
		3b. Review journal work with client on a regular basis.

(continues)

Standard of Care for the Client with a Dissociative Disorder *(continued)*

NURSING DOMAIN	CLIENT OUTCOME	NURSING INTERVENTIONS
		3c. Review nursing care plan and sleep patterns with client on a regular basis.
		3d. Assess client for what, if any, grounding techniques she currently uses.
		3e. Support client in use of following client-appropriate grounding techniques: Going to safe place Holding ice in hands Placing feet on the floor and grasping a chair Wrapping self in blanket Staying out of the room Blowing her nose Listening to tapes that provide pleasant memories Washing face Counting forward or backward Requesting quiet room Requesting p.r.n. medicines Requesting restraints
Therapeutic milieu	1. Client identifies triggers in environment that lead to dissociation.	1a. Educate client about concept of trigger. 1b. If client switches rapidly, start flow sheet to identify pattern of triggers. 1c. Provide client with feedback about when dissociation was observed.
	2. Client participates in promotion of safe milieu.	2a. Explore with client how the need to feel safe is met. 2b. Educate client about the need to not allow own behavior to become alarming to other clients (abuse is unacceptable). 2c. Develop plan with client to contain violent or self-destructive alters when and if they come out. 2d. Encourage client to have child alters come out only in privacy of her room. 2e. Support client in stating when another client's behavior seems similar to past abuse.

(continues)

Standard of Care for the Client with a Dissociative Disorder *(continued)*

NURSING DOMAIN	CLIENT OUTCOME	NURSING INTERVENTIONS
Activities of daily living	1. Client maintains a structured day.	1a. Assess client's ability to make up a daily schedule. 1b. Support client in keeping appointments by providing positive feedback. 1c. Provide client with unit-restricted schedule if she is being kept on the unit. 1d. Actively support client in adhering to schedule. 1e. Document any dissatisfaction client expresses with schedule. 1f. Assist client in structuring time for alters to come out.
	2. Client participates in development of safe nighttime environment.	2a. Help client identify her patterns of sleep and wakefulness. 2b. Problem-solve periods of wakefulness. 2c. Encourage identification and use of specific self-soothing techniques as a part of bedtime preparation.
Health teaching	1. Client verbalizes purpose, side effects, and dose of medication.	1a. Provide client with appropriate information about medications. 1b. Explain the value of consistent medication dosage. 1c. Encourage client to identify which alters, if any, are resistant to medication. 1d. Problem-solve resistance to use of medication.
	2. Client verbalizes understanding of nursing care plan development and implementation.	2a. Explore understanding of nursing care plan in development of care plan. 2b. Identify with the client the value of participating in development of care plan. 2c. With client, practice identifying problem goal and intervention.
	3. Client demonstrates use of journal as tool to facilitate continuity of experience.	3a. Assess client's experience with journal writing: how often: _____ technique: _____ tools: _____

(continues)

Standard of Care for the Client with a Dissociative Disorder *(continued)*

NURSING DOMAIN	CLIENT OUTCOME	NURSING INTERVENTIONS
		3b. Teach client journal structure and value of using journal consistency.
		3c. Review client's journal writing with her.
		3d. Encourage journal writing as a substitute for acting out and as method to self-soothe.
	4. Client demonstrates use of safe place.	4a. Assess client's history of using safe place: where: _____ when: _____ how long: _____
		4b. Teach client value of still using safe place as an adult.
		4c. Encourage client to identify safe place on the unit.
		4d. When client appears overstimulated, remind her of safe place.
		4e. If client harms self or others in safe place, repeat b and c.
		4f. Encourage client to use safe place for alters via imagery.
Somatic therapies	1. Client adheres to prescribed medication regimen.	1a. Encourage client's input regarding most effective time structure of doses.
		1b. Assist client in encouraging resistant alters to help take care of the body.
		1c. Teach client to use p.r.n. medication as a preventive basis using warning signs.
	2. Client uses self-soothing techniques for grounding.	2a. Assess client's repertoire of self-soothing techniques.
		2b. Encourage attendance at group activities promoting body awareness.
		2c. Assist client in use of grounding techniques listed under Psychotherapeutic interventions.
Discharge planning	1. Client develops relapse prevention plan for triggers that lead to dissociation.	1a. Review relapse prevention plan with client.
		1b. Practice prevention plan with client.
		1c. Help client identify people with whom she will share plan after discharge.

DISSOCIATIVE FUGUE

Cause

The origin of dissociative fugue is usually the desire to withdraw from emotionally painful experiences (Coons, 2000).

Symptoms

Dissociative fugue is a dissociative process that results in an identity and memory disturbance manifested by sudden travel away from the home or work environment along with confusion about personal identity or, rarely, the assumption of a new identity. The travel may be brief or extensive. These patients appear normal, not attracting the attention of others.

DISSOCIATIVE IDENTITY DISORDER

Cause

Dissociative identity disorder is most likely caused by a severe childhood trauma. The trauma is usually severe sexual abuse that overwhelms the child's nondissociative defenses.

Symptoms

Dissociative identity disorder was previously known as multiple personality disorder. It is considered the most serious of the dissociative disorders. Clients have two or more distinct personalities, each with its own behavior and attitudes (APA, 2000).

The following are the signs and symptoms of dissociative identity disorder:

- Unremembered behaviors
- The discovery of items in the client's possession for which she cannot account
- Loss of time
- Behavior characteristics that represent distinctly different ages
- Changes in appearance and dress
- Use of different voices

TREATMENT

It should be noted that the alters of the client with dissociative identity disorder may have varying degrees of responsiveness to neuroleptics. This is not manipulation, but a basic difference in psychological responsiveness.

The nurse's role in pharmacotherapy is to educate the client about the medication, including the purpose of the medication, the dose schedule, and possible side effects. The nurse must assess the client for medication adherence, which can be disrupted by dissociative episodes. An emphasis on client responsibility, especially persons with dissociative identity disorders, is paramount for medication adherence and safety.

Intensive psychotherapy is probably the most effective treatment for the dissociative disorders, particularly dissociative identity disorder. The psychotherapy will be long term in nature. Hypnosis is also a technique that has been found to be useful in treating these disorders. The advanced-practice nurse may be involved in these treatment modalities.

Additional psychosocial interventions include assessing and monitoring the client's risk of danger to self and others, assisting in developing adaptive coping skills, and providing opportunities to succeed in activities that increase self-esteem.

RESOURCES

Please note that because Internet resources are of a time-sensitive nature and URL addresses may change or be deleted, searches should also be conducted by association or topic.

Internet Resources

http://www.healinghopes.com   Support forum for abuse/trauma survivors

http://www.issd.org   International Society for the Study of Dissociation

http://www.sidran.org   Traumatic Stress Foundation

9 Eating Disorders

• Key Terms

Alexithymia: Refers to a lack of introceptive awareness, mistrust of self and others, cognitive dysfunction, and starvation-induced depression.

Anorexia Nervosa (AN): Self-induced starvation resulting from fear of fatness; not caused by true loss of appetite.

Body Image Disturbance: Refers to a distortion in the image of the body that is of near or actual delusional proportions; may include strong feelings of self-loathing projected onto the body, body parts, or perceived fat.

Body Mass Index (BMI): Refers to a mathematical formula that is highly correlated with body fat. It is weight in kilograms divided by height in meters squared (kg/m^2). In the United States and in the United Kingdom, people with BMIs between 25 and 30 kg/m^2 are considered overweight and those with BMIs of 30 kg/m^2 are categorized as obese.

Bulimia Nervosa (BN): Binge eating followed by self-inflicted vomiting, laxative or diuretic abuse, or starvation.

Eating Disorder (ED): A general term for abnormalities in behavior toward food, growing out of fear of fatness and pursuit of excessive thinness.

Purge: Self-induced vomiting or misuse of laxative, diuretics, or enemas.

Eating disorders (EDs) are a significant health problem among children, adolescents, and young women. Western society places an emphasis on physical attractiveness, and, in this century, there is an extreme emphasis on thinness as the epitome of feminine beauty. Cultural values, particularly since the 1970s, have promoted images of willowy, gaunt young women as the ideal female form. Simultaneously, there has been an explosion in the number and variety of high-fat, high-calorie fast foods as well as in food advertising, and there is an increase in the number of markedly obese people of all ages, except for the elderly. The rate of obesity among children has doubled in the last decade (DHHS, Mental Health of the Surgeon General, 1999).

EATING DISORDERS— GENERAL

Causes

Obsessive-compulsive traits are observed and documented in the eating disorder population, particularly related to the obsessive drive toward thinness at all costs and the compulsive nature of the binge-purge or food-restricting behaviors. Eating elicits the anxiety (or morbid fear of weight gain), and purging reduces the anxiety. Binge eaters who do not vomit or purge, sometimes referred to as compulsive eaters, also experience a drive to eat, accompanied by anxiety reduction as they "fill the emptiness." This is in contrast to clients with bulimia, whose anxiety level rises with the sensation of fullness. Anxiety disorders, including obsessive-compulsive disorder and generalized anxiety disorder, are positively associated with AN (Fairburn, Cooper, Doll, & Welch, 1999; Klump, Kaye, & Strober, 2001).

Fairburn et al. (1997; 1999) found an association with substance abuse in eating-disorder behaviors. Brewerton (1995) reviewed the relationship of serotonin (5-HT) in the development of alcoholism and other addictions and looked at a unified theory of 5-HT dysregulation to eating and other disorders. The relationship of problems of impulsive control leads

the client with bulimia to experience the uncontrolled eating as more ego dystonic than the client with anorexia and more likely to seek help (Kaplan & Sadock, 1998).

Brewerton's extensive research (1995) postulates a unified theory of 5-HT dysregulation in clients with eating and related disorders. Clients with ED exhibit several clinical features and biologic findings indicative of 5-HT dysregulation as well as a failure of neurotransmitter regulation, rather than a simple increase or decrease in activity. These include feeding disturbances, depression and suicidal behavior, impulsivity and violence, anxiety and harm avoidance, obsessive-compulsive features, substance abuse, seasonal variation of symptoms, disturbances in neuroendocrine and vascular tissues, and neurochemical systems linked to 5-HT such as temperature. Research review supports a 5-HT dysregulation hypothesis and that a variety of psychobiological stressors, such as dieting, binge eating, purging, drug abuse, photoperiodic changes, as well as psychosocial-interpersonal stress, perturb a vulnerable 5-HT system. The interaction with a variety of psychobiological stressors perturbs the vulnerable 5-HT system, leading to further dysregulation. See Table 9–1 for the interaction of stressors with vulnerable 5-HT system.

Table 9–1 • 5-HT Dysregulation
Hypotheses of Eating Disorders:
Interaction of Stressors with
Vulnerable 5-HT System

- Dieting; fasting
- Binge eating
- Purging; dehydration
- Compulsive exercising
- Alcohol and drug use
- Photoperiodic changes
- ED clients exhibit disturbances in other neurochemical systems linked to 5-HT, including:
  - Hypothalmic-Pituitary Adrenal (HPA) axis
  - Noradrenergic system
  - Dopaminergic
  - Isatin, an endogenous MAO-like compound
  - Neuropeptides, e.g. β-endorphin, dynorphin, cholecystokinin, neuropeptide Y and YY, galanine, arginine, vasopressin
  - Leptin

5-HT, serotonin. MAO, monoamine oxidase.

Note. From *Serotonin Dysregulation in the Eating Disorder Adolescent,* by T. D. Brewerton, 1997, paper presented at Eating Disorders at AACAP, Toronto, Ontario, Canada.

Minuchin, Rosman, and Baker (1978) identified characteristics often present in the families of children with eating disorders as enmeshment, overprotectiveness, rigidity, and lack of interactions of the child and the family. Finally, Minuchin et al. (1978) addressed the *rigidity* within these families, which refers to their inflexible nature and their desire to maintain the status quo. The *lack of conflict resolution* refers to the family's inability to negotiate any type of compromise or any kind of solution to an identified problem. Family conflicts are usually polarized into a "win or lose" situation, with no one wanting to be on the losing end. Transgenerational perspectives take into account the transmission of anxiety and dysfunctional patterns that the family system has of relating over generations, with

the triangulation of symptoms onto one or more vulnerable family members. Usually there is a pattern of poor differentiation from grandparents and difficulty in the parental marriage. These "family legacies" can be viewed as the experiential portion of family belief systems that evolved because family organization shifts and changes over time. In the bulimic family, the multigenerational legacy revolves around weight, attractiveness, fitness, success, and eating of food. Usually there is a pattern of poor differentiation from grandparents and a belief in filial loyalty coupled with success (Roberto, 1986; 1992).

Obviously, we live in a diet-conscious society in which thinness is viewed as attractive and healthy. Images and messages, both blatant and subtle, bombard young girls and women, promoting thinness, dieting, and weight loss as attractive and associated with sex appeal and achievement.

It has been thought in the past that certain sociocultural groups, specifically white females, were at highest risk for these disorders; however, current clinical practice indicates that the most assimilated minority cultures are at as great risk as white females. This incorrect perception, that EDs are mainly a disease of white females, has led to a general lack of awareness among clinicians and subsequent failure to diagnose disturbed eating behaviors in minority clients. African American women report laxative and diuretic abuses as well as fasting behaviors to avoid weight gain. Research indicates that younger, more educated, and perfection-seeking African American women were most at risk for succumbing to these disorders. Among Latinos, EDs are also directly related to acculturation (Fitzgibbon & Stolley, 2001). Models, actresses, and others in the entertainment industry have a high frequency of EDs. Gymnasts and ballet dancers are at extremely high risk.

In addition, there is tremendous pressure on women today to achieve in separate arenas simultaneously. They must be successful, independent, and competitive professionally while competently maintaining their traditional role as wife, mother, and homemaker. The stressors inherent in this situation may be overwhelming to those women who may be predisposed to EDs.

Issues of disturbance in sexuality and intimacy have been associated with EDs. The early experiences of sexual and physical abuse may affect the libido, and the association with mood disorders may decrease the libido. Persons who restrict food intake appear to have decreased libido and be less interested in sex, whereas those who binge or binge and purge seem to have more frequent sexual activity and interest.

The clinical picture presented by the adolescent also needs to be considered within a developmental framework. Central to the ED are those issues relative to puberty, such as increased independence from the family and increased autonomy in problem solving; family and peer pressures, including sexuality; and initiation in the process of major life choices.

Researchers believe that diabetes may predispose one to the development of an ED, because a person can attempt to control weight by manipulating an insulin dosage (Colton, Rodin, Olmsted, & Daneman, 1999; Rydall, Rodin, Olmsted, Devenyi, & Daneman, 1997). Many women with diabetes equate insulin usage with weight gain and therefore reduce their insulin dosage to decrease their weight. This method results in glycosuria and the life-threatening consequence of diabetic ketoacidosis (DKA). An ED should be suspected in a female with diabetes who presents with a history of multiple incidents of DKA and unexplainable difficulties in the regulation of blood glucose levels.

Symptoms

The client with a coexisting personality disorder and ED presents unique challenges for nurses and therapists. Clients with personality disorders and EDs can be considered aggressive toward others and toward themselves. They share characteristics of impulsivity, self-mutilation,

and disinhibition. They may evidence frequent suicide attempts, drug and alcohol use, and angry behavior, and the health care team may be challenged by the manipulative or immature qualities evidenced in behaviors (Klump et al., 2001).

Most clients with ED experience shame and disgust with their bodies, whether they are obese, of normal weight, or very thin. These feelings obviously interfere with any enjoyment or pleasure in physical touching or joining. Additional intimacy issues include hiding or not showing their bodies to partners or spouses and projecting feelings of disgust when looked at or touched.

The young child with an ED is one who is in a prepubertal stage of development and is considered to be preadolescent—classic DSM criteria may not be applicable. However, *DSM-IV-TR* now addresses feeding disorders that occur in childhood before the age of 6 years (see the display on diagnostic criteria for feeding disorder of infancy or early childhood). For instance, a child does not have to lose the percentage of weight appropriate for an adult with an ED.

EDs typically present in the male with the same core psychopathological features as in the female; however, there are some unique features. According to Anderson (1984), males tend to be less focused on their exact weight and more intent on attaining the idealized masculine shape of large shoulders and narrow waist and hips.

In addition, males tend to exhibit more sexual anxiety related to issues of homosexuality and bisexuality. A variation of extreme body awareness seems to be occurring among young men who do not meet the "idealized" masculine image of hypermuscularity promoted by the media.

Key Facts

Studies have shown that from 30 to 50 percent of adult women with EDs also report unwanted sexual experiences as children or adults. The literature is just beginning to explore this link, and the cause-and-effect relationship remains unclear (Fairburn et al., 1997; 1999).

TREATMENT

The care of the person with an ED is complex and multifaceted. The optimal form of treatment is via the team approach. This method helps diffuse the heavy burden of dealing with these clients and their families. Essential members of the team include a family physician or pediatrician, a psychotherapist from one of the designated mental health professions, a dietician, a consulting psychologist to administer standardized tests, and a consulting psychiatrist to assess the need for psychotropic medication. During inpatient hospitalization, the nursing staff plays an integral role in the care also.

It is essential that team members communicate and firmly abide by the boundaries of their particular role; otherwise, the goals of treatment may be sabotaged. A major function of the team is to provide support, clarification, and feedback to the mental health professional acting in the role of primary therapist. Team conferences may be held frequently and regularly to optimally aid the client and family being treated. Changes in reimbursement for inpatient treatment have resulted in the development of intensive outpatient programs (IOPs) for ED treatment.

Multiple diagnoses in the same person are commonly anecdotally identified in psychiatry and are just now receiving attention. See Table 9–2, Mental Status Examination and Comorbid Psychiatric Conditions with Eating Disorders.

Recognition of the patterns and risk factors of ED is crucial for early identification and school and parental education about these serious comorbid disorders. Nurses are in pivotal positions to provide health education and primary prevention in vast practice settings.

Because of the unique biological and life-threatening challenges presented by the client with an ED, special circumstances must be considered in the treatment plan based on the development needs of the client. See Table 9–3 for an overview of when specific EDs occur in relation to the life stage.

Prepubertal children have a lower percentage of body fat. A child who is thin at the start of the weight loss process may reach an unhealthy state quickly. In addition, children tend to eliminate fluids, including water, as well as food. It is helpful to continually plot out the child's progression on the growth chart, accounting for both height and weight. This important tool quickly shows developmentally inappropriate positions on the chart that need specific attention. In addition, both boys and girls present with infantile or childhood anorexia, whereas bulimia is extremely unusual. Symptoms of depression are also usually present and need to be addressed.

Within the psychotherapeutic process, developmental theory continues to be of great importance. Infants or younger children are still very involved in the family and may react strongly to changes within the household and stressful family events. The infant who refuses food or fails to thrive is a medical and life-threatening emergency. Immediate and accurate assessment must be done quickly before permanent damage occurs. A major component of treatment should be family education and individual treatment for the caregiver as well as family therapy. A child protective services referral, with a service plan instituted for the family, may need to be instituted. Individual therapy for the child, depending on age, may also prove helpful.

The adolescent with an ED will benefit from a variety of therapies, including individual, family, and group work.

The registered nurse may plan to monitor the results of the glycosylated hemoglobin tests. This blood test monitors the glucose levels of the client with diabetes over the past 3 months. The normal values for this test range from 4 to 8 percent, so a result between 12 and 20 percent would indicate uncontrolled blood glucose levels. In other words, if a client with diabetes claims to have had normal blood glucose levels at home, a glycosylated hemoglobin test will validate or

(continues)

Table 9–2 • Mental Status Examination and Comorbid Psychiatric Conditions with Eating Disorders

Mental Status Examination	Variable affective range cheerful and hyperactive to hypomanic
	Sad and hypoactive to depressed; generally, affect restricted
	Limited capacity for self-observation, insight, psychological mindedness
	Resistance to treatment and denial of disorder
	Body image disturbance: cognitive distortion that client is fat in spite of emaciation
	All or nothing thinking: " If I am not perfect I am a complete failure"
	Faulty perception of inner sensations: unable to identify inner sensations of hunger with constant thoughts of food
	Sense of personal ineffectiveness
Personality Characteristics	Obsessional traits, insecurity, minimization of emotional expression, perfectionism, excessive conformance, rigid impulses control, highly industrious, competitiveness, enviousness, and responsible
Comorbidity	Depressive disorders
	Anxiety disorders, including dissociative disorders
	Substance abuse
	Obsessive-compulsive disorder
	Personality disorders: commonly avoidant, schizoid, borderline, narcissistic
	Psychosis
	Sexual abuse history
	Impulse control disorders: shoplifting, compulsive shopping, and spending

Note. From *Practice Guidelines for the Treatment of Patients with Eating Disorders* (2nd ed., Compendium 2000, pp. 627–697), by the American Psychiatric Association, 2000, Washington, DC: Author; "Toward a Unified Theory of Serotonin Dysregulation in Eating and Related Disorders," by T. D. Brewerton, 1995, *Psychoendocrinology, 2016*, pp. 561–590; "Eating Disorders in Males: A Report on 135 Patients," by D. J. Carlat, C. A. Carmago, Jr., and D. B. Herzog, 1997, *American Journal of Psychiatry, 154*, pp. 1127–1132; and "Epidemiology and Mortality of Eating Disorders," by S. Nielsen, 2001, *Psychiatric Clinics of North America, 24*, pp. 201–214. Adapted with permission.

Table 9–3 • Occurrence of Eating Disorders Throughout the Life Span

	Anorexia	Bulimia	Obesity	Rumination Disorder	Pica	Binge Eating Disorder
Infant (Birth–1 yr)				X		
Toddler (2–5 yr)			X		X	
Early School Age (6–9 yr)			X			
Late School Age (10–12 yr)	X		X			
Adolescence (13–18 yr)	X	X	X			X
Adulthood (18 yr +)	X	X	X			X

TREATMENT *(continued)*

invalidate this claim. Most important, appropriate control of the diabetes must be the first goal of treatment.

The use of psychotherapy in treatment may take more than one form—many clients benefit from a combination. Many clients with EDs, especially bulimia, seem to benefit from group work. It is essential that the group therapist have advanced preparation in group leadership skills as well as in ED treatment because of the issues mentioned previously. The primary goal of any therapeutic relationship is the establishment of trust (George, 1997). The issue of confidentiality should be addressed early in therapy. However, any indication of an issue involving self-harm (or maltreatment in the case of a child) needs to be addressed with family members. This should be explicitly shared with the identified client, and the family, if appropriate.

Solution-focused approaches have shown a degree of success over older, traditional forms of psychotherapy. Cognitive behavioral treatment emphasizes changing old patterns that maintain the illness. Emphasizing change instead of illness is especially important with clients with ED for two reasons:

1. Because the client with ED experiences low self-esteem, which is a factor in developing and maintaining the disorder

2. The tendency for clients with ED to engage in all-or-nothing thinking in which they view themselves as all good or all bad, and discount any progress that is not absolutely perfect

Another behavioral approach to EDs, particularly when they are comorbid with borderline personality disorder, is dialectical behavior therapy (DBT) (Linehan, 1993). Studies show that DBT reduced relapse in clients with BN and other EDs. Major behavioral changes and benefits involved enhanced coping skills, modulation of distress and emotions, and a decrease in binge-purge behaviors (Safer, Telch, & Agras, 2001; Swenson, Torrey, & Koerner, 2002).

Halmi (1997) developed an outpatient treatment protocol using cognitive-behavioral therapies and psychopharmacologic treatments. This approach involves a treatment plan that identifies problems and client-generated solutions. The client identifies and selects coping strategies, defines steps for coping, carries out the strategy, and evaluates the process. The goal is to overcome the food phobia, restore weight, and restructure the cognitive operations. This takes place for approximately 37 sessions over a 12-month period with more intensity initially, then tapered in an intensive outpatient format.

Transgenerational family therapy moves beyond present issues to exceed symptomatic relief and emphasizes restoring familial resources for growth and strength to cope with future stress. The family of origin consultation may be used to elicit multiple perspectives on the problem. Transgenerational issues involve using a genogram to create a "map" of the structure and interrelationships over generations, while providing an analysis of the family structure, life cycle, and multigenerational patterns over at least three generations (Roberto 1986; 1992; Dave & Eisler, 1997). Family therapy may be used to educate members about the disorder, support the family as they deal with guilt and stigma about having a member with the disorder, and focus on fostering open, healthy interaction patterns (Benjamin-Coleman, 1998).

Leadership, power, autonomy, and decision-making issues may need further exploration within the privacy of marital sessions. A transgenerational focus may also be used in assisting each member of the marital dyad to recognize how each brings unresolved issues from their parents' marriages to their marriage. Marital therapy may focus on the messages or pressure that the spouse may be projecting onto the ED partner to maintain a certain weight and appearance, while at the same time denying the existence of a life-threatening ED.

(continues)

TREATMENT *(continued)*

Group work can be an effective tool in the treatment of clients with an ED. Clients with bulimia especially seem to benefit from the support of a group. Clients with anorexia may have difficulty with the group setting because it may be too threatening to speak so openly about relevant issues. The group leaders must be aware of the potential for competition in the group. The groups need the supervision of highly skilled professionals who are knowledgeable about group dynamics. The advanced-practice nurse can be an effective member of the team in providing care for this population (Cummings et al., 2001; George, 1997). Chapter 26 of the core text provides a comprehensive discussion of group therapy principle.

Ideally, an outpatient regimen is the method of choice when treating a person with an ED. After the initial evaluations with the EDs team, the client may carry on with usual daily activities. Concurrently, she meets regularly with the therapist, dietician, family physician, and psychiatrist as needed. In this way, progress is monitored closely, and any indication of need for hospitalization will be noted quickly and acted on accordingly. Seriously ill or emaciated clients may need to be hospitalized when seen for the first assessment on an outpatient basis. Involuntary commitment, to stave off further deterioration or possible death, may be initiated; however, the establishment of trust following the decision to ask for detention may be counterproductive. See Table 9–4, Physiological Assessment in Eating Disorders.

The medical management of the client with an ED is critically important. Along with the history, laboratory examination should augment the physical examination. Laboratory tests include determination of the following:

- Complete blood count
- Renal function
- Thyroid function
- Electrolytes
- Blood glucose
- Trace minerals
- Cholesterol and triglycerides
- Hepatic profile
- Muscle enzymes
- Urinalysis may be used to detect the use of stimulants, laxatives, or

(continues)

Table 9–4 • Physiological Assessment in Eating Disorders

Anorexia

Clients with anorexia will present themselves as "fine," although that is a far cry from reality. There is often a history of lethargy or frenetic energy, or both.	*Gastrointestinal* symptoms, including emptying, constipation, bloating, and abdominal pain are frequent.
	Cardiovascular symptoms such as bradycardia, orthostatic hypotension, mitral valve prolapse, and electrocardiographic (ECG) abnormalities.
	Endocrine abnormalities include amenorrhea, osteoporosis, hypothermia, elevated growth hormone levels, and changes in thyroid function. During fluid restriction there may be changes such as an increased blood urea nitrogen (BUN) level, decreased glomerular filtration rate, renal calculi, and edema.
	Dermatological abnormalities include hair loss, dry skin, and development of lanugo hair. Metabolic changes include trace mineral deficiencies (e.g., zinc), osteopenia, and increased plasma cholesterol and triglyceride levels. The client with anorexia may show signs of anemia, leukopenia, and thrombocytopenia.

(continues)

Table 9–4 *(continued)*

Bulimia

Clients with bulimia also present a complex clinical picture.	*Gastrointestinal* symptoms include constipation, bloating, abdominal pain, and nausea owing to delayed gastric emptying. Chronic laxative abuse can result in the loss of normal peristalsis, and recurrent vomiting of stomach acid can result in esophagitis. Forceful vomiting can cause tears in the esophagus (Mallory-Weiss syndrome) and possible gastrointestinal bleeding—esophageal rupture is a life-threatening situation. Chronic vomiting causes salivary and parotid gland enlargement.
	Cardiovascular symptoms include dehydration, orthostatic hypotension, arrhythmias owing to electrolyte imbalance (e.g., potassium), bradycardia, myocardial changes related to ipecac poisoning, and possible congestive heart failure.
	Endocrine changes include irregular menses.
	Pulmonary complications usually take the form of aspiration pneumonia secondary to vomiting. Fluid and electrolyte imbalance is extremely serious and results in dehydration, hypokalemia, hypochloremia, metabolic acidosis and alkalosis, hypophosphatemia, hyponatremia, and hypocalcemia. Vomiting induced with the use of a finger produces calluses and abrasions on the fingers and knuckles. The teeth are eroded by stomach acid, and there may be increased dental caries.
	Renal symptoms such as an elevated BUN level is usually noted owing to fluid restriction and loss. Another renal symptom includes a reduced glomerular filtration rate. There may be polydipsia and polyuria.

TREATMENT *(continued)*

diuretics. An electrocardiogram (ECG) may also be helpful.

The main goal of a medical admission is emergent medical stabilization.

During hospitalization, the dietician plays a major role in the rehabilitation process. Using a nonjudgmental approach enables the dietician to provide support and establish rapport. The dietician supplies nutritional education, helps the client explore extreme misperceptions and use of food, and recommends realistic goals to the client and the treatment team. The dietician attempts to reestablish regular eating patterns with the client. Dieticians use the BMI as a measure of nutritional status (Table 9–5).

(continues)

Table 9–5 • **How to Calculate Ideal Weight Using the Body Mass Index**

Body mass index (BMI) is a measure of relative body weight, in which the weight in kilograms (2.2 pounds) is divided by the square of the height in meters (39.37 inches). For example,

$$\frac{\text{Weight (kg)}}{\text{Height (m)}^2} = \frac{35 \text{ kg}}{(1.54 \text{ m})^2} = \frac{35 \text{ kg}}{2.37 \text{ m}} = 14.76 \text{ BMI}$$

This is an example of an woman with anorexia who is approximately 5'½" tall and weighs 77 lbs. A desirable BMI is in the range of 19 to 23. As can be seen, her BMI is far lower than would be expected for a healthy woman.

Note. From "Definition, Measurement and Classification of the Syndromes of Obesity," by G. A. Bray, 1978, *International Journal of Obesity, 2,* pp. 99–112. Adapted with permission.

TREATMENT *(continued)*

The treatment of a person with an ED is challenging for all involved, and considerable knowledge, skill, and energy are required. The ED team meets with the nursing staff to review treatment and facilitate clear communication among the members of the team. The primary nurse assumes responsibility for the care plan.

Generalist nurses have an important role to play because they enforce the therapeutic milieu of the unit. They must be empathic and supportive but clearly able to define boundaries and set appropriate limits with these clients. It is essential that the nursing staff is well versed in nutritional and physiological information relative to EDs. Most generalist nurses are invaluable in their ability to establish trust within the therapeutic relationship. In order for the nurse-client relationship to be effective it must be empathic with unconditional positive regard and acceptance; the nurse must be warm and committed as well as nonjudgmental (George, 1997). Nurses need ongoing support and preparation in order to deal effectively with this population (King & de Sales, 2000). Their conversations and exchanges with the client with ED may serve to strengthen and augment the relationship between the client and the primary psychotherapist.

In addition, it is essential that the nurse explore feelings about clients with EDs. These include the following: sharing society's obsession with thinness, revulsion at the binge-purge behavior, and envy of the client (especially one who is "model thin"). The nurse with eating or weight problems must be prepared to deal with his own issues relative to weight through supervision or therapy when working on an ED unit in order to be able to deal with these issues in a nondefensive way. The generalist nurse also provides client teaching to the client with ED regarding medication actions, side effects, and encourages family support of medicine, as well as clears up misconceptions about medicine. The nurse provides physical assessment and implements the weight management program, while stressing to the client with ED that the primary concern is regaining health through better nutrition.

The advanced-practice registered nurse (APRN) may participate in a variety of roles. The APRN with prescriptive authority may provide medication management in an outpatient setting, either while providing psychotherapy or in conjunction with another psychotherapist. The advanced-practice nurse may participate as part of the specialized ED team as a primary psychotherapist. The APRN is also responsible for individual, family, marital, or group therapy. Additional responsibilities may include being the program director of an ED team, which involves coordination of services and consultation to facilitate restoration of health and an optimal level of functioning for clients with EDs.

Psychosocial assessment begins with establishing a trusting relationship with the client and family members. Major components of the psychosocial assessment include identifying the client's reasons for seeking treatment, present and past history of impaired eating and coping patterns, family involvement, and the impact of family members on the client's well-being. A complete family assessment is a critical part of assessing clients with EDs.

The client's medical condition must be assessed to determine the extent of nutritional deprivation and potential complications. A complete physical examination includes laboratory tests and cardiac evaluation.

Other aspects of the assessment process include the following:

- Mental status examination
- Substance abuse history
- Family and social history, including employment history
- Academic achievement and performance
- Present and past psychiatric and medical treatment
- Current and past medications; drug and other allergies

(continues)

TREATMENT *(continued)*

- Quality of support system and other resources
- Level of danger to self or others
- Individual and family strengths
- Current stressors

Major nursing diagnoses for clients with EDs include:

- Imbalanced Nutrition: Less than Body Requirements related to dysfunctional eating patterns
- Disturbed Body Image related to fear of weight gain
- Powerlessness related to lack of control over food avoidance
- Anxiety related to fear of weight gain as evidenced by rituals associated with food intake
- Constipation related to erratic eating patterns
- Decreased Cardiac Output related to inadequate caloric and fluid intake
- Ineffective Coping related to feelings of lack of control, fears of growing up, denial of the severity of the ED and symptomatic response to family stress
- Compromised Family Coping: Disabling related to impaired interactions, poor conflict resolution and ineffective management of stress

Medical interventions depend on the extent of nutritional alterations. Major interventions focus on restoring fluid and caloric intake while monitoring for medical complications such as cardiac arrhythmia. Furthermore, close monitoring of laboratory studies, cardiac status, intake and output, and vital signs enables the health care team to assess responses to treatment.

Psychosocial interventions include solution-focused approaches, cognitive-behavioral interventions, assertiveness techniques and family therapy, as well as psychoeducational approaches. Cognitive-behavioral techniques increase self-awareness, including realization of low self-esteem and maladaptive coping patterns. Relapse prevention should include coping strategies, identifying triggers, developing support systems, distracting activities, contacting friends, and anticipating problem situations in advance.

ANOREXIA NERVOSA

Causes

Bruch believed that anorexia and bulimia were related to "underlying deficits in the individual's sense of self-identity and autonomy" (1982, p. 1532). She was the first to formally suggest that there was an actual disturbance of body image in AN.

The issue of sexuality is noteworthy because clients with anorexia tend to have difficulty with interpersonal intimacy and closeness. Both groups of clients with anorexia and bulimia may reveal a history of childhood sexual trauma, which would have implications for future sexual relationships.

Symptoms

Anorexia nervosa (AN) refers to a syndrome manifested by self-induced starvation resulting from fear of fatness rather than from true loss of appetite. Persons with AN continue to feel hunger but persist in denying themselves food. The onset is usually in an adolescent female who perceives herself to be overweight.

Features of anorexia nervosa include amenorrhea, an intense fear of gaining weight or becoming fat, refusal to maintain a normal body weight (e.g., less than 85 percent of expected weight for age and height, or **body mass index** [BMI] less than 17.5 kg/m^2), failure to gain expected weight during growth (Treasure & Schmidt, 2001), and a distorted body image. Other psychological characteristics include fear of loss of control, **alexithymia**, lack of introceptive awareness, mistrust of self and others, cognitive dysfunction, and starvation-induced depression (George, 1997).

Physiological findings present as a result of the severe starvation and weight loss (Table 9–6).

Table 9-6 • Physiological Findings in Eating Disorders

Physical Symptoms	Cold intolerance, constipation, abdominal discomfort, dizziness, bloating, and hyperactivity
	Lethargy is worrisome because it may indicate cardiovascular compromise
Physical Examination	Appearance is younger than chronological age
	Multiple layers of clothing, cachexia, and breast atrophy
	Dry skin, bradycardia, hypotension, hypokalemia, lanugo, alopecia, edema of the lower extremities, and dental enamel erosion
Medical Complications	Cardiovascular, hematologic, gastrointestinal, renal, neurologic, endocrine, and skeletal
Cardiovascular Complications	ECG abnormalities
	Prolonged QT intervals, and emetine-induced myocardial damage may be life threatening
	Long-standing bradycardia due to regular exercise
Hematologic Changes	Mild anemia 30% of cases
	Leukopenia up to 50% of cases
Gastrointestinal Complications	Decreased gastric motility and delayed gastric emptying
Renal Abnormalities	Dehydration results in increased levels of blood urea nitrogen
	Polyuria due to decrease in renal concentrating capacity and abnormal vasopressin secretion producing partial diabetes insipidus
	Peripheral edema in 20% of cases
Neurologic Abnormalities	Rarely found
Endocrine Complications	Amenorrhea is hallmark of anorexia, due to starvation-induced hypogonadism
Skeletal Complications	Osteopenia; skeletal fractures

ECG, electrocardiogram, the portion of the cardiac complex on the electrocardiogram that extends from the beginning of the Q wave to the end of the T wave.

Note. From *Kaplan and Sadock's Synopsis of Psychiatry* (8th ed.), by H. Kaplan and B. J. Sadock, 1998, Baltimore: Williams & Wilkins. Adapted with permission.

Body image disturbance is an essential characteristic of AN. Although it is related to a more generalized misperception of internal states, such as hunger and emotions, it specifically involves the inability of the client with anorexia to identify her appearance as abnormal. This misperception can be extremely dangerous because it can become almost delusional as the client with anorexia defends an emaciated body shape.

Clients with AN are described by clinicians as having specific personality characteristics, as shown in Table 9–7.

TREATMENT

Fluoxetine (Prozac) has been shown to reduce the obsessive-compulsive behavior, anxiety, and depression seen in

(continues)

Table 9–7 • Personality Factors

Anorexia Nervosa (AN)

- Resistance to acknowledging they have a problem
- Obsessional thoughts about doing things right
- Hyper-rigid behaviors
- Difficulty learning from experience
- Greater risk avoidance (compared to controls)
- Emotionally restrained
- Conformity to authority
- Trait obsessionality
- Inflexible thinking
- Social introversion
- Limited social spontaneity

Bulimia Nervosa (BN)

- Problems identifying internal states contributing to feelings of helplessness (self-regulation)
- Variable moods: fatigue and depression to agitation, which contribute to impulse control difficulties
- Sense of loss of control related to bodily experience (probably related to early experiences with abuse/trauma; children of alcoholic parents)
- Low self-esteem, personal efficacy, leading to self-doubt and uncertainty
- Highly self-critical and punitive in self-evaluation
- Self-conscious, sensitive to rejection from others

TREATMENT *(continued)*

classic anorexia symptoms, carbohydrate craving, and other pathologic eating behaviors (Walsh, Agras, & Devlin, 2000). Halmi (1997) recommends a protocol for anorectic treatment of liquid chlorpromazine (Thorazine) for severely delusional, overactive, hospitalized clients, and liquid cyproheptadine (Periactin) for severely overactive clients who do not binge or purge. They suggest using fluoxetine (Prozac) after weight restoration because of its tendency for inducing arousal for severe obsessive-compulsive disorder (OCD) behaviors and depression, clomipramine (Anafranil) for OCD, and the tricyclics antidepressants for severe depression. Mirtazapine (Remeron), an atypical antidepressant, because of its well-known tendency to quickly add weight, shows promise as a medicine that may be helpful for clients with anorexia whose health status is severely compromised.

Correction of the body weight of the client with anorexia is of supreme importance. Liquid supplements or tube feedings may be employed along with intravenous fluids. Extreme care is needed to prevent fluid overload that may possibly result in congestive heart failure.

Milieu interventions for AN include:

- Weighing the client at specific intervals
- Providing for safety and physical needs
- Sitting with and observing during and 1 hour following meals
- Encouraging the client to share feelings with the staff
- Teaching relaxation techniques
- Discussing factors interfering with client's inability to eat
- Educating the client about the negative effects of dietary restriction and low weight and the rationale for maintaining a normal weight
- Documenting intake and output
- Instructing the client on how to increase caloric intake and developing strategies for coping with anxiety associated with such eating behaviors
- Validating the client's fear of relinquishing anorexia and the challenges associated with behavioral changes

BINGE EATING DISORDER

Symptoms

Binge eating disorder (BED) is a disorder newly described in the *DSM-IV-TR* (APA, 2000). See the display on research criteria for BED. Clients with BED experience recurrent binge eating but do not regularly engage in the purging behaviors or compulsive exercise that clients with bulimia use to avoid weight gain.

Characteristics of the BED population include impairment in work and social functioning; preoccupation with weight and shape; general psychopathology; significant time and energy devoted to dieting; and a history of depression, alcohol, or drug abuse and treatment for emotional problems (Spitzer et al., 1993).

BULIMIA NERVOSA

Causes

BN usually begins in late adolescence or early adulthood, and the disorder can follow a chronic and intermittent course over many years. Parents of clients with this disorder may be obese or markedly underweight, and there is a higher rate of major depression than expected in first-degree relatives. The families may be overly preoccupied with food and appearances. Clients with bulimia themselves commonly have a depressive disorder and may concurrently abuse psychoactive substances, most frequently alcohol, sedatives, or stimulants. They tend to have less superego control than their counterparts with anorexia. Disorders of impulse control such as compulsive shopping and shoplifting have been associated with bulimia. Persons with bulimia also reportedly have increased rates of obesity, parental problems, disturbed family dynamics, histories of sexual and physical abuse, parental weight or shape concern, anxiety disorders, low self-esteem, mood disorders, substance abuse, perfectionism, bipolar I disorder, and dissociative

disorders (Fairburn, Welch, Doll, Davis, & O'Connor, 1997).

Symptoms

Bulimia nervosa (BN) is more prevalent than AN. This disorder appears to have a later onset than AN. The term *bulimia* is translated as "ravenous appetite" and refers to a syndrome of episodes of binge eating, followed by self-induced vomiting, or **purge** behavior, accompanied by an excessive preoccupation with weight and body shape.

There is a feeling of a lack of control over eating behavior when binging, and the measures to prevent weight gain include use of laxatives, cathartics, enemas, and diuretics; periods of strict dieting or fasting; and strenuous exercise.

Clients with bulimia may have a normal weight, be overweight, or be underweight. Clients with this disorder characteristically have a thin body with swollen cheeks, owing to enlarged salivary glands, and exhibit signs of fluid retention. The skin tends to be dry with cuts and abrasions, particularly over the knuckles, owing to the repeated trauma of putting the fingers down the throat to induce vomiting (Russell's sign). The repeated vomiting causes erosion of the dental enamel, and any of the purging mechanisms may lead to dehydration and electrolyte imbalance, particularly of potassium. The condition is often first discovered by dental examination. Blood-streaked vomitus is not unusual, but frank bleeding may signal a life-threatening gastric or esophageal tear. Serious complications may also include cardiac arrhythmias owing to electrolyte imbalances, which can cause sudden death (Agras, 2001).

The most common ED is bulimia nervosa in women who maintain normal weight. These women exhibit symptoms usually found in women with AN, such as disturbed appetite, abnormal body image, depression, and neuroendocrine changes that precipitate menstrual irregularities. However, because these women are of normal weight, the changes cannot be attributed to weight loss.

Key Fact

About 10 percent of clients with bulimia are men (Hay & Bacaltchuk, 2001), whereas 2/100,000 a year of clients with anorexia are males (Treasure & Schmidt, 2001).

TREATMENT

In the client with bulimia, the focus may be on the interruption of the binge-purge cycle and the associated abuse of laxatives, diuretics, and ipecac. The abrupt cessation of laxatives results in constipation, whereas the discontinuation of diuretics may result in reflex edema. The constipation may be handled through the use of roughage intake, exercise, and hydration. The normalization of fluid imbalance will usually occur spontaneously.

The following are nursing interventions that are used during the hospitalization of a client with anorexia or bulimia (Benjamin-Coleman, 1998).

1. Implement behavioral protocol for gradual weight gain.
2. Supervise meals to ensure adequate intake of nutrients.
3. In collaboration with the dietician, determine the number of calories required to provide adequate nutrition and weight gain.
4. Sit with the client during mealtime for support and to observe amount ingested.
5. Strictly document intake and output.
6. Weigh client daily on arising.
7. Once the nutritional status is stable, explore with client feelings associated with fears.
8. Observe weighing activity to ensure that the client is not secreting weights to falsify data.

Milieu interventions for BN include:

- Behavioral diaries
- Encouraging the expression of feelings
- Reinforcing healthy coping
- Teaching recognition of cues for hunger and satiation

- Education about physical consequences of binging, self-induced vomiting, and laxative or stimulant abuse
- Limiting exercising
- Limiting food records, frequent weighing, obsessive calorie counting, cooking for others, reading recipes
- Providing nutritional consultation to the client
- Monitoring fluid and electrolyte status
- Teaching the client to reduce caloric anxiety with staff support and coaching
- Use rational statements and positive affirmations (Benjamin-Coleman 1998; Cottrell & McMahon 1997; Cummings et al., 2001; King & de Sales, 2000)

OBESITY

Causes

Some obese women have reported much anxiety when dieting in the context of becoming more attractive and thus sexually appealing. It would appear that the ED syndrome might provide comfort, safety, and anxiety reduction when the client is presented with the fears and conflicts of intimacy.

Symptoms

Obesity is recognized as a serious health problem but is not classified by itself as an eating disorder, at least in the *DSM-IV-TR* (APA, 2000). Many medical diseases and complications are associated with obesity, including hypertension, gallbladder disease, diabetes, trauma to weight-bearing joints, and increased risk of cardiovascular disease, especially when there is an excess accumulation of fat in the abdominal region. A precise measure of obesity is the amount of fat in the body or the BMI, which is calculated by the following formula:

BMI = [body weight in kg] ÷ [height in m^2]

BMI correlates with morbidity and mortality (Kaplan & Sadock, 1998).

TREATMENT

In spite of the widespread popularity of weight loss programs, most studies from the 1970s have shown that significant weight loss is rare and losses that do occur are not well maintained. Evidence is overwhelming that restrictive dieting serves to actually trigger weight gain once normal eating resumes.

Although obesity is not yet considered an ED in the psychiatric nomenclature, it is considered a risk factor for AN and BN. With the new category of BED, people with simple obesity must be differentiated from those with the more complex features of that disorder.

PICA

Causes

Pica is believed to result from iron and zinc deficiencies or related to lack of stimulation and adult supervision. Medical complications include lead poisoning from the ingestion of paint or paint-soaked plaster. *Toxoplasma* or *Toxocara* infections may result from the ingestion of feces or dirt. Hair-ball tumors may cause intestinal obstruction.

Symptoms

Pica refers to the persistent eating of a nonnutritive substance. The name is derived from the Latin word for magpie, a bird known to eat a variety of objects.

Infants with this disorder may eat hair, cloth, plaster, paint, or string, and older children may eat sand, leaves, insects, pebbles, or animal droppings. Almost all children occasionally ingest such substances, and the behavior is not considered abnormal in children 18 months of age and younger. Pica is common in children as old as 6 years of age, with greater occurrence in severely mentally retarded or children with psychosis (APA, 2000). Pregnant women may also exhibit pica.

RUMINATION DISORDER

Symptoms

Rumination disorder is a rare phenomenon, seen equally in male and female infants. It usually appears between 3 months and 1 year of age but may show up later in children who are mentally retarded or in adolescents. This disorder can be serious, with a reported 25 percent mortality rate from malnutrition. Even when children with this disorder survive, the failure to gain expected weight and malnutrition may lead to general developmental delays and severe impairment.

This disorder is marked by repeated regurgitation of food, with resultant weight loss or failure to gain expected weight (see the display on diagnostic criteria for rumination disorder of infancy). It develops following a period of normal functioning. There is no accompanying self-disgust, nausea, vomiting, or other associated gastrointestinal disorder. Ruminating infants typically regurgitate milk and partially digested food either spontaneously or after inserting their fingers into their mouth. They may chew and reswallow the regurgitated food, or they may vomit the food. The characteristic posture is described as straining and arching the back with the head held back.

TREATMENT

Rumination disorder must be differentiated from other disorders that cause regurgitation, such as pyloric stenosis and infections of the gastrointestinal system.

RESOURCES

Please note that because Internet resources are of a time-sensitive nature and URL addresses may change or be deleted, searches should also be conducted by association or topic.

Internet Resources

http://www.anad.org National Association of Anorexia Nervosa and Associated Disorders (ANAD)

http://www.overeatersanonymous.org Overeaters Anonymous, Inc.

http://www.acadeatdis.org The Academy for Eating Disorders

Personality Disorders

10

• Key Terms

Boundary: Refers to rules defining who and how members participate in a subsystem or a relationship. The clearer the boundary, the healthier the relationship.

Ego Dystonic: Discomfort in the presence of a disordered mental state.

Ego Syntonic: Personal comfort with symptoms that create discomfort in others.

Splitting: The internal mechanism wherein the person is unable to evaluate, synthesize, and accept imperfections in others so that a significant other is viewed as all good or all bad, and causing the phenomenon of setting persons up against each other.

Personality is reflected by a person's capacity and skill for managing activities of daily living. Individual responses and interactions to internal and external environmental demands (pressures) are influenced by the constant interplay of genetic, neurobiological, and psychological factors.

PERSONALITY DISORDERS—GENERAL

Causes

The exact cause of personality disorders is complex. Most data point to an array of factors stemming from environmental factors, such as early childhood trauma to neurobiological modifications in complex biochemistry and neuroanatomical structures, to genetic predisposition.

Neurotransmitters such as serotonin and dopamine have been implicated in impulsivity, aggression, and suicidal gestures manifested in disordered personalities, especially borderline and antisocial types (Oquendo & Mann, 2000). In addition, clients with borderline and antisocial personality disorders have been found to have low platelet levels of monoamine oxidase (the metabolizer of dopamine), resulting in higher than normal levels of dopamine, an arousal neurotransmitter. Abnormal testosterone circulation is considered influential in the production of antisocial aggressive behavior that may be impulsive and violent (Black, 1999).

Neuroendocrine studies using the dexamethasome suppression test and the thyrotropin-stimulating hormone test used to diagnose depression have recently been applied to clients with personality disorders and have shown abnormalities that suggest a relationship between disordered personality and depressed mood (Soloff, 1998). Additional neurobiological evidence includes a higher incidence of abnormal electroencephalographic waveforms in the temporal and frontal lobe regions in clients with borderline personality disorder when compared with control subjects.

Temperament appears to underlie general medical conditions in children who manifest personality disorders or behavioral problems. Specific behaviors include hyperactivity, or distractibility.

Data from genetic studies also associate temperament with a variance between the child and the environment (Comings et al., 2000; Dadds, Barrett, Rapee, & Ryan, 1996). Inadequacy in early caregiver roles often results in chaotic and inconsistent family systems. Children from these families often experience intense outbursts of anger, abuse, and abandonment.

Major stressors for adolescents include authority and control (separation-individuation issues). The younger adolescent is shifting from parents to peers in preference, and the older adolescent may be dealing with intimacy and sexual issues. Positive self-esteem is the core struggle in concert with the search for identity (Kalogerakis, 1992).

Impairments in ego and superego development are considered to be the major cause of maladaptive behavior. Erikson (1963) contended that if the adolescent were unable to attain a healthy identity, the result would be role confusion that then leads easily into problem behavior.

Clients with these disorders generally tend to be influenced by internal and external stimuli. Older adults are challenged to use their previous life experience to cope with biological and neurological changes associated with the aging process. In some instances, however, despair rather than integrity is the outcome because the person does not perceive himself to have had any or many positive experiences for which to be proud; in effect, the task of generativity was not accomplished and probably neither were other earlier tasks.

Symptoms

The *DSM-IV-TR* (APA, 2000) delineates clinical features of personality disorders as an enduring pattern of feeling (emotions), thinking (cognitive distortions), and behaving (maladaptive in nature) that become rigid and stable over time. Features of personality disorders appear to emerge during adolescence or early adulthood.

Behavioral features of personality disorders tend to be rigid and inflexible, resulting in distress or maladaptive coping skills. Some clients experience lifelong difficulty adapting to change, tolerating frustration and crises, and forming healthy relationships.

Clients often deny their existing problems and usually lack insight into the maladaptive behaviors that create even more problems for them. These behaviors are symptoms that are described as **ego syntonic** (i.e., comfortable for the individual but usually uncomfortable for others) and thus acceptable to them because they represent aspects of the clients' personality that have become typical and gratifying for them. Clients with personality disorders differ from other clients experiencing anxiety, depression, or other emotional disorders because the latter experience an uncomfortable and unacceptable **ego dystonic** state that forces them to seek psychotherapeutic assistance. Because clients with personality disorders are usually comfortable with themselves and their behaviors, they do not recognize or accept the need for a change in the way they behave, and they tend to use displacement or projection to aid their coping. These clients usually tax the mental and physical resources of the health care team. They often display an uncanny ability to create crisis and uproar.

The 10 personality disorders are listed as follows: paranoid, schizoid, schizotypal, antisocial, borderline, histrionic, narcissistic, avoidant, dependent, and obsessive-compulsive. The three clusters under which various personality disorders are placed are depicted in Table 10–1.

Clients with personality disorders are often labeled as difficult because of their need for immediate gratification, their lack of empathy, and the intense affect they use in their frequent hostile outbursts and attacks, either verbal or physical. Persons with borderline personality disorder are noted for **splitting**—a behavior that involves setting up conflicts between others, almost as though saying, "Let's you and he/she fight." It is not uncommon for these clients to create splitting situations among staff members such that the staff become engaged in serious conflict concerning the appropriate management of the client.

Children with early faulty development frequently maintain primitive defense mechanisms such as projection, ambiv-

Table 10–1 • **Personality Disorders Organized By Cluster**		
	Type of Disorder	**Description**
Cluster I	Paranoid Schizoid Schizotypal	Clients are withdrawn and engage in odd, eccentric behavior.
Cluster II	Antisocial Borderline Histrionic Narcissistic	Clients seek attention and engage in erratic behavior.
Cluster III	Avoidant Dependent Obsessive-compulsive	Clients seek to avoid or minimize the experience of anxiety or fear.
Personality Disorders NOS	Passive-aggressive Masochistic	Clients are covertly aggressive against others or themselves.

NOS, not otherwise specified.

alence, regression, splitting, acting out, and denial. These mechanisms often represent the child's survival tools, and they often persist throughout the life span. These early defense mechanisms are used to ward off bad feelings, depression, anxiety, rage, and intense emotional pain.

These youngsters are frequently bored and frustrated, and they often experience difficulty dealing with intense feelings such as anxiety, fears, and intimacy (Mishne, 1986; Moss, Kevin, Lynch, Hardie, & Baron, 2002). They also have distorted cognitions (impaired reality testing) and low self-esteem. Other maladaptive behaviors include using primitive defense mechanisms such as acting out and expressing extreme hostility or aggression toward authority figures. Their ability to solve problems and control immediate gratification needs (impulsivity) is impaired. Adolescents with personality disorders experience bouts of depression and anxiety and turn to risky tension-reducing activities, including substance abuse, sexual promiscuity, suicidal behaviors and attempts, and various other antisocial acts to help in coping with their distress (Moss et al., 2002).

Clients with personality disorders often perceive crises or change as overwhelming. Their lack of internal and external resources compromises their ability to use adaptive coping methods to reduce or eliminate intense feelings. These persons often experience feeings of emptiness and loneliness in spite of their numerous efforts to form relationships in some cases. They also may be extremely demanding of the relationships that they do have, and this is representative of the unmanageable anxiety that they may have but fail to acknowledge because many or most tend to remain in an ego-syntonic state.

Older adults who have never developed healthy ego functions, as well as those with physical and mental problems, are at risk for experiencing despair (Erikson, 1963). Lacking accomplishment, the person may face what is left of life with hopelessness and helplessness. He may believe that any chance to make anything out of life is gone and that there is no reason to be cheerful or ambitious about anything. Because of the numerous losses in this period, there is a vulnerability to depression, and the rate of suicide among men is high (Berezin et al., 1988).

TREATMENT

Clients with personality disorders such as borderline and antisocial types exhibit a wide variety of maladaptive behaviors such as substance abuse, suicidal gestures, and other self-destructive behaviors. Nursing implications for working with these types require attention to the following:

- Understanding factors associated with personality development
- Recognizing the impact of early childhood traumas on coping styles
- Dealing with intense reactions that occur when working with these clients

- Working with other mental health professionals to develop consistency and prevent splitting of staff
- Recognition of the need to maintain boundaries that are extremely clear. **Boundary** means rules defining who and how members participate in a subsystem or a relationship. For example, it is important for the nurse to maintain a professional boundary between self and the client.

Understanding the origins of these behaviors can play a key role in minimizing negative reactions toward these clients, who are experts in evoking tension in nurses and other professionals. Working with these clients needs to be perceived as a challenge rather than a burden because nurses are challenged to sharpen their skills in patience, self-awareness, creativity, and nonjudgmental approach. Above all, the staff must develop treatment plans that do not allow for splitting of staff; to accomplish this, they must confer frequently.

Understanding key concepts in personality formation such as ego development and organization is crucial for nurses who must assess the meaning of their own, as well as of clients' maladaptive behaviors, facilitation of adaptive coping behaviors and evaluation of client responses to interventions.

Understanding ego development or organization is fundamental to the capacity for aiding effective adaptation to internal and external stressors. Evaluating ego function is a major aspect of the nursing process because it provides data that assist in making accurate diagnoses, planning psychotherapeutic interventions, and bringing about therapeutic outcomes. Table 10–2 provides a framework for assessing ego function.

Table 10–3 provides a list of unhealthy ego functions and their probable causes. Features of personality disorders seem to emerge during adolescence or early adulthood.

Assessing the adolescent's level of dangerousness is the same as for adults.

(continues)

Table 10–2 • Comparison of Healthy and Unhealthy Ego Functions

	Healthy Ego Functions (Mature)	Unhealthy Ego Functions (Primitive)
Defense Mechanisms (conflict resolution)	Repression Sublimation Rationalization Displacement Reaction formation Undoing	Denial Projection Splitting Dissociation Isolation Regression Avoidance Conversion reaction
Modulation of Affect (impulsivity)	Postpones gratification needs Tolerates frustration and stress Maintains gratification through sublimation	Low frustration and stress tolerance Poor impulse control Need for immediate gratification
Self-Esteem (competence)	Mastery of environment Sense of worth and confidence	Poor self-esteem Fluctuation in self-worth
Relationship to Others (depth of relationships)	Capacity for object relations Empathic Stable, lasting relationships Capacity to mourn and move on to form new relationships	Places own needs before others Lack of empathy Chaotic relationships Inability to relate to others
Reality Testing	Accurate perceptions and appraisal of inner mental state (insight) Intact ego boundaries Sense of reality	Distorted perceptions Depersonalization Lack of insight into present Fluid ego boundaries Derealization
Cognitive Processes (thinking, learning, judgment)	Tolerates stress Capacity to integrate new experiences Tolerates inconsistency and incongruency in others	Poor tolerance to stress Low capacity to integrate new experiences Rigid, inflexible thinking

TREATMENT *(continued)*

Suicidal adolescents present clinicians with a serious emergency situation. Assessing current stressors, the suicide plan, the available means for carrying out the act and previous personal or family history of suicide and gestures can assist the health care team in determining appropriate interventions.

Hospitalization of adolescents for spe- cific personality disorders is indicated when they exhibit destructive behavior toward themselves, toward others, or toward property. These may be suicidal acts or threats to self, eating disorders, substance abuse, homicidal acts and threats to others, or destructiveness to property. Failure to respond to treatment, severe depression, psychosis, or severe

(continues)

Table 10–3 • **Manifested Maladaptive Coping Behaviors Arising from Early Developmental Periods and Continuing across the Life Span**

	Maladaptive Behavior	Possible Cause
Infancy	Withdrawal, refusal to enter relationships	Absence of nurturing caregiver
Childhood	Projection, ambivalence, regression, splitting, acting out, denial	Faulty ego development
Adolescence	Boredom, frustration, difficulty dealing with intense feelings, distorted cognitions (impaired reality testing), low self-esteem, acting out, expressing extreme hostility toward authority figures, impaired ability to solve problems, impulsivity, risky tension-reducing activities (e.g., substance abuse, sexual promiscuity, self-destructive and suicidal behaviors)	Impairments in ego and superego development, role confusion
Early and Middle Adulthood	Feelings of emptiness, loneliness, and distress; extremely demanding of relationships; low self-esteem; intense but unacknowledged emotional pain; substance abuse; suicide attempts; destructive relationships and behaviors	Lack of healthy ego functions
Older Adulthood	Intensification of earlier behaviors, suicide, feelings of despair, hopelessness, and helplessness	Nondevelopment of new ego operations; exaggeration of existing defense mechanisms to cope with increased stress associated with loss, retirement, or illness

TREATMENT *(continued)*

family dysfunction may require inpatient care (Mishne, 1986; Rinsley, 1982).

Short-term treatment focuses on crisis resolution, and long-term care focuses on the facilitation of attitudinal and behavioral change in the adolescent and his family. The overall aim of care is to minimize acting-out behaviors and to increase ego strength. Egan (1986) stated that the following purposes are served when the adolescent's ego is strengthened:

• Increased impulse control

• Delayed need gratification
• Improved self-esteem
• Decreased dysphoric feelings (sadness) and anxiety
• Increased problem-solving skills

An array of therapeutic modalities are available to treat clients with personality disorders and include psychotherapies, group, and milieu; activity and educational therapies; behavior modification; and pharmacology. Perhaps the most useful modality for staff nurses is milieu therapy because a major function is to maintain

(continues)

TREATMENT *(continued)*

an environment that is safe, accepting, and therapeutic.

If the youth presents with symptoms of depression, such as dysphoric mood and sleep and appetite disturbances, antidepressants may be prescribed. Symptoms such as aggressive or impulsive acting out may respond to carbamazepine (Tegretol), lithium, divalproex sodium (Depakote), haloperidol (Haldol), or some of the newer antidepressants that also help calm anxiety. Lithium seems to be the drug of choice for treating children or adolescents with aggressive-hostile behaviors because it has fewer adverse side effects (Hollander et al., 2001; Kavoussi & Coccaro, 1998; Links, Steiner, Boiago, & Irwin, 1990). Psychopharma-cologic agents are used as an adjunct to behavioral and psychosocial interventions to maximize the treatment.

The care of clients with a personality disorder is difficult and often frustrating because they demonstrate behaviors that challenge even the experts. Interventions must be specific to the behaviors, which can vary widely from time to time and from client to client. Overall, however, some of the behaviors of clients with a personality disorder can be categorized using the *DSM-IV-TR* (APA, 2000) personality disorders' section. Table 10–4 outlines the diagnoses and some of the typical behaviors that have prevented these clients from establishing or maintaining meaningful relationships throughout their lifetime.

Table 10–4 • Typical Behaviors of Clients with Personality Disorders According to *DSM-IV-TR* Diagnostic Groupings and Suggested Interventions

Diagnosis	Typical Behaviors	Suggested Interventions
Avoidant	Anger	1. Offer self on a regular basis without intrusion
Obsessive-compulsive disorder	Dysfunctional independence	2. Acknowledge observed behaviors with the client
Paranoid	Isolation	3. Be particularly attentive to trust building
Passive-aggressive	Mistrust and suspicion	4. Work at drawing the client into one-on-one interactions that promote enjoyment of a relationship
Schizoid Schizotypal	Withdrawal	5. Involve the client in establishing at least one relationship and in working to increase the number of social involvements
Borderline	Attention-seeking	1. Assess the type and frequency of demands for attention
Dependent	Dependence	
Histrionic	Neediness	2. Establish a trusting relationship that allows confrontation of behaviors, and assist in acknowledging the behavior
Narcissistic (sometimes)		3. Set specific goals and methods for achieving greater independence
		4. Provide reinforcement of independent functioning

(continues)

Table 10–4 *(continued)*

Diagnosis	Typical Behaviors	Suggested Interventions
Antisocial Narcissistic (dishonest at times)	Aggression Entitlement Manipulation Risk-taking	1. Provide and maintain a team-developed set of rules that are reasonable and strictly followed 2. Remind the client of expectations before the temptation sets in to deviate 3. Develop an atmosphere of trust in which sincere confrontation is possible 4. Provide pleasurable activities that serve as a substitute for the previous deviant activities no longer permitted 5. Recognize that many of these clients have operated for a long time and have a pattern of behavior that is difficult, if not impossible, to change

Note. Adapted from *Diagnostic and Statistical Manual of Mental Disorders* (4th edition Text Revision) (*DSM-IV-TR*), by American Psychiatric Association, 2000, Washington, DC: Author. Adapted with permission.

ANTISOCIAL PERSONALITY DISORDER

Causes

Brain imaging studies have implicated brain anomalies in persons with antisocial personality (ASP) disorder. Another biological theory implies that one with antisocial personality disorder has a nervous system that is "strangely unresponsive, rendering him chronically underaroused and needing a 'fix' of sensory input to produce normal brain function" (Black, 1999, p. 115). It is suggested that underarousal is the factor that keeps individuals with antisocial personality disorder so calm under pressure, giving the appearance that they do not experience anxiety (Raine, 2002a). It remains evident, however, that there is no single cause of ASP disorder and some of the other disorders.

The literature suggests that there are genetic links for certain personality traits such as criminality and other antisocial behavior. Adoption and twin studies suggest a genetic base for antisocial personality (Cadoret, Yates, Troughton, Woodworth, & Stewart, 1995). Some twin studies have demonstrated higher incidences of personality disorders among monozygotic twins than dizygotic twins, suggesting a genetic basis for personality disorders (Jang, Livesley, Vernon, & Jackson, 1996; Livesley, Jang, & Vernon, 1998).

A recent study by Raine, Lencz, Bihrle, LaCasses, and Colletti (2000) provides "the first evidence for a structural brain deficit" in persons with antisocial personality disorder. The deficit is a prefrontal structural one that underlies characteristic features of low arousal, poor fear conditioning, lack of conscience, and decision-making deficits.

Symptoms

Typical characteristics of Antisocial Personality Disorder include the following (Brooner, Greenfield, Schmidt, & Bigelow, 1993; Gunderson, 1988):

- Failure to learn from experience
- Regular engagement in impulsive and risky behavior

- Lack of guilt demonstrated toward repetitive misbehavior
- Exploitation of others
- Chronic disregard for the rights of others
- Lack of fidelity, loyalty, and honesty

insecurity; preoccupation with criticism and rejection; interpersonal inhibition based on a sense of inadequacy; a view of self as unappealing, inept, and inferior; and a reluctance to engage in new activity because of a potential risk of embarrassment (APA, 2000).

TREATMENT

Clients with antisocial personality disorders tend to participate in high-risk behaviors involving substance abuse. The rate of intravenous drug use is estimated to range from 35 to 54 percent in this population (Khantzian & Treece, 1985; Rounsaville, Weissman, Kleber, & Wilber, 1982). These clients present several treatment problems in that treatment successes are low and risk is increased so that workups are needed to assess behavioral style and resulting illnesses. Other necessary preventive measures include education regarding high-risk behavior and the facilitation of more adaptive coping skills.

Although these clients have long been considered to be poor candidates for treatment, some studies have given some hope for success in developing insight. The studies have demonstrated that structure in confined settings, along with peer pressure and confrontations, are essential aspects of treatment (Frosch, 1983; Perry, Banon, & Ianni, 1999). Professional nurses must learn to approach these clients in a sensitive and nonjudgmental manner to facilitate trust and rapport because they fear and mistrust intimacy and closeness.

TREATMENT

These conditions of distrust make it imperative that nursing interventions facilitate the establishment of trust through the formation of reliable and dependable nurse-client alliances. This helps to minimize anxiety sufficiently to permit the exploration of old behaviors and to consider ways to change and feel better. Specific attention needs to be given to relaxing, because mistrust causes hypervigilance, and to developing other relationships in which trust can be expected.

AVOIDANT PERSONALITY DISORDER

Symptoms

Major manifestations of avoidant personality disorder are avoidance of activity based on fears of criticism, disapproval, or rejection; unwillingness to be involved without guarantees of acceptance; restraint within intimate relationships because of

BORDERLINE PERSONALITY DISORDER

Causes

Recent data support the role of temperament, character, and attachment patterns in borderline personality disorder (Fossati et al., 2001).

A number of studies have found a high prevalence of child abuse in the histories of clients with maladaptive behaviors. Clients with borderline personality disorders have a high rate of early childhood traumas (Gibb, Wheeler, Alloy, & Abramson, 2001). Several studies have demonstrated a significant prevalence of sexual abuse among female clients diagnosed with borderline personality disorders.

Meares, Stevenson, and Gordon (1999) hypothesized that symptoms found in BPD result from the maturation failure cascade of neural network connections in the prefrontal area that are dependent on experience. In some instances, these become active rather late in development and are then limited in coordinating disparate elements in the central nervous system.

Numerous factors have been associated with the development of borderline personality such as attachment problems, early childhood traumas or abuse (emotional, physical, or sexual), genetic predisposition, and various neurobiological causes.

Symptoms

Borderline disorder refers to people who have poorly integrated and fragile ego structures. Their dysfunction manifests itself in the lack of a sense of self-identity, the use of primitive defense mechanisms, and impairment in reality testing. They tend to regress during stressful times and often resort to splitting, denial, and projection. Gunderson (1988) stated that the essential feature of the disorder is fear of and intolerance for aloneness, and clients frequently report intense and excessive feelings of loneliness, emptiness, and rage. Their rage is often translated into self-abusive behaviors such as hitting walls; head-banging; skin scratching and tearing; and suicide attempts, gestures, or threats. Relationships are often unstable and are manifested by devaluation, manipulation, dependency, and self-denial. They may, at times, have psychotic-like perceptual distortions, become dissociative, or experience paranoid episodes (Gunderson, 1988). The *DSM-IV-TR* (APA, 2000) lists the following behaviors:

- Attempts to avoid abandonment, either real or imagined, that are frantic
- Alternating extremes of idealization and devaluation leading to relationship instability
- Poor and unstable self-image and sense of self
- Self-damaging impulsivity in at least two areas such as spending, sexual behavior, substance abuse, reckless drinking, or binge eating
- Gestures, threats, self-mutilation, or actual suicidal behavior that is recurrent

- Marked mood reactivity, lasting a few hours to days
- Chronic feelings of emptiness
- Anger that is inappropriately intense, uncontrolled, and frequent
- Stress-related paranoid thinking or severe dissociative symptoms that are transient

TREATMENT

Nursing interventions must center on assessing the meaning of crises, identifying current stressors and coping behaviors, and minimizing self-destructive behaviors. A preferable method of intervention is related to a careful consideration of the client's developmental level and experience. The need for psychopharmacologic intervention must also be considered as treatment for the affective components that frequently accompany this condition. The client is assisted to identify the reasons for the present hospital or outpatient experience; the coping methods used in the present situation and the alternative behaviors that might work better; and past coping methods and their outcomes. Because these clients are likely to resort to the use of substances and to attempt suicide, it is important to assess and discuss these issues as unproductive coping methods during therapeutic encounters.

Inpatient treatment typically focuses on crisis stabilization. The challenges in working with these clients has already been described, but it must be stressed that the ego development of these clients is insecure and a great deal of structure, gentle confrontation, and limit setting similar to that used with the antisocial client is needed.

Johnson and Silver (1988) stressed that the treatment of persons with borderline personality disorder is a stressful experience potentially full of conflict between clients and staff. They suggest that these clients probably evoke more intense staff reactions than other clients do. Some

(continues)

TREATMENT *(continued)*

methods for minimizing conflict and promoting growth in clients are suggested as follows:

- Identify and state the treatment, although not necessarily the goals, from the outset
- Use staff development meetings to discuss conflicts and problem-solving methods
- Seek and use professional staff supervision
- Help create an environment for the honest expression of feelings regarding unit conflicts

Antimanic agents (e.g., carbamazepine [Tegretol] and lithium [Eskalith, Lithobid]) and neuroleptics are used to control impulsivity (Kavoussi & Coccaro, 1998; Links et al., 1990). Other clients have responded favorably to antidepressants (e.g., tricyclics and the newer agents such as sertraline [Zoloft] and paroxetine [Paxil]). A number of studies have demonstrated increased effectiveness of combined psychotherapy and pharmacologic treatment (Livesley, 2000; Soloff, 1998; 2000).

CONDUCT DISORDERS

Causes

The causes of conduct disorder fall into the following categories (Kay & Kay, 1986):

Family dynamics—chaotic family dynamics, faulty ego structure (superego) (Keith, 1984), and a lack of parental empathy and affection

Neurobiological—includes temperament, alterations in central nervous system (Zubieta & Alessi, 1993), increased slow wave activity on EEG (Raine, Venables, & Williams, 1990), and genetics (Cadoret et al., 1995)

Sociological—consists of disturbed parent-child relationships marked by rejection and chaotic interactions, social deprivation, substance-related

disorders, early rejection, and lower socioeconomic status (Dadds et al., 1996; Widom, 1999).

Table 10–5 depicts the causes and characteristics of conduct disorders.

Children with faulty ego structures or maladaptive coping patterns often present with behavioral symptoms or conduct disorder. Their histories are frequently dominated by chaotic or dysfunctional family systems. Some psychodynamic theorists suggest a parallel between early childhood traumas and early object losses as common factors in the histories of clients with personality disorders (Freud, 1957; Kernberg, 1984; Masterson, 2000).

Table 10–5 • Causes and Characteristics of Conduct Disorders

CAUSES

Psychological
Chaotic family dynamics
Lack of parental empathy/affection
Faulty ego structure (superego)
Learned behavior

Neurobiological
Genetics
Temperament
Neurological dysfunction, including neurochemical

Sociological
Low socioeconomic status
Media environmental violence
Substance abuse
Disturbed parent-child relationship (rejection, chaotic interactions, inconsistency)

CHARACTERISTICS

- Stealing
- Lying
- Running away from home (history of several instances)
- Truancy
- Disrespect for others
- Fire setting
- Cruelty or violence to others and/or animals
- Early experimentation with substances
- Early sexual experimentation

Many of these losses are attributed to mental illness, substance abuse, and indifference in primary caregivers (Parker, 1984).

Symptoms

The *DSM-IV-TR* (APA, 2000) identifies the essential feature of a conduct disorder as a repetitive and persistent pattern of behavior that violates the basic rights of others or major age-appropriate norms or rules. Certain specific behaviors (at least three) such as lying, truancy, staying out after dark without permission, stealing, vandalism, forced sex, physical cruelty, and use of weapons must have been present during the previous 12 months with at least one criterion present in the past 6 months. The behaviors are grouped according to severity levels of mild, moderate, and severe. These behaviors are also manifestations of antisocial personality disorder in those 18 years of age or older.

TREATMENT

Psychodynamic theorists agree that children with faulty ego function have a developmental arrest that begins in early childhood. The role of psychiatric nurses includes assessing areas of impairment, and the process begins by approaching clients and their significant others in a caring nonjudgmental manner. This approach facilitates trust building and enhances the potential success of treatment plan outcomes. Many of these children have disruptive behavior disorders that set the stage for future problems as well. The *DSM-IV-TR* lists the following diagnoses in this category:

- Conduct disorder: Childhood-onset type and adolescent-onset type
- Disruptive behavior disorder not otherwise specified

The following are desired outcomes:

- Establishing rapport
- Completing a comprehensive diagnostic workup (neurobiological, psychological, sociological)

- Understanding the meaning of behaviors and associated thoughts and feelings
- Maintaining a safe, supportive environment
- Improving ego function

Establishing rapport and trust is extremely difficult, but it is crucial if work with these youngsters is to progress. Nurses must form an alliance with such children and the parents (if possible), even though the parent-child relationship is often tenuous.

DEPENDENT PERSONALITY DISORDER

Symptoms

The hallmark of dependent personality disorder is the pervasive pattern of dependency and submissiveness. These clients rely on others exclusively for their support. They rarely make their own decisions, and they place tremendous demands on others for reassurance and advice. They attach and cling tenaciously to anyone who will take care of them, tell them what to do, or make their decisions for them. They are fearful of many things and become the willing shadow of anyone who will take care of them. Their behavior is often childlike in their hesitation to stand on their own as responsible adults.

TREATMENT

In all therapeutic endeavors, the most apparent need is the reduction of anxiety, and in nearly all instances, a concomitant need for increasing self-esteem. This is no less true for dependency. A skillful balancing act is needed to provide enough but not too much in the process of helping clients grow into a more adaptive lifestyle. The nurse-client relationship may be the only place in which this is given an

(continues)

TREATMENT *(continued)*

opportunity to begin. Nurses are urged to consider the dependent-independent-interdependent need construct of themselves and their clients (Whiting, 1994).

Psychotherapeutic intervention may take place through individual therapy that fosters the development of insight and individual change. The techniques may be interpersonal, behavioral, analytical, or cognitive. Other appropriate modalities include group therapy, family therapy, and psychoeducation to provide decision-making models and assertiveness training.

it also is necessary to gain understanding about infantile fantasies (feelings). As these tasks are accomplished, the client can be helped to develop more adaptive coping skills by finding alternatives to previous destructive behaviors. Encouragement and assistance in developing and recognizing how new behaviors will lead to increased self-worth will be needed. The nurse who is skillful in helping the client accomplish these outcomes also needs to recognize how extremely sensitive to rejection and depressive moods and episodes these clients tend to be. A detailed discussion of treatment strategies are similar to that found in the section on BPD.

HISTRIONIC PERSONALITY DISORDER

Symptoms

Symptoms of histrionic personality tend to be manifested by attention-seeking behaviors in which clients exhibit the following behaviors (APA, 2000):

- Discomfort in situations where he is not the center of attention
- Inappropriate sexually seductive behavior with others
- Rapidly shifting and shallow emotional expressions
- Excessively impressionistic style of speech that lacks detail
- Self-dramatization, theatrics, or exaggerated emotional expressions
- Suggestibility
- Attitude that relationships are more intimate than they are

TREATMENT

Treatment is similar to that of some other personality disorders and focuses on consistency, understanding, managing countertransference issues, and providing an environment that minimizes maladaptive coping patterns.

In addition to the trust and rapport-building activities and identifying the client's particular maladaptive behaviors,

NARCISSISTIC PERSONALITY DISORDER

Causes

Children whose parents are aloof, aggressive, rejecting, and emotionally cold are at risk for developmental arrest at the early narcissistic stage because the person is prevented from achieving a sense of self-worth and value.

Symptoms

Narcissistic individuals are independent, not easily intimidated, and quite aggressive. They prefer loving to being loved and enjoy serving as champions to others (Freud, 1957).

The *DSM-IV-TR* (APA, 2000) states that five or more of the following characteristics must be present to diagnose this disorder:

- Has a grandiose sense of self-importance (e.g., exaggerates achievements and talents, expects to be recognized as superior without commensurate achievements)
- Is preoccupied with fantasies of unlimited success, power, brilliance, beauty, or ideal love
- Believes that he is "special" and unique and can only be understood

by, or should associate with, other special or high-status people (or institutions)

- Requires excessive admiration
- Has a sense of entitlement, that is, unreasonable expectations of especially favorable treatment or automatic compliance with his expectations
- Is interpersonally exploitive, that is, takes advantage of others to achieve his own ends
- Lacks empathy; is unwilling to recognize or identify with the feelings and needs of others
- Is often envious of others or believes that others are envious of him
- Shows arrogant, haughty behaviors or attitudes

TREATMENT

As with other personality disorders, nursing interventions first require that the nurse be aware of his own reactions around clients who evoke a great deal of tension in their demands for attention. Kohut (1971) contended that the establishment of therapeutic alliances is important for increasing self-esteem. The nature of narcissism is such that these clients are preoccupied with themselves and need assistance in understanding and valuing events that occur outside their internal environments. To do this, they must first begin to view themselves from a different perspective, and this demands therapeutic intervention requiring much time and effort. Other nursing interventions are the same as those listed in the section on BPD.

It may be necessary to provide a period of individual psychotherapy either before or concomitant with a lengthier period of group therapy to achieve the greatest benefit. Individual psychotherapy is often the treatment of choice and allows clients an opportunity to introject or incorporate the adaptive aspects of the therapist (Meissner, 1988) and to avoid the regressive use of primitive defenses such as rage, splitting, and projection.

OPPOSITIONAL DEFIANT DISORDER

Causes

Recent data indicate that oppositional defiant disorder is more a family characteristic than a child disorder (Fletcher, Fischer, Barkley, & Smallish, 1996). Several theories about this disorder concerning family dynamic and psychosocial issues are emerging (Fletcher et al., 1996):

- Parental discord (too harsh or lacking)
- Overidentification by the child with the parent who has an impulsivity disorder
- A lack of attachment owing to the parent or guardian's lack of emotional and physical warmth

Although psychosocial and family dynamics play key roles in oppositional defiant disorder, neurobiological and temperamental factors may also contribute to this disorder.

Symptoms

The primary manifestations of oppositional defiant disorder (APA, 2000) are negative, hostile, and stubborn behaviors such as:

- Difficulty in controlling temper
- Frequent arguing with adults, including parents and teachers
- Frequent refusal to follow rules or to do chores or homework
- Frequently being purposely annoying to others
- Being easily agitated or upset by others
- Frequent use of profanity

TREATMENT

As with other psychological conditions of childhood, medical and neurological examinations are suggested to rule out neurological disorders or other illnesses that may contribute to the behaviors.

(continues)

TREATMENT *(continued)*

Psychosocial assessment should attend to the type and quality of parent-child interactions, parental skills in disciplining and rewarding, attachment behaviors, and the child's self-perception.

Nursing interventions need to focus on establishing rapport with the child and parents, teaching parental skills in child management, and promoting self-esteem in both child and parents. Realistic limits need to be set and consequences explained in an empathic manner. Therapeutic goals should be established as follows:

- Establishing trust through a therapeutic relationship
- Assisting parents to avoid the use of negative reinforcing behaviors toward the child
- Helping the child to understand the meaning of self-destructive behaviors and obtaining a "no suicide" pact
- Finding ways to build or restore self-esteem
- Building adaptive coping behaviors in children and their parents. See Chapter 19 of the core text.

- Is reluctant to confide in others because of unwarranted fear that the information will be used maliciously against him
- Reads hidden demeaning or threatening meanings into benign remarks or events
- Persistently bears grudges, that is, is unforgiving of insults, injuries, or slights
- Perceives attacks on his character or reputation that are not apparent to others and is quick to react angrily or to counterattack
- Has recurrent suspicions, without justification, regarding fidelity of spouse or sexual partner

TREATMENT

Interventions are planned to draw the client into a nurse-client relationship in which a measure of trust can be established.

The client with paranoid personality disorder needs the nurse to do the following:

- Establish rapport
- Minimize potential for aggressive behavior
- Support adaptive behaviors

PARANOID PERSONALITY DISORDER

Symptoms

People with pervasive distrust and suspiciousness of others such that their motives are interpreted as malevolent are more likely to develop this disorder, and it is the basis for *DSM-IV-TR* criteria for paranoid personality disorder. The following characteristics are defined in the *DSM-IV-TR* (APA, 2000):

- Suspects, without sufficient basis, that others are exploiting, harming, or deceiving him
- Is preoccupied with unjustified doubts about the loyalty or trustworthiness of friends or associates

SCHIZOID PERSONALITY DISORDER

Symptoms

Individuals with this disorder demonstrate a pervasive pattern of detachment from social relationships and manifest a restricted range of emotional expression with others. The pattern is apparent by early adulthood in a variety of contexts (APA, 2000). These loners choose solitary activities that do not require much participation with others. They may be very adept at computer or mathematical games. There is little interest in sexual activity with another person, and there is minimal pleasure sought from sensory, bodily, or interpersonal experience. There are generally no close friends except possibly a first-degree relative. There is no seeking out of approval from others and they seem oblivious to what others think of them.

SCHIZOTYPAL PERSONALITY DISORDER

Cause

Clients with this disorder usually have positive neurobiological and genetic markers similar to those found in schizophrenia. Gunderson (1988) stated that there may be greater differences between schizoid and schizotypal disorders than previously supposed.

Symptoms

Individuals with this disorder demonstrate a pervasive pattern of social and interpersonal deficits accompanied by marked discomfort with and limited capacity for close relationships along with cognitive and perceptual distortions and behavioral eccentricities (APA, 2000). They are poor candidates for treatment and are at risk for developing schizophrenia.

Isolation, limited peer relationships, social anxiety, school underachievement, hypersensitivity, peculiarities in thought and language, and bizarre fantasies are all characteristics often found in schizotypal personalities as early as childhood and adolescence (APA, 2000).

TREATMENT

Working with clients with schizotypal and schizoid disorders requires that nurses understand the need for establishing rapport and that the clients are difficult to engage and establish positive affective interactions. Feedback will be limited, but in addition to rapport, the nurse will need to work at establishing a reality base and developing adaptive behaviors.

- Approach the client in a calm manner
- Maintain a comfortable distance based on the client's verbal and non-verbal communication
- Administer psychotropics (e.g., risperidone [Risperdal], olanzapine [Zyprexa], and quetiapine [Seroquel]) and observe the client's responses— both desired and adverse
- Engage supportive groups to provide feedback on the client's behaviors
- Provide for structured social interactions

Sexual Disorders

• Key Terms

American Association of Sex Educators, Counselors, and Therapists (AASECT): A multidisciplinary national organization of professionals dedicated to the study, education, and role of spokesperson for sexuality.

Sexual Desire: One's internal psychological state of pleasure governed by sexual pleasure centers in the brain.

Sexual Health: Integration of the somatic, emotional, intellectual, and social aspects of sexual being in ways that are positively enriching and that enhance personality, communication, and love (WHO, 1975).

Sexual health is a lifelong process of awareness, exploration, growth, and development. Sexual relationships can propel an individual into new growth potential, create an ongoing laboratory for adventure and satisfaction, or at times become boring and lackluster. When the "sexual connection" is off balance, partners need to use communication skills to explore the lack of interrelatedness and create new opportunities for growth and sexual satisfaction.

SEXUAL DISORDERS—GENERAL

Causes

In clients with sexual problems treatment depends on the part of the central nervous system affected. Sexual desire also has a neurophysiological component.

The nervous system and sex hormones are important parts of sexual desire and behavior. The sex hormones, testosterone, an androgen secreted by the male testes, and progesterone, an estrogen secreted by the female ovaries, are regulated by the anterior lobe of the pituitary gland and the hypothalamus, located on the lower side of the brain. The hypothalamus, pituitary, gonads, testes, and ovaries work together in sexual functions such as the menstrual cycle, pregnancy, puberty, and sexual behavior (Hyde, 1986). The human sexual response is complex. Sexual disorders and difficulties can arise from multiple sources within this cycle.

Table 11–1 lists the sexual disorders recognized by the APA's (2000) *Diagnostic and Statistical Manual of Mental Disorders* (4th edition Text Revision) (*DSM-IV-TR*). These disorders are described next.

Life experiences and learning influence sexual behavior. A person whose first experience with sex-related activities was positive is more likely to increase the frequency of these activities than is a person whose first sex-related experience was not positive. If the first encounter with sex involves punishment, like the pain of rape or the guilt of being caught and severely punished for masturbating, the behavior is less likely to occur later or may occur in an altered form.

In the dominant American culture, social learning of sexual behaviors is not direct. Sexual activities occur behind closed doors and on the screen in movie theaters. Consequently, much learning about sex is through indirect example and innuendo, which open up the possibility of misunderstanding and lack of information. Children have five general resources for sexual learning: parents, spiritual centers, school, peers, and the media. Parents have the opportunity to be the primary sex educator for children and yet, all too often, because of poor or no role modeling, they abdicate this role (Caine & Caine, 1996; Dumas, 1996).

Humanistic psychologists, notably Maslow (1970) and Rogers (1951), view humans as growth oriented. Sex is viewed as one of many means of achieving self-actualization, one's human potential. Sex is not merely for reproduction, but rather a means of having fun, giving and receiving pleasure. For many, accepting pleasure can be difficult outside as well as inside the bedroom. Often an individual is more comfortable giving than receiving and may consistently place the needs of others before his own (Hooper, 1992).

The Internet has had a major impact on sexuality from a sociological basis. People use sex-related Internet sites for entertainment and recreation, much as they would use other materials such as magazines and videos. It has been noted that for those predisposed to sexually compulsive behavior, on-line sexual content is a more powerful trigger than traditional materials owing to the Internet's "Triple A"—access, affordability, and anonymity.

People's lack of knowledge about sex can give them problems. There has been great debate in America over the last

---

Table 11–1 • Sexual and Gender Disorders

Gender Identity Disorders

Sexual Dysfunctions

Sexual Arousal Disorders

Sexual Desire Disorders

Orgasmic Disorders

Sexual Pain Disorders

Sexual Dysfunction due to General Medical Condition

Substance-Induced Sexual Dysfunction

Paraphilias

Note. Data from *Diagnostic and Statistical Manual of Mental Disorders* (4th edition Text Revision) (*DSM-IV-TR*), by American Psychiatric Association, 2000, Washington, DC: Author. Adapted with permission.

several decades as to what children should be taught about sex, when, and by whom it should be taught. One segment of the population views sex and reproduction education as a private family matter, whereas another faction views sex and reproduction as a social issue that affects the population as a whole, thereby requiring public education. Some people believe that if adolescents have knowledge of sex and birth control, they will be promiscuous, leading to the breakdown of the social fabric of society. And yet, the opposite is true; when children have sexual information, can ask parents questions, and sexual conversations are given at different times about different subjects versus one "birds and bees" talk, they make wise choices for themselves (Haffner, 1999).

The failure to communicate is often the source of people's sex-related problems. Western culture does not openly discuss sex, and thus it does not encourage people, especially women, to ensure that their sexual needs are met through open discussion of problems with their partners. Several factors contribute to the lack of open discussion of sex. First, communication in general has not been stressed as a way to achieve human needs. Children are often told they are selfish or self-centered if they directly ask to have their needs met. Second, history has not helped. The Victorian era, in which men and women did not talk about their bodies at all, greatly influenced our thinking. "Nice" girls had no sexual feelings at all, so how could such a girl discuss her sexual needs? These taboos remain in some segments of our society today.

A person's body image may be the source of his sexual problems. We all have in our minds an ideal body image that has been shaped by our culture. Both male and female Americans have been found to be dissatisfied with some aspects of their bodies.

Spectatoring is when a person observes and judges his own sexual performance rather than living the sexual experience (Masters & Johnson, 1970). Body image distortions contribute to this problem. Spectatoring is when a person begins to ask "Is my stomach flat enough?" "Is my penis big enough?" or "Are my breasts large enough?" instead of experiencing the sensations of the sex act. People with disabilities can also suffer from body image problems that affect their sexual function.

Past experience of abuse can lead to sexual problems. Sexual abuse in childhood, inappropriate parent-child relationships, rape (both in and out of marriage), and other traumas can have lasting effects on sexuality. Sometimes, the experience of past abuse has been repressed to such degree that the abuse survivor has no awareness or memory of it. Sexual problems may appear bizarre and unexplainable or understandable.

Fear is yet another cause of sexual problems. For example, fear of pregnancy or STDs such as HIV infection can interfere with sexual satisfaction.

David Schnarch, a sex therapist (1997), described the concept of "wanting." One partner may "not want to want" the other, thus equating sexual closeness with fear.

Women's position in a Western dominant culture can interfere with their sexual activity. In a culture in which women are told their proper place is in the home raising children and keeping a husband happy, rebellion is a natural response. Add to this message that women are sex objects and the economic reality is that women must work, and it is easy to see why women's sex lives may suffer.

Aggression can be played out sexually in our culture. Rape is an example of using sex as a weapon in an aggressive act.

Sadomasochism is another form of aggressive sexuality practiced by couples. For some individuals, prior emotional, sexual, or physical abuse can contribute in some cases to a person's need to engage in this self-destructive behavior.

Sexual activity is a complex endeavor that involves many factors. The neurobiological aspects of sexuality are affected by age, genetic makeup, disease, use of mood-altering substances, nutrition, and many other variables.

Underlying depression may lead to fatigue and feelings of unworthiness. Lack of libido from dysregulation of various neurochemistry processes is probable. Depressed people often report no interest in sexual activity.

Use of mood-altering substances changes the neurochemistry of the brain and the rest of the nervous system (Crenshaw & Goldberg, 1996). Lack of libido, arousal disorders, and impotency in males have been noted with both short- and long-term substance use. Sexual themes and issues often emerge during recovery from addiction.

Stress has a physiological effect on the body. It changes a person's neurochemistry, and because mental processes and resultant neurochemistry define sex, sexual function may be altered. It is easy to see why sexual disorders may begin during periods of stress.

Sexual activity may decline somewhat in old age, but many people remain sexually active into their 80s and 90s. Decline in sexual activity may have more to do with attitudes about aging and the death of a spouse than with sexual dysfunction. Although physical changes do occur that make sex in old age different from sex in other periods of life (women experience less lubrication and elasticity and declining estrogen levels, resulting in thinner vaginal walls; men produce less testosterone, take longer to achieve an erection, and experience a longer refractory period), adjustments can be made for all of these changes so that sexual activity need not stop in old age.

Key Fact

Findings from the Kaiser Family Foundation/Children Now survey (1999) indicated that kids ages 10 to 15 want to know more about such things as how to handle pressure to have sex, how to know when they are ready to have sex, and how to prevent pregnancy. But the survey reveals that many parents do not talk about these issues with their young children. The survey illustrates that 62 percent of parents have not talked with their preteens about preventing pregnancy and STDs; 50 percent have never discussed how to know when one is ready to have sex.

TREATMENT

Any time a nurse and client interface, sexual concerns may be addressed. Regardless of practice setting, nurses need to create a safe and therapeutic environment that enables the client to express feelings and ask questions about sexual issues. For example, "One part of the nursing assessment is the sexual assessment. Are you sexually active? (If yes, then proceed. If no, ask what the concerns are for not having an active sex life at this time.) Often people describe their sexual relationship as unfulfilling. It may be caused by stress, exhaustion, disinterest, or even difficulties in the relationship. What concerns do you have in your sexual relationship?" Then the nurse must be willing to listen or must refer the client to someone who will. In this way, sexual issues and themes can be addressed openly in a way that gives comfort to the client.

The psychiatric-mental health nurse is in a key position to support sexual behavior changes in groups at risk for HIV infection and other sexually transmitted diseases (STDs). More effort in developing effective client-centered counseling and educational programs is needed. Psychiatric-mental health nurses are uniquely qualified to provide holistic care, counseling, and education to clients at risk for HIV infection. In addition, in an administrative role, the nurse can ensure that groups at risk are targeted for appropriate and effective services. In a scientific role, the nurse researcher can generate and test theories regarding interventions that may be used in clinical settings to support behavior changes in people at risk for HIV infection.

American Nurses Association's (ANA) *Scope and Standards of Psychiatric-Mental Health Nursing Practice* (2000) states that every nurse should own and use three essential documents: a copy of the nurse state practice act, the legal source that defines the scope and privileges of practice in which the nurse practices; the American Nurses Association Code for Nurses, which describes the

(continues)

TREATMENT *(continued)*

ethical responsibilities for conduct by nurses; the previously mentioned document because it sets the standards for a particular nursing specialty. The document can be purchased on-line on ANA's Web site at http:// www.Nursesbooks.org: nursingworld.org/anp/pcatalog.cfm

The generalist nurse addresses sexual themes and problems in the same way the nurse addresses other problems: through the nursing process. The nurse needs to feel comfortable asking about clients' sexual concerns and listening to their problems. After assessment, the nurse develops methods to increase the client's awareness of the problems and potential solutions. Increasing awareness involves education and counseling skills. The generalist nurse is responsible for knowing his personal limitations, because they lack knowledge of complex sexual issues, or lack of skill in these areas. The nurse can overcome limitations in knowledge, skills, and differences in values and beliefs by assisting the client through referral, consulting with appropriate professionals, and seeking continuing education opportunities or further education.

The advanced-practice psychiatric-mental health nurse (e.g., clinical nurse specialist, nurse practitioner) uses psychotherapy and may or may not specialize in sex therapy. Regardless of whether the advanced-practice nurse is a certified sex therapist, effort to determine the appropriate intervention is necessary for the client with a sexual problem. The psychiatric generalist nurse may seek wise counsel from these clinicians or choose to refer for client follow-up.

Sexual health promotion requires the client's active participation and, ultimately, assumption of responsibility for care. The client must use an organized, systematic process to choose a specific course of action for behavior change. Psychiatric clients may have difficulty with decision making. Being faced with choices for behavior change may create conflict within the person and the family. Feelings of helplessness in the client may encourage unnecessary dependence on the nurse. It is the nurse's job to enable the client to operate free of help as quickly as possible, while ensuring the client's self-care potential.

Facilitating sexual behavioral change begins with the nurse's assessing the meaning that the client attaches to sexual behavior. Interventions are then developed to help the client identify alternative sexual methods or nonsexual methods of finding meaning.

A sexual history includes all aspects of sexuality and therefore is holistic. Sexual influences are part of the evaluation—role modeling by parents; messages by parents, early exploration, masturbation, initial experiences with intercourse and religious influences encompass the assessment. In addition, levels of desire, arousal, orgasmic function, pain, and frequency of sexual activity should be discussed with the client. An overall health assessment, including a thorough physical examination, is basic to good problem identification, because sexuality includes neurological, vascular, muscular, hormonal, psychosocial, and other components. A sexual history should include the context in which the problem emerged and the context in which it currently exists, awareness of both the nurse's and client's underlying anxieties and prejudices, a description of the experience as it is lived by the client, the meaning of the problem from the client's perspective, and the support currently available to the client and the nurse. See Table 11–2, Comprehensive Sexual History.

American Association of Sex Educators, Counselors, and Therapists (AASECT) is a multidisciplinary, national association for sexology professionals. AASECT, along with Sexuality Information Education Council of the United States (SIECUS), have become one center for sexual public policy issues in the United States. AASECT provides standards and a credentialing process for professionals to advance their knowledge and skill levels, thus providing quality sexual care to clients.

(continues)

Table 11–2 • Comprehensive Sexual History

The nurse can formulate client questions related to the following categories: sexual development, current sexual function, and current sexual relationship to provide a comprehensive sexual history.

Sexual Development

Parental messages
Childhood experiences
Significant relationships
History of sexual abuse/trauma
Initial sexual experience
Religious influences

Current Sexual Function

Desire (how often felt)
Masturbation frequency
Ability to be aroused
Use of erotic material—video, books, magazines
Use of fantasy
Orgasmic function with partner
Orgasmic function with self
Sexual pain
Unpleasant sexual experiences
Sexually transmitted diseases
Birth control
Medical conditions
Medications
Alcohol, substance use
Menstruation history

Current Sexual Relationship

Who initiates
Foreplay
Frequency of sexual activity
Frequency of intercourse
Satisfaction with intercourse
Affairs
Repertoire of sexual behaviors
Ability to communicate sexual needs with partner

TREATMENT (continued)

Self-awareness and awareness of others regarding sexual issues or themes are key attributes nurses need to be most effective in their role of client advocate. First, nurses need to be aware of their own attitudes, values, and beliefs regarding sexual health. Second, nurses need to be aware of their clients' sexual issues. Third, nurses need to be aware of how their personal attitudes, values, and beliefs affect their ability to recognize and react to clients' sexual issues and themes.

It is important to know the different theoretical perspectives on sexuality. No theory can claim to be the real truth. In sexual health care, as in all nursing activity, the nurse's therapeutic use of the self is expected. The therapeutic interaction between nurse and client should never be underestimated. The nurse's concern for and acceptance of the client and the problem can have a profound influence on the health care outcome.

Punishment and reward must be immediate to shape behavior. If a person does something "bad" and is not caught and punished until time passes or is not punished every time the behavior is enacted, chances are the frequency of the behavior will not decrease. In fact, it may increase. Behavior modification, the use of operant conditioning to change behavior, has become popular in educational as well as therapeutic settings.

Aversion therapy was used years ago in work with sex offenders. In extreme cases castration was seen as an option. Today castration is seen as a violation of our sense of civilization. Relapse prevention treatment strategies and the "no cure" mind-set are predominate forms of treatment for sex offenders.

Feeling that one deserves pleasure is an essential element in a healthy sexual relationship and leads to higher levels of self-actualization. Learning to be comfortable with pleasure and pleasuring can be a challenge. It requires several things; first, one must learn what satisfies; second, one must have the ability to communicate this information to one's partner; third, be specific about sexual preferences; and last, learn to accept pleasure from a partner.

Nursing has traditionally supported knowledge as a method to empower indi-

(continues)

TREATMENT *(continued)*

viduals and groups. Sex education has become a part of nursing practice, whether the nurse works in a school, birth control clinic, and hospital or community system. Nurses need to be knowledgeable about sex and aware of a client's need for information. Getting in the habit of asking clients about sex-related issues or whether they have any questions about sex issues is a good idea. The nurse who cannot or is unwilling to address the client's sex-related questions is obligated to make a referral to a specialized sex educator or sex therapist.

Whether the message is about condoms or the failure to reach orgasm, communication is a fundamental aspect of sex. Nurses are well advised to learn to talk with their clients about the use of clear, direct communication and to role model it themselves.

Although nurses must encourage and explicitly teach clients avoidance of risky sexual practices, giving the idea that sex is dangerous and that all aspects of human closeness should be avoided is shortsighted and irresponsible. Sex is a basic human need that involves much more than intercourse. Nonrisky behaviors such as cuddling, necking, petting, and mutual masturbation can be encouraged as alternatives to risky behaviors. To encourage unattainable standards like total abstinence may lead to hopeless, helpless feelings that end in the client's abandoning any effort to control unsafe sex practices.

"Wanting to be wanted" demonstrates one's ability to experience sexual closeness as a positive aspect of the relationship, neither too close to fear engulfment by the other nor too far apart to feel rejected. This concept is helpful in working with clients to assist them in disclosing their feelings about sexual desire in relationship to their partner.

The selective serotonin uptake inhibitors (SSRI) medications available in the marketplace have led to speedy resolution of depressive symptoms. Examples of

SSRIs include fluoxetine (Prozac) and sertraline (Zoloft). These drugs tend to be the first line of treatment for depressive disorders because of their safer side profile and efficacy. However, a major drawback are the sexual side effects of these medications—for some individuals a decrease in sexual desire, for many, orgasmic retardation. Sexual side effects are a major reason for nonadherence to antidepressant medications and the major reason for nonadherence to medications in general. In addition, other medications, such as bupropion (Wellbutrin), nefazodone (Serzone) should also be considered because of fewer sexual side effects. Nurses working with clients who are depressed and are experiencing sexual problems need to inform them of these side effects and assist them in their decision making.

A person's ability to manage and cope with stressful situations is determined by the ability to mobilize internal and external resources. Positive coping skills for the same individual could be the following activities: exercise, relaxation activities or music, or talking to supportive people.

Nurses can empower clients to change their behavior by exploring the meanings attached to stressful experiences and by considering the possibilities for coping.

Sexual themes and issues are present throughout the life span. Nurses need to incorporate sexual histories in their assessments. See Table 11–3 for a summary of sexual issues across the life span.

An infertility support group led by a nurse with knowledge and experience in this area will help this couple share their experiences with others and learn they are not alone. It is important that a knowledgeable health professional be the group leader because misinformation is a real danger in leaderless support groups or psychotherapy groups led by someone who does not understand infertility and its treatment.

Although Viagra (sildenafil citrate) offers new options to enhance sexual

(continues)

Table 11-3 • Sexual Issues across the Life Span

Childhood:	Identification with gender
Adolescence:	Identity development vs. role confusion
Young Adulthood:	Intimate relationship development
Adulthood:	Generativity, guiding children
Middlescence:	Redefinition of identity and roles
Old Age:	Changing physical and mental conditions

Interventions should be aimed at (1) removal of the cause of the problem, (2) symptom management for problems that cannot be readily treated because their etiology is unknown or effective treatment is unavailable, (3) case management for the client with chronic problems, and (4) family support. Of course, intervention varies with each condition and client system.

The outcome of nursing interventions should be that the client reports satisfactory and socially appropriate sexual functioning within the context of his situation. Concern for the sexual partner if there is one is also an expected client outcome (NANDA, 2001).

TREATMENT *(continued)*

function, within the first year on the market, about 130 Americans who took Viagra died (Williams, 1999). The Food and Drug Administration issued warnings recommending that clinicians be cautious about prescribing Viagra. The new label states men who have had a heart attack, stroke, or life-threatening arrhythmia in the last 6 months, or who have significantly low blood pressure, significantly high blood pressure, a history of cardiac failure or unstable angina, or the eye disease, retinitis pigmentosa, not receive the drug. Research is also under way to evaluate the effectiveness of Viagra for women.

Working in partnership with the client, family, and interdisciplinary team to enable the client's sexual behavior change involves open communication and cooperation. All parties need to be aware of the nature of the problem and how to work toward a satisfactory change. This involvement is not always easy; conflict and discomfort may arise. Encouraging participants' expression of differences in values and beliefs while advocating acceptance of the client's wish to change should be the focus of nursing interventions.

AROUSAL DISORDERS

Cause

For a diagnosis of sexual arousal disorder in both men and women, no other Axis I diagnosis should be evident. For example, major depression, substance abuse, and sexual dysfunction related to a medical condition (e.g., spinal cord injury) all cause changes in a person's physiological ability for sexual arousal.

Symptoms

Sexual arousal disorders are primary disorders in people who have an inadequate physiological response during the period of sexual arousal. In women, the problem is a persistent or recurrent inability to attain or maintain lubrication and swelling of the vagina during the excitement phase. In men it is a persistent or recurrent inability to attain or maintain an erection.

DESIRE DISORDERS

Symptoms

Disorders in **sexual desire** are primary problems as identified by the person experiencing them or by the clinician during assessment. The disturbance must cause marked distress or difficulty in interpersonal relationships. Sexual desire may be hypoactive, or there may be an aversion to all sexual activity. Hypoactive desire disorder is marked by low or absent sexual fantasy or activities. The person's age, sex, and life context (culture, relationship, etc.) must be taken into account.

An aversion to sexual activity is a persistent and extreme avoidance of all or almost all genital sexual contact with a partner. The individual reports anxiety, fear, or disgust when confronted by a sexual opportunity with a partner. The presence of another Axis I diagnosis, such as depression or obsessive-compulsive disorder, must be ruled out before a sexual desire disorder diagnosis is made.

GENDER IDENTITY DISORDERS

Cause

Gender identity is defined by whether someone identifies as male or female. The culture in which the child grows up and relationships define and limit boundaries of sexual behavior. By the time the child reaches 3 years old, he or she proclaims to be a boy or a girl. Psychologists believe "gender constancy"—knowing one will always be a male or a female is developed by ages 5 to 7. There are some children who have gender disorders and for a variety of hormonal, prenatal, and, possibly, environmental factors, they do not feel that their actual physical sexual anatomy matches their gender.

Symptoms

Gender identity disorder is not allowing oneself to experience the role of the other; rather, it is a pervasive distress over being a boy or a girl. A child with a gender identity disorder may be preoccupied with the dress and behavior stereotypical of the opposite sex. In addition, the child persists in asserting that he or she will develop the sex organs of the other sex. In adulthood, this condition is referred to as transsexualism. The person is persist-

ently (for at least 2 years) preoccupied with getting rid of current primary and secondary sexual characteristics (Swaab, Jiang-Ning, Hofman, & Gooren, 1995).

Other identity problems are seen in children and adults who cross-dress, that is, wear culturally appropriate dress of the opposite sex. This cross-dressing is not to be confused with wearing clothes of the opposite sex for the purpose of feeling sexual arousal known as transvestic fetishism.

ORGASMIC DISORDERS

Symptoms

An orgasmic disorder for both men and women is a persistent or recurrent delay in or absence of orgasm following a normal sexual excitement phase. The disorder may be further categorized as generalized (occurs every time) or situational (orgasm may occur with self-stimulation or occurs with only a particular partner) (APA, 2000).

Premature ejaculation is another type of orgasmic disorder. The condition can be persistent in nature or recurrent, in that ejaculation may occur with minimal sexual stimulation before, on, or shortly after penetration and before the person wishes it.

TREATMENT

Behavior modification is a common modality used in treatment of male orgasmic disorders or premature ejaculation. Clients are taught to identify the "point of inevitability"—that moment in time when one knows orgasm is imminent. Masturbation exercises are the framework in which the man identifies the point of inevitability, withholds further stimulation, desensitizes his body to acute pleasure, and choreographs a new pleasure threshold for sexual activity with his partner.

The nurse must consider issues like the duration of the excitement phase, age, novelty of the sexual partner or situation, and recent frequency of sexual activity.

PARAPHILIA

Symptoms

Paraphilia is an umbrella term for variations in sexual behavior. Hyde's (1986) definition of abnormal sex may be used to give an overall framework to paraphilia. Sex is abnormal when it (1) is uncomfortable for the person doing it, (2) is inefficient in that it causes problems in that person's life (e.g., results in arrest), (3) is viewed by the person's culture as bizarre, and (4) does harm to the person and others. Table 11–4 presents a list of the paraphilias and their definitions.

SEXUAL DYSFUNCTION CAUSED BY A GENERAL MEDICAL CONDITION

Cause

There are times when a general medical condition such as hypertension interferes with sexual function, thus causing a great deal of distress, disruption of sexual functioning, and interpersonal problems (Fogel & Lauver, 1990; Lubkin, 1986). The sexual dysfunction may result in secondary male erectile disorder, secondary dyspareunia, secondary vaginismus, or another secondary sexual dysfunction. Table 11–5 lists nonpsychiatric medical conditions that affect sexual functioning.

SEXUAL PAIN DISORDERS

Symptoms

Persistent or recurrent genital pain in men or women before, during, or after intercourse that cannot be explained by other medical or psychiatric conditions is called dyspareunia. Vaginismus refers to an involuntary spasm of the musculature of the outer two thirds of the vagina that interferes with vaginal penetration with penis, finger, tampon, or speculum. Like other sexual conditions identified in the *DSM-IV-TR* (APA, 2000), the sexual pain

---

Table 11–4 • Definitions of Paraphilia

Exhibitionism: exposure of one's genitals to strangers

Fetishism: sexual fixation on an object to which erotic significance is attached

Frotteurism: sexual fantasies involving touching and rubbing against a nonconsenting individual

Pedophilia: sexual fantasies and activities with prepubescent children

Sexual masochism: sexual fantasies comprising being humiliated, beaten or bound, or made to suffer

Sexual sadism: sexual fantasies, behaviors, or acts that generate psychological or physical suffering of another person

Transvestic fetishism: recurrent and intense sexual urges and sexual fantasies involving cross-dressing

Voyeurism: sexual arousal at secretly viewing the nude body

Paraphilia not otherwise specified include the following:

> *Telephone scatalogia:* obscene phone calls
>
> *Necrophilia:* sexual fantasies and acts involving corpses
>
> *Partialism:* exclusive sexual focus on a part of the body, for example, the feet
>
> *Zoophilia:* sexual fantasies and acts with animals
>
> *Coprophilia:* feces hold sexual meaning for the individual
>
> *Klismaphilia:* sexual fantasies and arousal involving enemas
>
> *Urophilia:* urine produces sexual response

Note. Data from *Diagnostic and Statistical Manual of Mental Disorders* (4th edition Text Revision) (*DSM-IV-TR*), by American Psychiatric Association, 2000, Washington, DC: Author. Reprinted with permission.

---

disorders must be persistent or recurrent to warrant diagnosis and treatment. Both sexual pain disorders must cause a problem for the person individually and interpersonally.

Table 11–5 • Medical Conditions That Affect Sexual Function

Neurological	Pulmonary disease
Spinal cord injury	Arthritis
Cervical disc	Cancer
problems	**Genital Disease in**
Multiple sclerosis	**Females**
Vascular	Infections
Atherosclerosis	Cancers
Sickle cell anemia	Allergies to
Endocrine	spermicide
Addison's disease	**Genital Disease in**
Cushing's syndrome	**Males**
Hypothyroidism	Prostatitis
Diabetes mellitus	Orchitis
Systemic Disease	Tumor
Liver disease	Trauma
Renal disease	**Surgical Procedures**

Note. From *Sexual Health Promotions*, by C. I. Fogel & D. Lauver, 1990, Philadelphia: W.B. Saunders. Reprinted with permission.

SUBSTANCE-INDUCED SEXUAL DYSFUNCTION

Cause

In substance-induced sexual dysfunction, a prescription or recreational drug causes sexual dysfunction (Lehne, Moore, Crosby, & Hamilton, 1998). Usually, the substance was ingested within 6 weeks of the sexual problem's appearance.

TREATMENT

The specific substance should be identified as the etiology of the problem. Table 11–6 lists drugs that are known to affect sexual function.

RESOURCES

Please note that because Internet resources are of a time-sensitive nature and URL addresses may change or be deleted,

Table 11–6 • Drugs That Affect Sexual Function

Prescription drugs

Antianxiety agents
  Alprazolam (Xanax)
  Diazepam (Valium)

Anticholinergic agents
  Homatropine methylbromide (Homapin)
  Mepenzolate bromide (Cantil)
  Methantheline bromide (Banthīne)
  Propantheline bromide (Pro-Banthīne)

Anticonvulsant agents
  Phenytoin (Dilantin)

Antidepressant agents
  Most can cause changes

Antipsychotic agents
  Most can cause changes

Antiarrhythmic agents
  Disopyramide (Norpace)

Antihypertensive agents
  Beta blockers
  Diuretics
  Sympatholytics

Others
  Cimetidine (Tagamet)
  Sulfasalazine (Azulfidine)
  Over-the-counter drugs with anticholinergic properties

Social drugs

Alcohol	Marijuana
Amyl nitrate	Heroin
Cocaine	Methadone
Lysergic acid	

searches should also be conducted by association or topic.

Internet Resources

http://www.aasect.org   American Association of Sex Educators, Counselors, and Therapists (AASECT)
http://www.cdc.gov/hiv/stats   Centers for Disease Control and Prevention (CDC)
http://www.siecus.org   Sexuality Information Education Council of the United States (SIECUS)

12 Sleep Disorders

• Key Terms

Advanced Sleep Phase Syndrome (ASPS): A circadian rhythm disorder common in the older adult, with early bedtime and related early rising time, inability to remain asleep during the night, and the perception of being "out of sync" with the rest of the population. Associated with napping, which worsens the problem.

Cataplexy: Sudden loss of motor control while awake, usually occurring with strong emotions, associated with narcolepsy.

Chronic Insomnia: Refers to insomnia that lasts more than 3 weeks.

Circadian Rhythm: The variation in sleep tendency over a slightly greater than 24-hour period, associated with core temperature control, neurotransmitter and hormone secretion, and light or dark exposure.

Delayed Sleep Phase Syndrome (DSPS): A circadian rhythm disorder, common in adolescence, with late sleep onset, and resultant desire to oversleep.

Enuresis: Bedwetting after having been toilet trained; generally resolves by school age.

Hypersomnia: Excessive daytime sleepiness, associated with disordered, non-restorative sleep.

Insomnia: The perception of not sleeping well, including difficulty in falling asleep, early awakening, and disrupted sleep; includes a perception of inadequate sleep quantity as well as quality.

Narcolepsy: A rare disorder of chronic daytime sleepiness, cataplexy, and sleep paralysis. No amount of normal sleep ameliorates the disorder; individuals have disturbed nocturnal sleep, including vivid dreams, nightmares, or night terrors, or both.

Non-Restorative Sleep: Associated with fatigue, difficulty awakening, poor concentration, and low productivity.

Psychophysiologic Insomnia (PI): Refers to complaints of difficulty attaining or maintaining sleep during a normal sleep period.

Sleep Deprivation: Chronic lack of sleep, but may occur acutely, inability to get the needed 8.3 hours of sleep nightly.

Sleep Paralysis: Associated with narcolepsy, inability to move or speak just after or before awakening; breathing is not affected.

*Healthy individuals generally sleep well and wake up feeling refreshed. Normally, **restorative sleep** is controlled by homeostatic sleep processes, circadian rhythm, and sleeping environment. Generally, the circadian rhythm opposes the homeostatic sleep drive for about 16 hours daily, facilitating the wakeful state (Spitzer et al., 1999).*

SLEEP DISORDERS

The *Diagnostic and Statistical Manual of Mental Disorders* (4th edition Text Revision) (*DSM-IV-TR*) (APA, 2000) for sleep disorders include the following:

- Primary sleep disorders—includes dyssomnias and parasomnias
- Sleep disorders related to another mental condition
- Other sleep disorders
- Sleep disorders due to a general medication condition
- Substance-induced sleep disorders

Causes

Human behavior has a major impact on the normal sleep process and can disrupt sleep even when homeostasis, circadian rhythm, and environments are normal. In addition, normal circadian temperature curve governs sleep because during this period, the body temperature is at its lowest setting then rises on awakening (Spitzer et al., 1999). The relevance of body temperature and sleep is the time that most nurses measure the clients' temperature.

Individuals with health problems, either psychological or biological, often have disturbed or **non-restorative** sleep. Sleep patterns are often linked to disease and those who have sleep problems often eventually become ill, or existing chronic illness can become more severe. See Table 12–1, Non-rapid Eye Movement Sleep Stages.

Regardless of sleep stage, disruption often results in negative physiologic results such as various psychiatric and medical disorders.

Insomnia is incredibly prevalent in psychiatric disorders.

Biochemical process involving various neurotransmitters such as serotonin and norepinephrine play roles in sleep regulation. Drugs and medical or psychiatric conditions that alter brain chemistry contribute to sleep disorders.

Neuroanatomical studies also link sleep disorders to dysregulation in the hypothalamic-pituitary-adrenal (HPA) axis, which plays a role in cortisol release

Table 12–1 • Non-rapid Eye Movement (NREM) Sleep Stages

Stage	Physiological Process
Stage I: light sleep (falling asleep); (alpha waves interspersed with low-frequency theta waves; slow eye movement (transitional stage between wakefulness and sleep)	• Inhibition of the reticular formation (arousal mechanism) in the cerebral cortex occurs. • Basal metabolic decreases. • Cerebral blood flow to brainstem and cerebellum decreases. • Heart rate, respirations, temperature, and muscle tone decrease. • Pupils constrict.
Stage II: high K-complexes, sleep spindles, and slow eye movements (light voltage sleep)	• Cerebral blood flow to brainstem and cerebellum decreases.
Stage III: (slow sleep or "delta sleep"); slow waves on EEG; low-frequency delta waves with occasional sleep spindles and slow eye movements (restorative sleep)	• Blood flow to cortex decreases.
Stage IV: delta waves (restorative sleep)	• Blood flow to cortex decreases. • Growth hormone is released and cortico-steroid and catecholamines decrease.

EEG, electroencephalogram.

Note. Data from "Sleep disorders," by T. C. Neylan, C. F. Reynolds, and D. F. Kupfer, 1999, in *American Psychiatric Textbook of Psychiatry* (3rd ed., pp. 955–982), by R. E. Hales, S. C. Yudofsky, and J. T. Talbott (Eds.), Washington, DC: American Psychiatric Press. Adapted with permission.

(Yehuda, 1998). These data consistently indicate that low cortisol levels are found in post-trauma clients, whereas depressed clients are likely to have high cortisol levels (Yehuda, 1998). Sleep deprivation is associated with increased slow wave sleep, resulting in significant reduction in cortisol and growth hormone (GH) secretion the following day. Some researchers suggest that reduced cortisol levels arising from sleep deprivation may provide a temporary relief from depression. These data also strongly suggest that deep sleep has an inhibitory effect on the HPA axis, whereas it enhances the activity of the GH axis. These findings are consistent with data concerning idiopathic hypersomnia and HPA axis and activation of chronic insomnia (Leproult, Copinschi, Buxton, & Van Cauter, 1997; Redwine, Hauger, Gillin, & Irwin, 2000).

Data also indicate a familial incidence of insomnia. Clients with sleep disorders often report a positive history of sleep disturbances, particularly in women (Bastien & Morin, 2000). A genetic locus on chromosomes 8q, 12q, 13q, and 22q11 is also linked to the etiology of enuresis (Arnell et al., 1997; Elberg, 1998). Likewise, **narcolepsy** has a genetic etiology, and, recently, researchers from UCLA and Stanford discovered that individuals with narcolepsy have missing critical cells in the hypothalamus. These cells secrete a hormone called hypocretin, previously known as orexin, which is involved in the regulation of sleep. The researchers feel that the cells have been destroyed, most likely because of some autoimmune process.

Mood, anxiety, and substance-related disorders often result from insomnia. In addition, dementia is highly associated with disrupted sleep and, in fact, is a hallmark of Alzheimer's dementia (Hauri & Cleveland-Hauri, 1999). Other mental illnesses that affect, and are affected by, sleep include schizophrenia and other psychotic disorders (Hauri & Cleveland-Hauri, 1999).

Seasonal affective disorder (SAD) (APA, 2000) is another psychiatric disorder that is associated with prolonged days without sunlight. It can result in **hypersomnia**, depression, and a cycle of worsening sleep until sunlight returns. Hypersomnia is excessive daytime somnolence, associated with non-restorative sleep (APA, 2000). Seasonal changes and sleep disturbances tend to occur in global regions where there is prolonged darkness and days of light. These factors have a biological effect on sleep quality.

Somatic illnesses, once thought to be purely psychiatric disorders, include chronic fatigue syndrome and fibromyalgia, which are both strongly associated with sleep disorders. In fact, lack of Stage IV non-REM sleep is used to help make the diagnosis of fibromyalgia as well as symptoms of fatigue and reduced physical endurance (Dambro, 1998).

Psychophysiologic factors, such as anxiety about not sleeping, may result when there is a temporary cause of insomnia. Then the poor sleep patterns may be continued by the individual long after the original cause of the insomnia has disappeared. This is called **psychophysiologic insomnia**. Poor sleep hygiene is a major factor in this situation. In this type, the cause of the sleep disorder is the client's behaviors (Hauri & Cleveland-Hauri, 1999).

Many medical disorders affect sleep. Some of the most common are thyroid disorders, hypothyroidism (excessive sleep) and hyperthyroidism (sleep deficit), and any pain syndrome. Chronic obstructive pulmonary disease (COPD) and coronary artery disease (CAD) are both associated with sleep apnea. The sleep apnea increases the risk of a major cardiovascular event occurring in this population.

Another major medical condition that impairs sleep is nocturia or urinary frequency (Brown, 1999). Nocturia can occur in the form of enuresis in children and occasionally continues into young adulthood, but nighttime awakening to void is more common in the middle-aged and older adult. Individuals who are taking diuretics or who have osmotic diuresis, such as diabetics in poor control,

have frequently interrupted sleep. Men with benign prostatic hypertrophy often have nocturia as a classic symptom, with multiple awakenings to void. The seriousness of these problems is related to the individual's ability to return to deep sleep within a reasonable period of time. However, clients who are awakening three or four times a night are almost guaranteed to have non-restorative sleep. See Table 12–2 for the major medical conditions associated with sleep disorders.

Cognitive factors associated with sleep disorders often parallel other psychiatric disorders such as anxiety and mood disorders. Frequently, the inability to sleep stems from worrying about staying awake or faulty distortions, such as "I need to get 8 hours of sleep every night."

There are many behavioral factors associated with sleep disorders. Most commonly, it is associated with self-induced sleep deprivation because of stress and hectic irregular schedules. Many feel that this is a state to be expected and never seek help for their poor sleep or their exhaustion. Choices may be made that interfere with getting adequate restorative sleep. Even if more hours of sleep are achieved, the quality of the sleep is often impaired owing to stress and worry or other behavioral choices.

Individuals who worry excessively and have difficulty "shutting down" to sleep, may tend to have sleep disturbances. Any major stressor can disrupt sleep; for example, starting college, moving, marrying, a new job, a new baby, or the loss of a loved one. Other stressors include significant losses, pain, illness, development of health problems, or need for surgery, all of which have the potential to disrupt sleep.

Oftentimes clients resort to using various sleep aids, such as OTC medications that contain diphenhydramine (Benadryl), or have an alcoholic beverage. Alcohol relaxes the individual, increasing drowsiness and the ability to fall asleep. However, with more than two drinks, and especially if they are ingested within a couple of hours of bedtime, alcohol interferes with normal sleep architecture so that the quality of sleep is impaired. In addition, OTC sleep preparations containing diphenhydramine

Table 12–2 • **Common Medical Conditions, Psychiatric Disorders and Medications That Cause Insomnia**

Medical Conditions	Psychiatric Disorders	Medications
Cardiovascular diseases	Major depressive episode	Diuretics
Chronic obstructive pulmonary disease	Bipolar I and II disorders	Alcohol
Endocrine disorders, such as diabetes and thyroid disease	Seasonal affective disorder	CNS stimulants
Dementia	Post-traumatic stress disorder	Diphenhydramine (Benadryl)
Menopause	Obsessive-compulsive disorder and other anxiety disorders	Caffeine
Pain		Theophylline
Nocturia		Selective serotonin reuptake inhibitors (e.g. fluoxetine [Prozac])
Periodic limb movement disorder	Schizophrenia and other psychotic disorders	
Restless leg syndrome		Antipsychotic agents
Fluid and electrolyte imbalance	Substance-related disorders	Cortisone
Delirium		Thyroid replacement hormone
Allergies—rhinitis, sinusitis	Somatoform disorders	
Bronchitis	Personality disorders	
Gastroesophageal reflux disease (GERD)		
Peptic ulcer disease		
Malignant tumors		
Fibromyalgia		

Note. Data from "Sleep Problems Associated with Mood and Anxiety Disorders," by R. Benca, 1999, *Primary Psychiatry, 6*, pp. 52–60; "Diagnosing and Treating Insomnia," by P. Hauri and C. Cleveland-Hauri, 1999, *Primary Psychiatry, 6*, pp. 61–71; "Sleep Patterns of Sheltered Battered Women," by J. C. Humphreys, K. A. Lee, T. C. Neylan, and C. R. Marmar, 1999, *Image: Journal of Nursing Scholarship, 31*, pp. 139–143; and "Management of Insomnia: A Meta-analysis of Treatment Efficacy," by D. J. Kupfer and C. F. Reynolds, 1997, *American Journal of Psychiatry, 336*, pp. 341–346. Adapted with permission.

(Benadryl) may also produce paradoxical side effects that disturb sleep.

Caffeinated drinks are known causes of sleep disruption. Various dietary and nutritional preparations contain caffeine, including chocolates and certain teas. Women taking female hormones also clear caffeine much more slowly, so they may have to limit caffeine much earlier in the day to achieve sleep after initiating hormone therapy. Many people who "sleep fine" after caffeine are really not achieving the deep sleep needed for normal physiological processes. Also, use of any headache medicines that contain caffeine, which may help relieve the headache, but interfere with sleep.

Environmental factors that contribute to

sleep disorders include noise in the sleep setting, inability to achieve a dark room, and season of the year. Likewise, admission to a health care facility interferes with sleep through many of the mechanisms above, especially environmental changes, including having a roommate and having strangers and nurses entering the sleep environment, sometimes without warning. Administration of medications, treatments, and taking of vital signs and blood all interfere with sleep. The more disruptive and frequent the intrusion, the more difficult to return to a state of sleep that is restorative.

Polysomnographic studies indicate that sleep and fragmentation are common in acutely ill clients. Of particular interest are clients with acute MI and neurological and respiratory conditions (Freedman, Kotzer, & Schwab, 1999; Kahn et al., 1998; Knill, Moote, Skinner, & Rose, 1990).

Other environmental factors that contribute to sleep disturbances arise from alterations in the circadian rhythm. **Circadian rhythm** is the variation in sleep tendency over a period slightly greater than 24 hours. The core body temperature, neurotransmitter and hormonal secretion, and light and dark exposure modulate circadian rhythms. Circadian rhythm sleep disorders arise from various causes, including *delayed sleep phase type, jet lag type,* and *shift work type.* Delayed sleep phase type is marked by sleep and wake times that are considerably later than desired, with a resultant difficulty in falling asleep and awakening at a desired time. Jet lag type normally occurs when people cross various time zones that are different from their normal zone time. This sleep disorder usually spontaneously corrects itself after several days. Shift work type occurs in people who repeatedly and rapidly change work schedules. The effects of these disorders vary among individuals and reflect alterations in one's normal sleep-wake cycle.

In adolescents, major physiological and hormonal changes are occurring, including major growth spurts, voice changes, and secondary sexual characteristic development. In and of themselves, these changes are stressful; however, in the face of sleep deficit, these processes are impaired, and sleep deprivation at this time increases the stress, and thus a vicious cycle ensues. In addition, repeated nights of impaired sleep are linked to psychosis and other mental illnesses.

As individuals take on the tasks of adulthood, sleep, or lack of it, may have a serious impact on the activities of daily living. Marriage and learning to live and sleep with another individual may be a challenge that has negative consequences if coping skills are lacking. Managing to attend work in a timely fashion, staying employed, and dealing with shift work, all become tasks adults must strive to complete successfully.

Once adults begin to deal with the challenges of adding children to the family, sleep deficit can become a serious issue, especially for the primary caregiver(s).

Work and financial stressors also contribute to sleep problems. These worries are common in adulthood, as individuals are striving to manage the tasks of achieving a successful career, maintaining financial stability, and planning for the future.

Older adults tend to go to sleep earlier and arise earlier. If an individual plans to sleep at 8 P.M., then it would be reasonable to arise at 4 A.M. This tends to be perceived as abnormal by many clients. If the individual then goes to sleep later, but continues to awaken at 4, sleep deficit will result (Neubauer, 1999). These changes are called **advanced sleep phase syndrome (ASPS)** and are common in the older adult. Daytime napping may worsen the problem, with delayed onset of nighttime sleep, further decreasing restorative deep sleep.

In addition, older adults are more prone to the sleep disorders such as restless leg syndrome, sleep apnea, or snoring. If the older adult has a partner with any of these problems, then both partners will need to be treated to resolve the issues. Disorders of mental health can cause or exacerbate sleep, and the neurodegenerative disorders such as Alzheimer's disease commonly result in disordered sleep (Neubauer, 1999).

Older adults are particularly prone to be receiving medications that result in sleep alterations. Common suspects should include the selective serotonin reuptake inhibitors (SSRIs), decongestants, bronchodilators, diuretics, antianxiety agents, and many OTC "sleep aids." Diphenhydramine (Benadryl) is a common active ingredient in many OTC sleep products, and although it does create drowsiness, it also contributes to falls from the sedation. It also has drying effects that may cause further problems in this age group. In addition, diphenhydramine does not support normal sleep architecture, so it is a poor choice if there is an ongoing sleep disorder, especially in older adults.

Symptoms

Although the term **insomnia** is often used to describe sleep problems, there is general lack of its meaning among clinicians. Generally, this term refers to a subjective description of inadequate sleep. Most complaints of inadequate sleep range from difficulty falling asleep, staying asleep, early morning wakening, and resultant daytime sleeping caused by insomnia (Walsh & Unstun, 1999). **Chronic insomnia** refers to sleep disturbances lasting more than 3 weeks.

Sleep deprivation is a chronic lack of sleep but may vary according to the person's normal sleep requirements. Sleep deprivation is pervasive and often goes unrecognized. Common consequences of sleep deprivation include decreased job performance stemming from concentration and memory difficulties, increased health care costs, and poorer general health (Leger, Scheuermaier, Philip, Paillard, & Guilleminault, 2001).

Primary symptoms of narcolepsy include chronic daytime sleepiness or "sleep attacks," abnormal REM sleep manifestations, including *hypnagogic hallucinations*, **cataplexy**, and **sleep paralysis** (APA, 2000). Sleep paralysis is associated with narcolepsy and an inability to move or speak just before and after awakening. Hypnagogic hallucinations refer to a misinterpretation of sensory perception occurring while falling asleep and are normally not associated with a mental disorder.

Restless leg syndrome (RLS), and periodic limb movement disorder (PLMD) interfere with the quality of sleep, and further affect daytime quality of life through continued limb symptoms. These include a classic "creepy-crawly" feeling, deep-aching, inability to sit still, and a deep powerful aching in the legs (APA, 2000; Hauri & Cleveland-Hauri, 1999).

Common complaints from clients include "not feeling rested" or complaints of poor quality sleep and increased requests for sleeping aids.

Primary insomnia is diagnosed when other causes of insomnia are eliminated. The *DSM-IV-TR* diagnosis of primary insomnia requires that a client has difficulty falling or maintaining asleep or has non-restorative sleep, and experiences marked distress or social, occupational, or other area disturbances (APA, 2000). Moreover, this sleep disturbance is not related to other psychiatric or medical conditions previously listed under these criteria (APA, 2000).

In terms of psychiatric illness, children more commonly have a disorder within the parasomnias, such as nightmares, sleep terrors, talking in their sleep, and sleepwalking (APA, 2000).

Unfortunately, instead of exhibiting excessive daytime sleepiness, they often appear to be hyperactive, or irritable, preventing correct diagnosis (Kushida, 1999). Children also suffer more from **enuresis** (refers to bedwetting after being toilet trained), with concurrent psychological stresses associated with parental sleep deficit and disapproval and fear of peer knowledge of the disorder. These children may develop social isolation when they do not interact with other children, attend or host sleepovers, or have school-associated problems owing to the stress and sleep issues.

Teenagers are particularly prone to **delayed sleep phase syndrome (DSPS)**, with difficulty or delay of falling asleep, and thus difficulty waking (Spitzer et al., 1999).

In the older adult, almost 40 percent have some type of sleep disorder, with complaints of early morning awakenings, disturbed sleep, and daytime sleepiness (Vitiello, 1999). The sleep pattern in the older adult commonly results in a decrease in deep sleep cycles, with an increase in wakefulness.

Observing the client is essential, and, typically, the sleepless client presents with apparent fatigue, dark circles under the eyes, yawning, or even dozing while waiting to be seen. Sleepless clients can be irritable and impatient as well. Many of the signs of sleeplessness also are seen with anemia, hypoxia, cognitive deficits, and mental illness. A complete physical examination is always useful to rule out other, or concurrent, disease.

Key Fact

Common psychiatric disorders (e.g., anxiety disorders, dementia, mood disorders) and psychosocial factors, such as job-related stress and family and interpersonal stressors account for about 50 percent of all insomnia complaints (Folks, & Fuller, 1997; Hauri, 1998; Humphreys, Lee, Neylan, & Marmar, 1999; Kupfer & Reynolds, 1997).

TREATMENT

Because of the profound impact that sleep has on mental and physical functioning, nurses need to develop assessment skills that enable them to evaluate sleep disturbances and develop a plan of care that restores health. A review of basic sleep physiology is helpful in understanding the significance of restorative sleep and the potential health risks associated with non-restorative sleep.

Because of the profound impact that sleep has on mental and physical functioning, nurses need to understand its relevance when caring for the client who presents with psychiatric and medical conditions. In addition, nurses must recognize intricate factors that prevent normal or restorative sleep and develop a plan of care that restores it.

A thorough nursing assessment or evaluation is crucial to making an accurate diagnosis of a sleep disorder. By asking questions, such as the client's current sleeping patterns, family history, substance abuse history, caffeine consumption, current medications, both prescribed and over-the-counter (OTC), the nurse can make an accurate diagnosis.

Assessing the client's sleeping patterns need to be an integral part of treatment planning beginning with an initial assessment and throughout treatment. The nurse must collaborate with the client and family and identify effective measures to restore and maintain restorative sleep. See Table 12–2, Common Medical Conditions, Psychiatric Disorders, and Medications That Cause Insomnia.

An important part of the nursing assessment is identifying the cause of the clients' distress. Questions concerning the meaning of sleep and excessive worrying can provide invaluable information about the client's coping skills. Health education about exercise, diet, and maladaptive behaviors reduces stress and restores normal sleeping patterns.

Sometimes questions concerning OTC medications, dietary preparation, and beverages are overlooked during the nursing process. Because these agents interfere with normal sleeping patterns, nurses need to ask about them and provide appropriate health teaching to address these concerns.

Because sleep deprivation produces significant stress during acute illness, nurses must identify these high-risk groups, modify environmental factors, and promote rest and sleep. Nurses need to initiate interventions such as active listening, music, back rubs, and therapeutic touch that reduce pain and anxiety and promote a relaxation response.

Making a diagnosis of insomnia requires a complete physical and psychiatric evaluation to rule out medical and psychiatric conditions. Psychiatric nurses play key roles in the data collection process and must ask questions that elicit relevant data concerning the client's sleeping pattern, current medication, substance abuse, and family history of sleep disorders. The assessment process helps the nurse and other clinicians uncover causative factors and initiate appropriate treatment planning.

The most common pharmacologic interventions are the most common treatment strategy for primary insomnia (Kupfer & Reynolds, 1997). Symptoms of primary insomnia may respond to various medications, such as hypnotics. Hypnotics are the mainstay treatment for acute insomnia and play a limited role in chronic insomnia (Langer, Mendelson, & Richardson, 1999). Examples of common hypnotics include benzodiazepines (e.g.,

(continues)

TREATMENT (continued)

temazepam [Restoril]) and nonbenzodiazepines (zolpidem [Ambien], zaleplon [Sonata]).

See Table 12–3, Pharmacologic Agents Used to Treat Insomnia and Specific Medical Conditions.

Specific treatment should be initiated for disorders that are associated with sleep, such as RLS and PLMD, Parkinson's disease, and other dementias. Parkinson's disease, RLS, and PLMD generally respond to dopaminergically active medications such as pergolide (Permax), bromocriptine (Parlodel), and carbidopa/levodopa (Sinemet). Other choices include medications such as clonazepam (Klonopin, a controlled substance), gabapentin (Neurontin), or pain medications (Bexchlibynk-Butler & Jeffries, 2000).

Regardless of the pharmacologic agent, psychiatric nurses must assess their clients for desired and adverse side effects associated with these medications. Pharmacologic considerations for older adults taking sleep agents include monitoring their blood pressure and asking them to rise slowly from lying and sitting positions to reduce orthostatic hypotension. Encouraging hydration and oral hygiene reduces dry mouth and oral care. Cautioning clients to avoid operating vehicles and machinery is crucial to reduce fatal or dangerous accidents. Because of the risk of suicide among clients with chronic medical and psychiatric conditions, nurses need to assess the client's risk of danger to self and others throughout treatment planning. Certain diagnostic studies are necessary before and during some treatments, specifically when tricyclic antidepressants are used.

The explosion of complementary or alternative therapies offers clients with various sleep disorders an array of preparations. Most of the agents are derived from the dietary supplement melatonin and plants and include valerian and kava (Schultz, Hansel, & Tyler, 1998). Likewise, foods such as turkey and potatoes and, of course, warm milk, have tryptophan, which may promote rest and sleep.

Regardless of the treatment approach, psychiatric nurses play key roles in providing pharmacologic and nonpharmacologic interventions. Nonpharmacologic nursing interventions include psychosocial approaches such as deep breathing exercises, sleep hygiene stress management (Antai-Otong, 2001), relaxation, and cognitive-behavioral therapies.

(continues)

Table 12–3 • Pharmacologic Agents Used to Treat Insomnia and Specific Medical Conditions

Medication	Side Effects	Nursing Implications
Benzodiazepines flurazepam (Dalmane) temazepam (Restoril)	Psychological and physiological dependence CNS sedation Rebound insomnia	• Provide health education about sleep disorders • Educate about sleep hygiene • Monitor for signs of dependence or abuse (increase dose to achieve same effects) • Encourage to use nonpharmacologic (adjunct) interventions, including relaxation techniques • Assess level of danger to self and others • Encourage to keep sleep diary

(continues)

Table 12–3 *(continued)*

Medication	Side Effects	Nursing Implications
Nonbenzodiazepines (short-term use with various psychiatric disorders; sleep latency problems) zolpidem (Ambien) zaleplon (Sonata)	Contraindicated in clients with substance-related disorders and pregnancy Nausea Drowsiness/daytime sedation Sleepwalking Delirium Headache Potential for abuse/dependence	• Same as above—particularly for signs of abuse and psychological dependence • Encourage to use nonpharmacologic (adjunct) interventions, including relaxation techniques
Antidepressants (tricyclic) doxepin (Sinequan), useful in the treatment of chronic pain syndromes imipramine (Tofranil), helpful in the treatment of enuresis	Anticholinergic: dry mouth, blurred vision, constipation, urinary retention Cardiotoxic (lethal in overdosing) Sedation Orthostasis Weight gain Delirium* Cognitive deficits*	• Health education, same as above • Assess for suicide throughout treatment • Provide health education that reduces anticholinergic side effects (e. g., high roughage diet and fluids [if not contraindicated]) • Encourage a regular exercise program (as medically safe) • Order baseline ECG prior to beginning tricyclics, including children • Instruct to rise slowly to reduce dizziness and falls—risks associated with orthostasis
Antidepressants trazodone (Desyrel), increases Stages III and IV nefazodone (Serzone)†	Anticholinergic properties Priapism Sexual dysfunction Daytime sedation	• Same as above, except encourage men to report erectile or sexual difficulties (women the latter) • Monitor liver enzyme levels; ask to report change in color of urine, stool, sclera, or skin
Anticonvulsants (restless leg syndome and pain syndromes) gabapentin (Neurontin)	Neurotoxic Sedation Ataxia Confusion Weight gain	• Same as above except for erectile problems and liver enzymes

ECG, electrocardiogram; *Higher risk in older adults; †FDA (black box warning concerning liver damage).

Note. Data from "Sleep Problems Associated with Mood and Anxiety Disorders," by R. Benca, 1999, *Primary Psychiatry*, *6*, pp. 52–60; "Management of Insomnia: A Meta-analysis of Treatment of Efficacy," by D. J. Kupfer and C. F. Reynolds, 1997, *American Journal of Psychiatry*, *336*, pp. 341–346; *American Hospital Formulary Service* (pp. 2311–2343), by G. K. McEvoy, 2001, Bethesda, MD: American Society of Health-Systems Pharmacists; and "Treating Insomnia in the Depressed Patient: Practical Considerations," by T. Roth, 1999, *Hospital Medicine*, *49*, pp. 23–28. Adapted with permission.

TREATMENT *(continued)*

Deep abdominal breathing exercises and stress management techniques help the client gain control of physiological manifestations of anxiety and stress. Brisk walks, regular exercise, and a balanced diet also promote health and promote rest. Stressing the importance and role of sleep in health promotion through health education using sleep hygiene and a sleep diary provides the client with a sense of control. Ultimately, health teaching and other psychosocial interventions return the client's normal sleeping patterns and improve quality of life. See Table 12–4, Behavioral Rules for Good Sleep Hygiene.

Cognitive-behavioral therapy is another psychosocial and behavioral intervention that is limited to the advanced-practice psychiatric nurse practice who is educationally prepared and nationally certified. Major goals of cognitive-behavioral therapy include reducing cognitive and biological arousal and helping the client challenge distorted cognitions, such as "all or none" thinking that generate distress. Clients presenting with various pain syndromes, anxiety, and mood disorders can benefit from cognitive-behavioral therapy (Antai-Otong, 2000; Currie, Wilson, Pontefract, & deLaplante, 2000).

Disorders such as post-traumatic stress syndrome, of which insomnia is a major manifestation, should benefit from ongoing therapy as well as a variety of medications that may be helpful, such as antidepressants and antianxiety agents. Clients with panic and anxiety disorders often benefit more from combination therapy, counseling, and medications than from medications alone, because triggering the episodes may be linked to specific stimuli that the client needs help to work through.

Health promotion is an integral part of nursing practice. Facilitating the clients' return to normal or restorative sleep is a major concern for psychiatric nurses. Health promotion begins by establishing a trusting relationship with the clients, families, and significant others.

Table 12–4 • Behavioral Rules for Good Sleep Hygiene

1. Avoid using bed for activities other than sleep.

2. If sleep does not occur after lying awake for 15 minutes (whether initially or on early awakening), get out of bed and do something that facilitates sleep, such as reading a boring book, until sleepiness occurs.

3. Avoid caffeine after 6 P.M. (some say noon, or no caffeine at all).

4. Use relaxation techniques.

5. Go to bed and arise at planned times on a daily basis.

6. Avoid worrying or trying to resolve issues before bedtime.

7. Avoid alcohol before bedtime.

8. Avoid napping during the day.

9. Eliminate pre-sleep activities that create arousal, such as exercise, watching violent television, work, or socializing.

10. Remove the clock from the bedroom, or face the numbers away from the bed.

11. Create a quiet, dark sleep environment.

12. Avoid nicotine.

13. Avoid large meals close to bedtime, but do not go to bed hungry.

14. If using diuretics, take them early in the day, and empty the bladder before going to bed.

15. If using a hypnotic or other medications for sleep, avoid using them on a daily basis.

16. Maintain a cool room temperature because it facilitates sleep if the individual has adequate covering; a room that is too hot or too cold will interfere with sleep.

The generalist nurse offers an array of health-promoting activities. This process begins by assessing the client's holistic needs and stressing the importance of health-promoting activities that restore

(continues)

TREATMENT *(continued)*

normal sleeping patterns. A thorough nursing assessment needs to include the client's normal sleeping patterns, duration of sleep disturbances, psychiatric and medical histories, level of danger to self and others, and cultural and personal preferences. The generalist nurse also collects data concerning the client's physical health, including vital signs, neurological status, and relevant aspects of the mental status examination. In addition, the generalist nurse reviews client data and synthesizes data that assist the mental health team in making a differential diagnosis. Once the diagnosis is confirmed, the nurse provides appropriate interventions such as crisis intervention, stress management, and relaxation techniques.

The role of the advanced-practice psychiatric nurse, like the generalist nurse, needs to focus on health promotions that facilitate restorative sleep. They promote sleep and quality of life by providing psychosocial and cognitive-behavioral therapies and pharmacologic interventions. Initially, the advanced-practice nurse performs a comprehensive mental status examination and orders appropriate diagnostic studies to rule out medical and psychiatric disorders. Once a differential diagnosis is made, the advanced-practice nurse will develop an individualized treatment plan.

Characteristics associated with sleep disorders are easily assessed through interviewing the client and her significant other(s). The individual can simply be asked if she sleeps well, for about 8 hours, and if she wakes up feeling refreshed, all of which are necessary components of restorative sleep. It assesses the likeliness of dozing in a variety of situations, such as while reading, sitting, and talking to someone, and at the extreme, in a car while stopped in traffic. Use of a scale in a clinical setting is very helpful, because it may help diagnose a problem initially (and provides documentation), and it can be reused to follow and document the course and treatment of a problem.

Other questions should address any difficulties falling asleep; early awakenings; sleep interruptions; the perception of not sleeping; falling asleep when not stimulated (as in a boring meeting); fatigue or lack of energy, difficulties with concentration and memory; and psychiatric symptoms such as anxiety and changes of mood.

Other diagnostic criteria include sleep studies and monitoring for abnormal laboratory results, which might indicate sleep problems such as an elevated or depressed thyroid-stimulating hormone (TSH), elevated or depressed potassium, calcium, or magnesium levels, which can lead to muscle spasms or somnolence. Other studies include complete blood count to rule out anemia and diagnostic studies to rule out arrhythmias.

The following are potential nursing diagnoses that can be considered for the client who presents with a sleep disorder (North American Nursing Diagnosis Association [NANDA], 2001):

- Disturbed Sleep Pattern
- Ineffective Coping
- Risk for Self-Directed Violence
- Fatigue
- Situational Low Self-Esteem
- Anxiety

The client's goals for sleep are often much different from the nurses' goals for the client. Client goals that facilitate major client outcomes include:

- The client will be able to express feelings rather than acting on them.
- The client will be able to express feelings appropriately and express that he feels in control of life again.
- Reduce the number of times the client gets up during the night from three to one.
- List two or three positive personal attributes.
- The client will express feeling less fatigue and be able to tolerate performing specific activities of daily living within 2 weeks.

The psychiatric nurse and the client need to collaborate a plan of care that *(continues)*

TREATMENT *(continued)*

reflects identified nursing diagnoses and outcome measures. Treatment considerations need to be evidence-based and client centered. In addition, nursing interventions need to integrate biological, psychosocial, and cognitive modalities that facilitate sleep restoration and help the client manage medical and psychiatric conditions. Family and significant others must be included in the treatment planning process, which can elicit the client's goals related to his personal needs for sleep and rest.

Implementing a plan of care for the client with a sleep disorder requires using an array of interventions that promote sleep. Depending on the practice settings, nursing interventions may range from structuring the client's environment by reducing noise or light, such as in an extended care unit, to teaching the client cognitive-behavioral techniques to reduce cognitive distortions. Medication administration and prescriptive authority reduce biological aspects of the sleep disorder, whereas psychosocial interventions can strengthen coping skills and increase self-esteem.

Evaluation focuses on client responses. In this case, major outcome measures and evaluation include the following:

- Develop adaptive coping skills to manage present stressors and restore confidence and self-esteem.
- Return to the prehospitalization sleeping patterns.
- Increase energy (self-report) and be able to perform designated activities (gradually) as medical condition permits.

RESOURCES

Please note that because Internet resources are of a time-sensitive nature and URL addresses may change or be deleted, searches should also be conducted by association or topic.

Internet Resources

http://www.aasmnet.org American Academy of Sleep Medicine
http://www.asda.org American Sleep Disorders Foundation
http://www.sleepfoundation.org National Sleep Foundation
http://www.rls.org Restless Leg Syndrome Foundation
http://bisleep.medsch.ucla.edu Sleep Home Pages

Somatization Disorders

13

• Key Terms

Body Dysmorphic Disorder: A chronic and debilitating mental health condition characterized by a preoccupation with imagined defect in appearance (e.g., a "large" nose, "thinning" hair, or facial "scarring").

Conversion Disorders: Refer to unexplained physical manifestations or deficits affecting voluntary motor or sensory function that suggest a neurological or other underlying medical condition.

Fibromyalgia Syndrome: A nonspecific condition whose primary symptoms include diffuse musculoskeletal pain, fatigue, distress, and sleep disturbances.

Hypochondriasis: Refers to persistent preoccupation with fears of having, or the idea that one has, a serious disease based on the person's misinterpretation or exaggeration of bodily functions.

Pain Disorder: Disorder whose major symptom is pain in one or more anatomical sites. It is the predominant focus of the clinical presentation and is of sufficient severity that necessitates clinical attention. It also produces significant distress that results in impaired occupational, interpersonal, and social performance.

Somatoform: Refers to a group of psychiatric disorders whose symptoms are severe enough to cause global impairment or functioning. Typically, these clients present with recurring, multiple, clinically significant somatic complaints. In addition, these complaints are colorful and exaggerated, but lack specific factual information to support the diagnosis.

According to the Diagnostic and Statistical Manual of Mental Disorders *(4th edition Text Revision)* (DSM-IV-TR) *(APA, 2000),* **somatoform** *refers to a group of psychiatric disorders whose symptoms are severe enough to cause global impairment or functioning.*

SOMATIZATION DISORDERS—GENERAL

Causes

The precise cause of somatoform disorders remains obscure, but many studies indicate various factors such as genetic, personality style, biological, neuroanatomical, culture, and psychosocial stressors. Many of these disorders occur comorbidly with other mental disorders, namely, anxiety and depressive disorders, and challenge nurses to address both their physical and mental conditions.

The psychoanalytic theory suggests that symptoms represent a substitution for repressed instinctual impulses and are best depicted by the concept of *hysteria.* Paul Briquet (1859) first recognized the syndrome characterized by multiple dramatic medical complaints in the absence of a physiological basis. Because of his noted observations, this condition was called *Briquet's syndrome* at one time. Later this syndrome would be referred to as somatization disorder. In comparison, Freud (Breuer & Freud, 1893–1895/1955) focused most of his work on the concept of hysteria and postulated that the mechanism of the ego defense mechanism of conversion represented hysteria. That is, this mechanism was conceptualized as converting "psychic energy" into physical manifestations. Briquet's hysteria concept was further refined by adding a quantitative perspective by Purell, Robins, and Cohen (1951) and further defined by Perley and Guze (1962). Eventually, major symptoms of hysteria involving varied somatic complaints were comorbid with anxiety and depressive symptoms.

Conversion stems from the premise that the person's physical manifestations depict a symbolic resolution of an unconscious psychological conflict, reducing anxiety and serving to hide the conflict from awareness. This manifestation is referred to as a primary gain. In contrast, secondary gain stems from the conversion symptom or external manifestation, and benefits involve evading negative responsibilities (APA, 2000).

There is prevailing evidence that somatization is associated with substantial emotional distress expressing underlying anxiety, depression, and stress-related disorders (e.g., adjustment disorders).

The literature consistently reveals that females are more likely to report ill health than males despite some controversy about the true excess prevalence or by female-specific patterns of health care utilization. The incidence of reporting physical symptoms seems even higher in women in low socioeconomic class and high emotional distress (Ladwig, Martin, Mittag, Erazo, & Gundel, 2001). The sick role is often accepted, validated, and reinforced within various social contexts as a coping response. Acceptance of the sick role suggests that they are more likely to frame their bodily changes as ill health. Consequently, women tend to respond more emotionally when their physical function is perceived to be or actually is impaired (Ladwig et al., 2001; Macintyre, Hunt, & Sweeting, 1996). Although women seem to be at a greater risk of developing these disorders, some data also indicate that social class and high emotional stress increase the risk in men (Ladwig et al., 2001).

Although the findings are inconsistent, some researchers have found an increased prevalence of childhood abuse in some cases of these disorders. Comorbid conditions associated with somatoform disorders include other somatoform disorders, depression, anxiety, and borderline personality disorders (APA, 2000; Arnold & Privitera, 1996; Lesser, 1996; Tojek, Lumley, Barkley, Mahr, & Thomas, 2000). A recent review of the literature concerning somatization disorders indicates that these behaviors may result from complex childhood experiences of illness and the responses of the person's social system to the adult behavior (Stuart & Noyes, 1999). These researchers also submit that early life experiences serve as diatheses, governing illness behavior and resulting in maladaptive coping or personality traits. Likewise, interpersonal stressors occurring during adulthood are likely to generate somatizing behavior in high-risk groups. Based on this premise, health-seeking behavior is synonymous with attachment behavior and assists in procuring or retaining "closeness" to another person for the purpose of receiving care. Unfortunately, this adult attachment behavior (Bowlby, 1973; 1977; 1988) is reinforced each time the client receives attention and "care" for somatization symptoms, thereby gratifying their attachment needs. Maladaptive attachment behaviors tend to be fixed and rigid, often resulting in the client being more sensitive to perceived or actual threats and persistently seeking help from others (Stuart & Noyes, 1999).

Because of the intimate relationship between the brain and complex physiological processes, it is conceivable that there is dysregulation in perceptions of an event and subsequent physiological responses. Exaggerated appraisal of risk, danger, and vulnerability to disease or illness may play key roles in the cognitive distortion of somatoform disorders (e.g., hypochondriasis).

Studies show an array of theories concerning the neurobiological causes of somatoform disorders, ranging from genetics to neurotransmitter dysregulation in pain disorders. According to the *DSM-IV-TR* (APA, 2000), many somatoform disorders have familial patterns and show that male relatives of women with these disorders are predisposed to the risk of personality disorders and other psychiatric conditions (APA, 2000). In addition, recent functional and brain imaging studies reveal that alterations in neuroanatomical structures and regional brain perfusion may accompany some disorders (e.g., conversion symptoms) (Yazici & Kostakoglu, 1998).

There is a plethora of strong empirical data concerning the substantial role of cross-culture transition and psychological distress in somatization. In addition, factors such as duration of immigration, self-reported health problems, and help-seeking behaviors appear to contribute to these disorders (Ritsner, Ponizovsky, Kurs, & Modai, 2000).

Prior studies also link other factors such as gender, age, marital status, low educational and socioeconomic status, and minority ethnicity (Escobar, Ribio-Stepec, Canino, & Karno, 1989; Ford, 1986). There are inconsistent data concerning gender issues (Ohaeri & Odejide, 1994; Piccinelli & Simon, 1997; Wool & Barsky, 1994).

Unquestionably, the precise causes of somatoform disorders remain obscure. However, most data suggest an association between underlying psychological distress, neurobiological processes, and symptomatology. These considerations strengthen the argument that these disorders are an integral part of anxiety and depressive disorders continuum.

These clients often grow up in families who are inconsistent, unreliable, and provide little or no emotional support.

Symptoms

Typically, these clients present with recurring, multiple, clinically significant somatic complaints. In addition, these complaints are colorful and exaggerated but lack specific factual information to support the diagnosis. Specific somatoform disorders include somatization disorder, conversion disorder, hypochondriasis, body dysmorphic disorder, and pain disorder.

Typically, these clients are vague historians, but their presentations are often dramatic and they report detailed and complicated medical problems. They are tenacious in seeking medical attention and are likely to be seeing more than one health provider at a time. Their histories also reveal chaos, impulsiveness, manipulative behaviors, suicidal threats or attempts, unstable occupational and social functioning, and turbulent interpersonal relationships (Bass & Murphy, 1995; Kaminsky & Slavney, 1976; Stuart & Noyes, 1999).

Key Fact

Recent studies of primary care clients show that the prevalence may be as high as 30 to 60 percent of symptoms that have no medical basis. Because of the high incidence of comorbidity with other psychiatric disorders, such as anxiety, depression, and personality disorders, some researchers believe that somatization disorders may manifest personality pathology with traits of histrionic, borderline, and antisocial personality disorders (Bass & Murphy, 1995; Lilienfeld, 1992; Stuart & Noyes, 1999).

TREATMENT

When working with clients with somatization disorders it is imperative for the nurse to understand the meaning of their symptoms. Notably, physical symptoms that cannot be explained by an underlying medical condition need to be explained as a coping mechanism that enables the client to respond to stressors, similarly to the way anxiety and depression reflect distress. Implications for nursing care include assessing the client's needs, setting firm and consistent limits, and balancing empathy with structure. It is crucial that nurses recognize manipulative behavioral patterns and avoid reinforcing dependency. Clients with somatoform disorders tend to be tenacious and use persistent complaints of pain and physical illness to elicit care from the nurse. Because of the self-defeating nature of these behaviors, nurses may reject clients, further reinforcing their somatic symptoms. Formulating nursing interventions that promote self-reliance, confidence, problem solving, and independence are crucial

aspects of treatment planning. Psychotherapy and other forms of cognitive therapy and pharmacologic interventions are indicated when the nurse assesses these maladaptive coping patterns.

During the data collection process, the psychiatric nurse needs to conduct a thorough family history of symptoms, treatment, and comorbid conditions. Assessment information is relative to understanding family coping patterns, motivation for treatment, and prior treatment outcomes.

Major components of the assessment include history, severity and duration of symptoms; level of functioning; present stressors; and coping patterns. The nurse needs to avoid confrontations, and provided instructions must be clear, direct, and respond to crises empathetically. Keep visits for medical complaints brief and assist the client in understanding the symptoms as emotional communication rather than an underlying medical condition.

An important part of the assessment process is the client's illness perception. Danish researchers Fink, Rosendal, and Toft (2002) developed a comprehensive treatment and assessment approach of functional (somatic) disorders and suggested the following questions for understanding the client's illness perception:

- Identify the illness: What does the client think is wrong?
- Cause: What does the client believe is the basis of her symptoms—physical or psychosocial?
- Duration: How long does the client believe present symptoms will last—acute or chronic?
- Consequences: What effects will the symptoms have on the client's ability to function?
- Recovery and self-efficacy: What are the client's prospects of recovering and what types of treatment are available? What kind of control does the client have over the illness, or how much control does the client have over present symptoms?

(continues)

TREATMENT *(continued)*

Despite the explosion of ethnocultural studies, nurses and other health care professionals may find it difficult to accurately interpret the meaning of a client's culture-bound syndromes. For instance, some cultures, such as Southeast Asia, may consider somatic symptoms rather than depressive feelings as a legitimate basis for seeking treatment (Kirmayer & Weiss, 1997; Kirmayer & Young, 1998). Understanding the meaning of the client's somatic symptoms and identifying underlying distress enable the nurse to distinguish culture-bound symptoms from somatization. This process requires asking questions that facilitate understanding of symptoms within a social and cultural context. Recognizing the high level of distress among immigrants and the need to strengthen their social networks and coping skills and understand the meaning of their symptoms from a cultural perspective are crucial to their care. In addition, psychiatric nurses need to understand the impact of their own culture and its effect on the analysis of the client's experience. These assessment data guide the assessment process, help make an accurate diagnosis, facilitate culturally sensitive nursing interventions, and promote positive outcomes. See Table 13–1, Cultural Expression of Somatization.

Most studies suggest that treating somatoform disorders is challenging and requires a diverse treatment approach that involves the following principles once the diagnosis is confirmed:

1. Establish a firm and therapeutic relationship with the client and family.
2. Differentiate manipulative and other maladaptive behaviors from cultural factors.
3. Provide health education concerning major symptoms (e.g., inform clients that they are not going "crazy," prognosis, treatment outcomes).
4. Be firm and consistent and provide reassurance.
5. When indicated, treat anxiety and depressive symptoms.

Predictably, these clients are difficult to manage in most practice settings and many clinicians find them difficult to engage in a therapeutic relationship. A major challenge for psychiatric nurses involves patience, empathy, and firm limit

(continues)

Table 13–1 • Cultural Expression of Somatization

Culture	Symptoms
Jewish immigrants to Israel	"Heart distress" associated with personal and social concerns related to grief and loss.
Korean	*hwa-byung.* Somatic expression of anger or rage found mainly in lower socioeconomic, married women: feelings of heaviness, epigastric burning or mass; headaches, muscle pain, sleep disturbances, palpitations, and indigestion. It also includes depressive symptoms, irritable mood, underlying resentment, despair, and interpersonal and social problems.
South Asia (India)	*dhat syndrome.* Associated with semen loss. Treatment of comorbid anxiety or depression may alleviate symptoms.

Note. The data in column 2 are from "Somatization in an Immigrant Population in Israel: A Community Survey of Prevalence, Risk Factors, and Help-Seeking Behavior," by M. Ritsner, A. Ponizovsky, R. Kurs, and I. Modai, 2000, *American Journal of Psychiatry, 157,* pp. 385–392; "Hwa-byung: A Community Study of Korean Americans," by K.-M. Lin, J. K. C. Lau, J. Yamamoto, Y. P. Zheng, H. S. Kim, K. H. Cho, et al., 1992, *Journal of Nervous and Mental Disorders, 180,* pp. 386–391; and from "The 'Dhat Syndrome': A Culturally Determined Form of Depression?" by D. B. Mumford, 1996, *Acta Psychiatrica Scandinavica, 94,* pp. 163–167. Adapted with permission.

TREATMENT *(continued)*

setting. Setting limits offers structure and facilitates a supportive environment that fosters a therapeutic nurse-client relationship. See Table 13–2, Diagnostic Criteria for Somatization Disorders.

It is very important to understand that the client with a somatization disorder may actually suffer emotionally because of their unyielding belief that they will not be cared for (Stuart & Noyes, 1999). Although there is no physical basis for these concerns, the thoughts of being ill and needing help often result in debilitat-

ing depression or anxiety, which need to be treated accordingly (e.g., antidepressants, psychotherapy). Working with the client with somatization disorder challenges the nurse to conduct thorough physical and mental status examinations that assist in making a differential diagnosis of a medical condition or comorbid mental disorder or factitious disorder.

It is imperative for the nurse to assess the role of the child's symptoms in the family and cultural factors. The complexity of childhood- and family-related issues concerning somatization require

(continues)

Table 13–2 • Diagnostic Criteria for Somatization Disorder

A. A history of many physical complaints beginning before age 30 years that occur over a period of several years and result in treatment being sought or significant impairment in social, occupational, or other important areas of functioning.

B. Each of the following criteria must have been met, with individual symptoms occurring at any time during the course of the disturbance:

- Four pain symptoms: a history of pain related to at least four different sites or functions (e.g., head, abdomen, back, joints, extremities, chest, rectum, during menstruation, during sexual intercourse, or during urination)

- Two gastrointestinal symptoms: a history of at least two gastrointestinal symptoms other than pain (e.g., nausea, bloating, vomiting other than during pregnancy, diarrhea, or intolerance of several foods)

- One sexual symptom: a history of at least one sexual or reproductive symptom other than pain (e.g., sexual indifference, erectile or ejaculatory dysfunction, irregular menses, excessive menstrual bleeding, vomiting through pregnancy)

- One pseudoneurological symptom: a history of at least one symptom or deficit suggesting a neurological condition not limited to pain (conversion symptoms such as impaired coordination or balance, paralysis or localized weakness, difficulty swallowing or lump in the throat, aphonia, urinary retention, hallucinations, loss of touch or pain sensation, double vision, blindness, deafness, seizures, dissociative symptoms such as amnesia, or loss of consciousness other than fainting)

  Either (1) or (2):

  1. after appropriate investigation, each of the symptoms in Criterion B cannot be fully explained by a known general medical condition or the direct effects of a substance (e.g., a drug of abuse, a medication)

  2. when there is a related general medical condition, the physical complaints or resulting social or occupational impairment are in excess of what would be expected from the history, physical examination, or laboratory findings

The symptoms are not intentionally feigned or produced (as in factitious disorder or malingering).

Note. From *Diagnostic and Statistical Manual of Mental Disorders* (4th edition Text Revision) (*DSM-IV-TR*), by American Psychiatric Association, 2000, Washington, DC: Author. Adapted with permission.

TREATMENT *(continued)*

family and other psychotherapies to address these issues. Health education is also an integral part of working with children and their families, and focusing on communication patterns and dysfunctional interactions may reduce tension and family stress.

Treatment considerations include client-centered and age-specific interventions. Many problems relating to somatoform disorders have their bases for development during childhood. The client's level of functioning and quality of life are bound to be impaired after years of these debilitating disorders. Efforts to assess the client's needs and preference and encouraging an optimal level of functioning are major treatment foci for the older adult.

The generalist needs to approach the client in a caring, nonjudgmental and firm manner that reduces manipulation or other maladaptive behaviors. Psychosocial stressors appear to exacerbate physical symptoms and emotional distress and must be assessed. Because of the high prevalence of mood and anxiety disorders, the nurse needs to assess the client's level of functioning, reasons for seeking treatment, and risk of dangerousness. Working with the interdisciplinary team enables the generalist nurse to provide structure and firm and consistent limit setting that enable the client to reach an optimal level of functioning and reduce preoccupations with health-seeking behaviors. The assessment process is ongoing and it is key to crisis resolution, symptom management, and appropriate illness perception. Cultural factors must also be assessed to determine their role in symptom manifestation. Stress management techniques, client and family health education, medication administration, and monitoring are important nursing interventions for the client and family presenting with a somatization disorder.

The advanced-practice psychiatric-mental health nurse is likely to collaborate with other health care providers and develop a holistic plan of care that includes pharmacologic and nonpharmacologic interventions. Pharmacologic interventions may include prescriptive authority and medication management. Oftentimes, the advanced-practice nurse coordinates with the medical team or acts as a psychiatric liaison consultant in various inpatient and primary care settings to address the client's physical and mental health concerns. Nonpharmacologic interventions include various psychotherapies, such as individual, family, and group, to improve or reduce cognitive distortions that perpetuate somatization.

BODY DYSMORPHIC DISORDER

Causes

A recent population-based study of BDD showed that it is significantly associated with comorbid major depression and anxiety disorder. The highest comorbid anxiety disorders include social phobia and obsessive-compulsive disorder (OCD). These data also demonstrate its overall prevalence of about 0.7 percent in women (Otto, Wilhelm, Cohen, & Harlow, 2001). Phillips and colleagues found a 13.8 percent lifetime history of BDD highest in clients with OCD (Phillips, Gunderson, Gophincth, & McElroy, 1998).

Symptoms

Body dysmorphic disorder (BDD) is a chronic and debilitating mental health condition characterized by a preoccupation with imagined defect in appearance (e.g., a "large" nose, "thinning" hair, or facial "scarring") (APA, 2000; Phillips, 1996). It often results in social isolation, unnecessary medical procedures, and occupational and interpersonal impairments.

Recent studies show that people with BDD have some cognitive and memory deficits demonstrated by poor performance on neuropsychological tests (Abbruzzese, Bellodi, Ferri, & Scarone, 1995; Hanes, 1998). Specific deficits seem to indicate poor performance on executive tasks such as learning, long- and short-term memory recall, and organization of verbal and nonverbal memory. Clinical symptoms that reflect these deficits may include preoccupations that result in obsessional thinking and compulsive behaviors and avoidance of various tasks, including work, school, and social interactions. See Table 13–3 for the *DSM-IV-TR* criteria for body dysmorphic disorder (APA, 2000).

Key Fact

A note of interest when dealing with clients with BDD is that a small percentage of them has a history of corrective surgeries ranging from plastic to dermatology (Phillips, 2000a).

TREATMENT

Currently, there is no mainstay treatment or best practice model for BDD. However, there are promising results from pharmacologic interventions such as the serotonin selective reuptake inhibitors (SSRIs). Clients with BDD seem to require higher doses that are useful in the treatment of BDD with comorbid OCD and depressive symptoms. A partial response of these agents with adjunct buspirone (BuSpar) offer improved treatment (Phillips, 2000b). Other studies indicate the efficacy of clomipramine (Anafranil), a tricyclic with potent serotonin properties (Hollander et al., 1999). Clomipramine is also indicated in the treatment of OCD. A combination of an SSRI medication and cognitive-behavioral therapy, to reframe negative thoughts and maladaptive behaviors,

have also demonstrated symptom reduction (Kroenke & Swindle, 2000; Phillips, 2000b; Phillips, Dwight, & McElroy, 1998).

Although the client with BDD presents a challenging clinical picture, psychiatric nurses need to use an empathic and sensitive approach and assess their preoccupations with personal appearance and resulting emotional distress. Areas of particular interest during the assessment and treatment planning include determining the level of global impairment owing to their preoccupations and excessive time spent worrying about their appearance.

CONVERSION DISORDER

Symptoms

Conversion disorders refer to unexplained physical manifestations or deficits affecting voluntary motor or sensory function that suggest a neurological or other underlying medical condition.

According to the *DSM-IV-TR* (APA, 2000), the criteria shown in Table 13–4 are necessary for a diagnosis of conversion disorders.

TREATMENT

Major treatment must avoid reinforcing maladaptive behaviors and focus on helping the client develop effective stress management and coping behaviors. If comorbid conditions, such as anxiety or depression, exist, they need to be treated accordingly with pharmacologic or nonpharmacologic approaches.

Table 13–3 • Diagnostic Criteria for Body Dysmorphic Disorder

A. Preoccupation with an imagined defect in appearance. If a slight anomaly is present, the person's concerns are even greater.

B. The preoccupation causes marked significant distress or impairment in social, occupational, or other important areas of functioning.

C. The preoccupation is not better accounted for by another mental disorder such as dissatisfaction with body shape and size as in anorexia nervosa.

Note. From *Diagnostic and Statistical Manual of Mental Disorders* (4th edition Text Revision) (*DSM-IV-TR*), by American Psychiatric Association, 2000, Washington, DC: Author. Adapted with permission.

Table 13-4 • Diagnostic Criteria for Conversion Disorders

A. One or more symptoms or deficits affect voluntary motor sensory function that suggest a neurological or other underlying medical condition.

B. Psychological factors are deemed to be associated with the symptom or deficit because the initiation or exacerbation of the symptom or deficit is preceded by conflicts or other stressors.

C. The symptom or deficit is not intentionally produced or feigned (as in factitious disorder or malingering).

D. The symptom or deficit cannot, after appropriate investigation, be fully explained by an underlying general medical condition, or by direct effects of a substance, or as a culturally sanctioned behavior or experience.

E. The symptom or deficit causes clinically significant distress or impairment in social, occupational, or other important areas of functioning or warrants medical evaluation.

F. The symptom or deficit is not limited to pain or sexual function, does not occur exclusively during the course of somatization disorder, and is not better accounted for by another mental disorder.

Specify type or deficit:

With motor symptom or deficit

With sensory symptom or deficit

With seizures or convulsions

With mixed presentation

Note. From *Diagnostic and Statistical Manual of Mental Disorders* (4th edition Text Revision) (*DSM-IV-TR*), by American Psychiatric Association, 2000, Washington, DC: Author. Adapted with permission.

FIBROMYALGIA SYNDROME

Although **fibromyalgia syndrome** (FMS) is not considered a somatoform disorder, it is a common and complex musculoskeletal pain disorder whose features are similar to various somatoform disorders, including comorbid and depressive features.

Causes

The exact cause of this pain disorder is unknown; however, the literature indicates that biological, psychosocial, and social factors may predispose, precipitate, and maintain symptoms (Demitrack & Abbey, 1996; Wessely, Hotopf, & Sharpe, 1998). Some clients with fibromyalgia report histories of varied forms of abuse, further strengthening the argument concerning the role of psychosocial factors and stress in this disorder (Boisset-Pioro,

Esdaile, & Fitzcharles, 1995; Taylor, Trotter, & Csuka, 1995).

Symptoms

The American College of Rheumatology (1990), whose Web site address is http://www.rheumatology.org/research/classification/fibro.html, established criteria for FMS as:

A. Widespread pain for at least 3 months and not localized in one area, with various area involvement, including both sides of the body, over and above the waist, and axial skeletal pain

B. Presence of 11 or 18 tender points, including:
Designated occipital sites
Lower cervical, trapezius, gluteal area
Greater trochanter and knees

C. Sleep disturbances during non-rapid eye movement (NREM) sleep, reduced delta sleep, and increased arousal—leading to sleep deprivation or unrestful sleep

D. Emotional distress, depression

E. Fatigue

Depressed states are considered universal among these clients.

Key Fact

The lifetime prevalence of fibromyalgia is about 2 percent in community samples, and it occurs twice as often as rheumatoid arthritis, constituting a major health problem (Walker et al., 1997).

TREATMENT

Like somatoform disorders, treatment planning should focus on an interdisciplinary and holistic approach. Pharmacologic interventions using tricyclic agents and other antidepressants (e.g., fluoxetine [Prozac], doxepin [Sinequan], nortriptyline [Pamelor]) (Arnold, Keck, & Welge, 2000) offer some relief from widespread pain and depression. Other nursing interventions include stress management, meditation and yoga, and sleep manipulation. Assessing the client's risk of danger to self and others is also an integral part of treatment.

HYPOCHRONDRIASIS

The prevalence of hypochondriasis in the general population is 1 to 5 percent. Among primary care populations, the estimates may range from 2 to 7 percent. Like other somatoform disorders, the onset of this disorder could begin at any age, but it is more likely to occur during early adulthood. It is chronic and has a waxing and waning course.

Symptoms

Clients with **hypochondriasis** often focus on their fears of having, or the notion that they have a serious disease owing to an exaggerated appraisal of risk or vulnerability to disease. Oftentimes, these clients sense imminent peril and vulnerability to disease. This sense of heightened physical risk is focused and limited to having a disease or disease-related fears. In addition, the client's history reveals a misinterpretation of benign bodily sensations that are mistakenly associated with a suspected and dreaded illness, health hazard, and physical preoccupation. See Table 13–5 for the *DSM-IV-TR* (APA, 2000) diagnostic criteria for hypochondriasis.

Table 13–5 • Diagnostic Criteria for Hypochondriasis

A. Preoccupation with fears of having, or the idea that one has, a serious disease based on the person's misinterpretation or exaggeration of bodily functions.

B. The preoccupation persists despite appropriate medical evaluation and reassurance.

C. The belief in Criterion A is not of a delusional nature (as in delusional disorder, somatic type) and is not restricted to a circumscribed concern about appearance (as in body dysmorphic disorder).

D. The preoccupation causes clinically significant distress or impairment in social, occupational, or other important areas of functioning.

E. The duration of the disturbance is at least 6 months.

F. Generalized anxiety disorder, obsessive-compulsive, does not better account for the preoccupation disorder, panic disorder, a major depressive episode, separation anxiety, or another somatoform disorder.

Specify if:

With Poor Insight

Note. From *Diagnostic and Statistical Manual of Mental Disorders* (4th edition Text Revision) (*DSM-IV-TR*), by American Psychiatric Association, 2000, Washington, DC: Author. Adapted with permission.

TREATMENT

Mental health professionals can help clients with hypochondriasis if they are encouraged to seek help. Various psychotherapies, such as cognitive-behavioral therapy can be useful. This treatment approach helps the client understand distorted or problematic thought patterns, beliefs about self and illness, and related emotional distress. When working with these clients the nurse needs to understand the chronicity of this disorder and its potentially disabling course. It is crucial for the nurse and other health care providers to conduct comprehensive mental and physical status examinations to rule out true physical illnesses. Because of their use of health care resources with little resolution, clients with hypochondriasis are likely to express frustration and discouragement about their symptoms. Nurses need to approach these clients with an accepting and nonjudgmental attitude, but should avoid reinforcing preoccupation with bodily functions and illness.

PAIN DISORDER

Symptoms

The hallmark of **pain disorder** is pain of sufficient severity that warrants clinical attention. The association between depression and medically unexplained pain is well documented (Dickens, Jayson, & Creed, 2002; Jorgensen, Fink, & Olesen, 2000; Maier & Falkai, 1999, von Knorring, 1994). Table 13–6 lists major criteria of pain disorder.

According to the *DSM-IV-TR* (APA, 2000), pain disorder is divided into acute and chronic categories.

Key Fact

Regardless of comorbidity with depression or anxiety, pain produces significant distress and disability in functioning.

Table 13–6 • Diagnostic Criteria for Pain Disorder

A. Pain in one or more anatomical sites is the predominant focus of the clinical presentation and is of sufficient severity that necessitates clinical attention.

B. The pain causes clinically substantial distress or impairment in social, occupational, or important areas of interest.

C. Psychological factors are judged to play an important role in the onset, severity, exacerbation, or maintenance of the pain.

D. The symptom or deficit is not intentionally produced or feigned (as in factitious disorder or malingering).

E. The pain is not better accounted for by a mood, anxiety, or psychotic disorder and does not meet the criteria for dyspareunia.

Specify as:

Acute: duration of less than 6 months

Chronic: duration of 6 months or longer

Note. From *Diagnostic and Statistical Manual of Mental Disorders* (4th edition Text Revision) (*DSM-IV-TR*), by American Psychiatric Association, 2000, Washington, DC: Author. Adapted with permission.

Annual estimates in the United States show that 10 to 15 percent of adults experience some form of occupational disability owing to back pain.

RESOURCES

Please note that because Internet resources are of a time-sensitive nature and URL addresses may change or be deleted, searches should also be conducted by association or topic.

Internet Resources

http://www.painmed.org   American Academy of Pain Medicine
http://www.info@ampainsoc.org   American Pain Society

14 Stress-Related Disorders

• Key Terms

Adaptation: Sustaining homeostasis; the ability to mobilize resources and adjust to demands of internal and external environments.

Hardiness: Refers to a personality trait that enables people to maintain health and cope with stressful events.

Psychophysiological Disorder: Denotes emotional states producing or exacerbating physical problems.

Stress: A stimulus or demand that has the potential to generate disruption in homeostasis or produce a reaction.

T-cells: Viral- and tumor-fighting lymphocytes (all called natural killer cells) of the immune system. They are referred to as "T" cells because they are processed by the thymus gland.

Type A Personality: A constellation of personality traits, such as highly driven, time-conscious, and competitive behavior, associated with high risk for coronary artery disease.

Type B Personality: A constellation of personality traits opposite from Type A and manifested by "easy-going, laid-back, and reposed" behavior.

Humans are holistic beings, and when stress affects one system, all other systems are influenced. Circumstances that threaten homeostasis activate complex neurobiological and psychosocial coping processes that arise from the autonomic nervous system.

STRESS-RELATED DISORDERS—GENERAL

Causes

Human responses to stress involve psychosocial and neurobiological processes. In stressful situations, the body switches on its autonomic nervous system and neurobiological processes in an attempt to maintain homeostasis. Psychosocial adaptive processes are mobilized and sustained by temperament and personality traits that help the person cope with stressful situations.

The complexity of psychobiological disorders requires an understanding of the intrinsic relationship between emotions and physiological processes. Physiological processes activated by emotions are both innate and necessary for human survival and adaptation. However, a failure to mobilize resources and manage emotions and physiological processes threaten individual health and integrity. Acute stress responses activate a cascade of intricate survival processes that generate the "fight or flight" response. Prolonged activation of the stress response has potentially deleterious impact on mental and physical health.

Alexander (1950) delineated seven psychosomatic disorders: essential hypertension, skin disorders, rheumatoid arthritis, hyperthyroidism, ulcerative colitis, peptic ulcer diseases, and asthma. He believed that visceral or organ dysfunction arose from primarily unconscious personality traits or inadequate coping behaviors that interfered with reduction of intense emotions, such as anger, or repressed, sustained fears, anxiety, and aggression.

Freud (1958) hypothesized that unreleased psychological tension was converted into symptoms such as paralysis or blindness. He termed this reaction *conversion hysteria* and suggested that it stemmed from the inability to express feelings.

Stress is an integral part of living, and it denotes a stimulus or demand that has the potential to disrupt homeostasis or produce a stimulus. Hans Seyle introduced the concept that a person's inability to manage stress effectively increases their vulnerability to illness (Seyle, 1976).

The premise of Seyle's theory, referred to as General Adaptation Syndrome, is that there is a relationship between stress and neurobiological changes that arise from stimulation of the hypothalamic-pituitary-adrenal axis. Effective mastery of stress restores homeostasis and allows adaptation. **Adaptation** refers to sustaining homeostasis, the ability to mobilize resources and adjust to demands of internal and external environments.

Stress can alter various immunological processes. The immune system mediates intricate neurobiological processes and behavior to maintain homeostasis. Several studies suggest a relationship between stress and a reduction in natural killer (NK) activity. NK cells are involved in immune responses against certain viruses, bacteria, and parasites (Biron, Nguyen, Pien, Cousens, & Salazar-Mather, 1999; Lanier, 2000).

More recent studies link immunological suppression with depression, maladaptive coping behaviors, social interactions, substance abuse, cancer, and other physical disorders (Fletcher et al.,1998; Olff, 1999). Inappropriate and chronic release of stress hormones (adrenocorticotropic hormone and cortisol) eventually damages the normal neural and physiological mechanisms that maintain physical and mental adaptation. Long exposure to cortisol has been shown to contribute to systems diseases such as hypertension, atherosclerosis, and myocardial infarction.

Cognitive and behavioral factors that derive from personality styles also affect responses to stress. There is a relationship between personality or coping style and predisposition to certain illnesses. Friedman and Rosenman (1974) introduced the **Type A personality** and **Type B personality** more than 20 years ago; these researchers suggested a positive relationship between Type A personality and heart diseases.

Research suggests that some people are more vulnerable to stress than others. Risk factors include personality traits, genetics, diet, and environmental stressors. A lifestyle of chronic negative emotions, such as hostility, seems to produce neurobiological changes that increase a person's vulnerability to stress.

An often overlooked area concerning psychophysiological disorders is the role of culture and its impact on the client, family, and communities.

Childhood psychophysiological disorders have been linked with the need for protection and attachment to primary caregivers. Separation anxiety plays a key role in formation and exacerbation of physical symptoms. Immature cognitive function and inability to express feelings often compel the child to communicate anxiety and stress through physical symptoms (Cassileth & Drossman, 1998; Garralda, 1992). Other childhood stressors include disabling disorders, abuse, family chaos, and unstable living conditions.

Adolescence represents a period of intense biological and psychosocial turmoil as the youth searches for a sense of identity and strives to separate from primary caregivers. Other psychosocial stressors are tremendous academic demands and interpersonal relationships, which emerge as important developmental tasks preparing the youth for adulthood.

Symptoms

A contemporary term for conversion hysteria is *conversion disorder*. The *DSM-IV-TR* (APA, 2000) categorizes these disorders as somatoform disorders and lists several criteria:

- The loss or change in physical function is initially associated with a physical cause.
- Later, psychological components, such as intense stress and anxiety, are linked to the physical symptoms.
- The phenomenon is unintentional and unconscious.
- The symptom is not part of cultural mores, general medical condition, or substance misuse.
- The symptom is not associated with pain or disturbance in sexual performance.
- The symptom interferes with the client's optimal level of function.

Type A was delineated by the following behaviors:

- Rapid speech
- Rapid walking
- Irritability
- Time consciousness
- Difficulty relaxing
- Persistent need to stay busy
- Attempts to do more than one thing at a time

Smith (1997) outlines traits with which successful coping are associated. These include general beliefs about the world and responsibility for life problems. These traits include an internal locus of control, a sense of coherence or a person's ability to manage his tensions and have a sense of belongingness, and **hardiness**, which is comprised of control, commitment, and challenge. Table 14–1 compares successful coping traits with illness traits.

People with Type B personalities are less driven than those with Type A and generally are more easy going, laid back, and reposed. Their lifestyles are relaxed and goal directed (Friedmann & Rosenman, 1974).

The inability to express their feelings is manifested by closed body language,

Table 14–1 • Comparison of Successful Coping Traits and Illness Traits

Successful Coping Traits	Illness Traits
Internal locus of control	Negative affectivity
Hardiness	Anxiety
Self-efficacy	Hostility
Hope	Introversion
Optimism	Type A behaviors
Problem-solving skills	
Constructive thinking	

Note. Data from *Understanding Stress and Coping,* by J. C. Smith, 1997, New York: Macmillan. Adapted with permission.

such as folded arms and poor eye contact, an overly appeasing attitude, and an anxious mood. Inability or unwillingness to express feelings has been associated with sustained arousal of the sympathetic nervous system.

Bodily reactions affected by adolescents in response to stressful situations include recurrent abdominal pain, headaches, chest pain, musculoskeletal pain, chronic fatigue, and nonspecific symptoms such as dizziness or tiredness (Greene & Walker, 1997).

The long-term effects of biological response to chronic stress have been well documented. Certain people seem to be at risk for developing psychophysiological disorders, or they are disease prone. Disease-prone behaviors include certain personality traits, chronic tension, and internalized emotions. Table 14–2 lists psychophysiological disorders that may be experienced in adulthood.

TREATMENT

Implications for the psychiatric nurse include identifying high-risk groups and behaviors, reducing stress, and strengthening the client's repertoire of coping skills. Nurses can work more effectively with the client who presents with a psychophysiological disorder by understanding causative factors such as psychodynamic, neurobiological, and cognitive.

Because of the dramatic demographic changes in this country and globally, assessing the role of culture, religion, and spirituality is critical to understanding the client's experiences and symptoms. Implications for nursing practice include self-awareness of one's own culture and its potential impact of perception of the client's experiences.

The primary roles of the psychiatric-mental health nurse are to assess clients' current and past coping behaviors, help clients resolve crisis situations, minimize exacerbation of symptoms, and strengthen and promote adaptive coping behaviors. Hospitalized clients experiencing

Table 14–2 • Specific Psychophysiological Disorders

System	Disorders/Symptoms
Cardiovascular	• Hypertension • Mitral valve prolapse • Myocardial infarction • Coronary heart disease • Migraine headaches
Pulmonary	• Hyperventilation • Asthma • Allergies
Immunological	• Certain cancers • Autoimmune disease, such as lupus • Herpes zoster • Herpes simplex • Rheumatoid arthritis • AIDS
Gastrointestinal	• Peptic ulcer disease • Crohn's disease • Ulcerative colitis • Irritable bowel syndrome • Gastroesophageal reflux disease (GERD)
Dermatological	• Rashes • Urticaria • Psoriasis • Alopecia • Warts
Endocrine	• Diabetes • Thyroid disorders

acute exacerbation of symptoms require close monitoring so that homeostasis is maintained. Interventions such as adequate dietary intake, hydration, and control of pain involve assessing client response and promotion of self-care. Psychoeducation, crisis intervention, and stress-reducing activities are major nursing interventions for clients experiencing psychophysiological disorders (Table 14–3).

(continues)

Table 14–3 • Health Teaching for the Angry and Tense Client with a Psychophysiologic Disorder

The next time you find yourself feeling tense and angry, consider using the following techniques:

1. Recognize your anger. Normally, anger and tension manifest as:
   - Increased heart rate and breathing
   - Increased blood pressure
   - Sweating
   - Muscle tension
   - Clenched jaw
   - Need to move around

2. Once-you recognize your anger, do the following:
   - Take a time out (get out of the area and away from the stress).
   - Take 10 deep breaths using your abdominal muscles in the following way: Take a deep and slow breath through your nose—as your chest rises, slowly push your abdomen out (this may feel awkward initially, but it is the normal breathing pattern when you are completely relaxed); next exhale slowly through your mouth or nose and gently pull in your abdomen (you should feel relaxed with each breath).
   - Once your body is under control (decreased heart and breathing rate and blood pressure)— your mind and thoughts are clear and focused: ask yourself, "What am I angry about?" If your anger is legitimate, follow up with the person or situation assertively. If it is not legitimate (maybe the feedback was correct and you are overreacting), LET IT GO!

TREATMENT *(continued)*

Nurses in advanced-practice also work with clients and families to minimize exacerbation of symptoms and promote self-care and adaptive coping skills. In addition, the advanced-practice nurse identifies complex problems and collaborates with clients to modify behavior and coping patterns. Major interventions include various psychotherapies such as cognitive-behavioral and psychodynamic approaches. Furthermore, prescriptive authority enables the advanced-practice nurse to prescribe various psychotropics that enhance other treatment modalities. Assessing client responses and participating in comprehensive planning in inpatient, community, or home health care settings are critical roles of the advanced-practice nurse.

In treating clients with a psychophysiological disorder, the nurse is challenged to integrate biological concepts to assess client symptoms, identify client outcomes, develop effective interventions, and evaluate responses. This process first requires establishing rapport by approaching the client in a caring and nonjudgmental manner; encouraging client and family participation in treatment; and gathering data on current stressors, substance misuse, psychiatric and medical history, present and past symptoms, and coping behaviors. Many clients presenting with psychophysiological disorders have experienced rejection of and skepticism toward their symptoms. In addition, being referred to psychiatry often makes clients feel as though their symptoms are "all in their head." This premise needs to be dispelled quickly to get beyond suspiciousness and anger and focus on building adaptive coping skills.

Inquiring about reasons for seeking treatment and about past treatments and whether they were helpful can reduce these feelings. When past treatment has been unsuccessful, the client's perception of reasons for the lack of success needs to be assessed. Clients with chronic pain disorders are often sensitive to criticism of their illness and may become defensive or argumentative when questioned about pain medication.

Complete physical and mental status examinations are critical components of

(continues)

TREATMENT *(continued)*

the assessment process. Age-appropriate tools can elicit information of life span factors. Children and adolescents must be assessed both individually and in the context of family to determine the significance of the sick role and its impact on homeostasis. Family organization may be tied to the development and maintenance of the child's illness. Assessment of the family's developmental stage and interaction, especially those associated with overprotectiveness, rigidity, and poor problem-solving skills, indicates the family's level of function. Data on the history of symptoms; precipitating stressors, both biological and psychosocial; and symptom maintenance can help the nurse surmise the child's role within the family function (Minuchin et al., 1975).

In general, major outcomes for clients with stress-related disorders include the following:

1. Development of adaptive coping behaviors
2. Crisis resolution
3. Strengthening and mobilization of support systems
4. Minimization of exacerbation of symptoms
5. Promotion of self-esteem

Evaluating client responses to interventions is a dynamic process based on outcome identification and includes feedback from the client, family, and other members of the health team. Adaptive behaviors must be strengthened throughout treatment.

CARDIOVASCULAR DISORDERS

Cause

It has been hypothesized that Type A behavior is associated with a higher risk of coronary heart disease. Research conducted since 1981 has had mixed results on this issue (Littman, 1998), with the finding that hostility is the specific component of the Type A personality that may be responsible for increasing the risk of heart disease. Coelho, Ramos, Prata, Maciel, and Barros (1999), in a study of psychosocial risk factors, found type A behavior, depression, and lower levels of well-being to be significant features of acute myocardial infarctions. Hendrix and Hughes (1997) found Type A personality increases coronary heart disease risk.

Who is at risk for hypertension? Individuals at risk for this disorder include those with family histories of heart disease, diabetes, and maladaptive personality or coping styles. Psychosocial stressors, such as impoverished living conditions, high-pressured jobs, and strained interpersonal relationships also play key roles in development of hypertension.

TREATMENT

Prevention is critical to the treatment of hypertension and other cardiovascular disorders. By assessing the client's present stressors and coping styles and developing individualized teaching plans, the nurse can help the client recognize and understand the maladaptive nature and consequences of disease-prone behaviors and explore adaptive ways to manage stress. An interdisciplinary approach is critical to the success of health education and restoration. Major interventions include smoking cessation, weight loss, administration of cardiovascular agents, and compliance with the medication regimen, diet restrictions and healthy eating habits, and stress management. Stress management, psychoeducation, cognitive-behavioral and various forms of psychotherapy can help clients express feelings and develop effective coping skills. See Table 14–4 for a description of stress-reducing techniques.

Table 14–4 • Therapeutic Measures for Stress-Related Illness

Biofeedback

Biofeedback is an electronic indication of a person's stress level that is provided by instrumentation that registers the person's psychophysiological responses. A tone or signal provides the client with immediate feedback. The goal is to keep the tone below a certain threshold for 15 seconds on four occasions. The client learns to observe and control subtle internal body responses (blood pressure, temperature, and muscle tension). This intervention enables clients to play an active role in the promotion of their own health.

Indications: Migraine headaches, hypertension, Raynaud's disease, chronic pain, gastrointestinal disorders.

Deep Muscle Relaxation

The client is taught how to achieve deep muscle relaxation, which is basic to all behavioral stress reduction techniques. The following instructions are given to the client:

• Find a quiet area away from distraction.
• If desired, use a relaxation tape.
• Get into a comfortable position, such as lying on your back.
• Close your eyes and inhale deeply through your nose, allowing your lungs to fill with air and feeling your chest expand. Then slowly exhale.
• Repeat.

The success of deep relaxation depends on daily practice. The goal is to decrease respirations, reduce blood pressure, and reduce peripheral vasodilation.

Indications: Tension headaches, muscle tension, hypertension.

Visual Imagery

Deep muscle relaxation is imperative during visual imagery. A pleasant, quiet, peaceful place is visualized to reduce stress or pain and to enhance relaxation. As with deep muscle relaxation, ongoing practice is necessary for successful use of this technique.

Indications: Childbirth, gastrointestinal disorders, chronic pain, cancer.

Self-Talk

In this form of cognitive therapy, clients provide themselves with evaluative statements and suggestions to reduce stress and promote relaxation.

Indications: To reduce anxiety, stress, and faulty cognitions.

Note. Definitions are from *The Relaxation Response,* by H. Benson, 1975, New York: William Morrow; and from *Biofeedback: Methods and Procedures in Clinical Practice,* by G. D. Fuller, 1977, San Francisco: Biofeedback Press. Adapted with permission.

CHRONIC PAIN DISORDERS

Causes

Psychosocial stress can exaggerate pain and mask depression, hypochondriasis, malingering, and other conditions that provide secondary gains (Weisberg & Clavel, 1999).

Symptoms

Chronic recurrent pain can be emotionally and physically incapacitating and create feelings of guilt, low self-esteem, and discouragement (Menninger, 1963).

TREATMENT

Major nursing interventions for chronic pain begin with approaching the client in a caring and nonjudgmental manner. This approach is critical to allaying fears of the pain being all in the client's head. Major therapeutic measures include hydrotherapy, massages, physiotherapy, and analgesics. Additional major interventions include behavioral-cognitive techniques, relaxation, distraction, biofeedback, and group psychotherapy (Cottraux, 1998; Hodges & Workman, 1998). Table 14–4 describes some of the therapeutic measures recommended for clients with stress-related illnesses.

DERMATOLOGICAL DISORDERS

The skin, like other major systems, responds to the environment and is responsive to various emotions such as anger, embarrassment, and terror.

Symptoms

The condition of skin often reflects health status. Clammy, cool skin may indicate a serious medical problem or intense fear and anxiety. A generalized rash suggests an allergic reaction or an intense emotional response.

TREATMENT

Dermatological or skin disorders considered to be psychophysiological conditions include alopecia, pruritus (itching), psoriasis, and urticaria (hives). Psychosocial stress tends to aggravate skin disorders. Nursing implications include identifying stressors and developing interventions that reduce the intensity of stressors and strengthen and develop effective coping skills. In addition, stress reduction interventions, such as cognitive-behavioral techniques and desensitization, provide relief for some clients suffering from stress-induced illnesses (Drossman et al., 2000).

GASTROINTESTINAL DISORDERS

Cause

Gastrointestinal (GI) disorders have long been associated with emotions. The GI tract is innervated by the autonomic nervous system and, like other major organs, is affected by stress and tension. Stress and other emotional reactions create tension in the gut and can produce nausea, vomiting, or diarrhea.

Symptoms

Overproduction of gastric secretion and disturbance in motility are major symptoms of GI disorders (Drossman, 1998). Major GI disorders include irritable bowel syndrome, peptic ulcer disease, ulcerative colitis, and Crohn's disease.

Irritable bowel syndrome has been aligned with several mood disorders, including panic, agoraphobia, and depression. People with this syndrome tend to be tense, anxious, depressed, and irritable, and they also tend to internalize feelings (Drossman, 1999).

TREATMENT

Major interventions for irritable bowel syndrome are relaxation techniques, stress reduction, assertiveness training, and biofeedback. Psychotherapy and psychopharmacology (e.g., anxiolytics or antidepressants) may be indicated for some clients. Major treatment goals focus on strengthening and improving coping behavior and communication skills and reducing psychological and biological stress.

IMMUNOLOGICAL DISORDERS

Cause

Stress alters people's immunological processes and resistance to illness. Inadequate cellular immune response or alteration in tumor and viral fighting **T-cells** compromises the immune system, increasing vulnerability to illnesses such as acquired immunodeficiency syndrome; cancer; and the common cold, flu, herpes simplex Type I, and Epstein-Barr viruses (Cohen & Herbert, 1996; O'Connor, O'Halloran, & Shanahan, 2000).

PULMONARY OR RESPIRATORY DISORDERS

Symptoms

Breathing patterns reveal emotions. Rapid breathing or hyperventilation is a common sign of anxiety attacks or intense fears. In contrast, shallow breathing or sighs may indicate distress. The parasympathetic (vagal) and sympathetic nervous systems innervate lung tissues. Stimulation of the parasympathetic nervous system, which may be precipitated by dust, cold air, or emotions, causes vasoconstriction.

Asthma is a Greek term that means panting, or labored breathing. It is a common respiratory disorder that has numerous causes and is associated with bronchoconstriction, which is the perva-

sive narrowing of air passages that results from vagal stimulation caused by stress, allergic reactions, cold, dust, or infections.

Major manifestations of asthma include coughing, wheezing, shortness of breath, and intense anxiety and fear. Although there is no evidence that stress causes asthma, there is considerable evidence that stress can exacerbate symptoms (Emmelkamp & Van Oppen, 1998).

TREATMENT

Asthma attacks are very distressful, and regardless of the cause, require immediate medical attention. Other interventions include approaching the client in a non-judgmental manner; identifying the precipitants of the attacks, such as stress, infections, or allergies; developing teaching plans that incorporate stress reduction; and strengthening coping skills.

RESOURCES

Please note that because Internet resources are of a time-sensitive nature and URL addresses may change or be deleted, searches should also be conducted by association or topic.

Internet Resources

http://www.stress.org American Institute of Stress

http://www.plainsense.com Key Web site for general health information

http://www.stressfree.com Stress Free Net

Substance-Related Disorders

15

• Key Terms

Abstinence: Refers to avoidance of all substances with abuse potential. It denotes cessation of addictive behaviors, such as substance abuse/dependence.

Addiction: A pattern of out-of-control or compulsive use of psychoactive substances in which use continues despite negative consequences; often used interchangeably with the terms *chemical dependency* or *substance dependence.*

Binge Drinking: Five or more drinks on the same occasion at least once in the past month (SAMHSA, 2000).

Chemical Dependency: A pattern of out-of-control or compulsive use of psychoactive substances in which use continues despite negative consequences; a popular term often used interchangeably with the terms *addiction* or *substance dependence.*

Heavy Drinking: Five or more drinks on the same occasion on each of 5 or more days in the past month (SAMHSA, 2000).

Recovery: A state of physical and psychological health in which abstinence from dependency producing drugs is complete and comfortable (American Society of Addiction Medicine, 1982).

Relapse: Use of psychoactive substances after a maintained period of abstinence.

Substance Abuse: Repeated intentional use or misuse of a psychoactive substance; use is modified or discontinued with the occurrence of significant adverse consequences.

Substance Dependence: The accepted diagnostic term for a pattern of out-of-control or compulsive use of psychoactive substances in which use continues despite negative consequences; often used interchangeably with the terms *addiction* or *chemical dependency.*

Tolerance: A pharmacologic property of some abused substances in which increased amounts over time are required to achieve similar results as in earlier use.

Wernicke's Encephalopathy: A reversible delirium seen in alcoholics; it is associated with thiamine deficiency.

Withdrawal Syndrome: Substance-specific signs and symptoms precipitated by the abrupt cessation or reduction of a substance that produces tolerance and dependence after prolonged use.

Advances in neurobiology are rapidly providing new and expanded knowledge of human behavior, health, and disease. The role of biochemical processes has enhanced our understanding of health maintenance, prevention, and treatment of many illnesses. Addictionology—the diagnosis and treatment of addictive disorders—has greatly benefited from this knowledge explosion. Nevertheless, disagreement exists among health professionals regarding the etiology, progression, and treatment of substance use disorders. Despite technology's advances, the specific causes continue to elude us. Treatment remains multidimensional as well with no one approach rigorously supported by research. Neither psychosocial or biochemical processes fully explain the complexities of substance abuse and dependence nor offer us the best answer to treatment.

SUBSTANCE-RELATED DISORDERS

Causes

Substance-related disorders have neurobiological foundations and should be seen as legitimate medical problems, not moral failings. Others may disagree as to the emphasis on biological explanations and see substance abuse or dependence as a disturbance more rooted in psychosocial or spiritual causes. The evidence is strong, nonetheless, that just about every substance of abuse shares common neurochemical processes and pathways and sets in motion a cascade of biochemical responses. These drive the compulsive use and loss of control that characterize addiction (Leshner, 1997).

Individual, environmental, and social factors are also important in understanding addictive disorders.

Ego defenses protect against anger, boredom, emptiness, rage, shame, guilt, and depression. From the psychodynamic perspective, persons with substance-related disorders lack mature ego defenses and thus do not cope well with painful or unpleasant emotion. Lacking more effective ego defenses, substance use is an effort to enhance pleasure or self-medicate to soothe emotional distress or pain. The roots of initial substance use lie in this basic unconscious underlying psychopathology.

Initial use of drugs or alcohol is influenced by many factors, such as peers and cultures. One's beliefs about the substance and perceptions about its effects and potential dangers may encourage or inhibit experimentation. Availability and cost are important considerations not only for initial but also continued use. Psychopathology and biological vulnerability appear to play a larger role in the development of dependence.

B. F. Skinner's theory of operant conditioning asserts that behavior that produces reward will continue. Rewards reinforce behavior so the likelihood of the behavior continuing can be predicted. Using drugs or alcohol can produce a "rush"—feelings of relaxation, euphoria, elation, and an enhanced sense of well-being. Anxiety, depression, shyness, and social awkwardness are relieved at least temporarily. In some groups social acceptance is gained and maintained by the use of drugs or alcohol.

Animal studies have provided compelling evidence that virtually all substances of abuse activate the brain's pleasure and reward mechanisms. The reward and pleasure systems reside in what is termed the "old brain," or "primitive brain." The median forebrain bundle is the major site of action of addicting drugs. Neurotransmitters are the chemical message carriers between neurons. They are released from the neuron, travel across the synapse (the space between nerve cells), and exert an effect in the next cell. Dopamine, serotonin, and norepinephrine are the neurotransmitters most understood in the process of addiction. Dopamine is the neurotransmitter most associated with the pleasure and reward system.

Mood abnormalities and anhedonia, particularly in opiate-dependent individuals, may prompt the urge to use again. The syndromes appear to be associated with neurobiological changes resulting from chronic substance exposure and the brain's impaired ability to maintain proper neurochemical balance. Inadequate amounts of gamma-aminobutyric acid (GABA) and dopamine are associated with increased anxiety and depression.

Family systems theory maintains that what affects one family member affects other family members. The system functions to maintain homeostasis even if pathological behavior is necessary to achieve and maintain this balance. Families in which addiction is present may deny or rationalize the problem in an effort to maintain homeostasis. This is often referred to as enabling behavior and can become a treatment issue.

Jaffe (2000a) describes similarities that have been observed in families with multigenerational substance dependence. These include absence of a parent, particularly from divorce, abandonment, or incarceration; an overprotective, overcontrolling parent; a cold or emotionally distant parent; and the presence of drug-using children who remain overly dependent on the family well into adulthood. The pain of unresolved grief associated with family of origin losses might be a factor in addictive behavior.

The potential for opioids to produce tolerance, dependence, and withdrawal has been recognized for centuries. Opioids have a high abuse potential because they produce sedation, euphoria, and, depending on the agent, a sudden pleasurable sensation (a "rush"). Heroin addiction is a serious public health problem with significant adverse effects for the individual and the community.

Dopamine is increased with nicotine use, and serotonin, epinephrine, and norepinephrine may also play a role in the reward and reinforcement processes that sustain dependence. Anger is decreased, mood is stabilized, hunger is decreased, and metabolic rate is increased. Nicotine may enhance performance on long, boring tasks (Hughes, 2000).

Genetic susceptibility to substance use disorders, parental psychopathology, and quality of parenting continues to be examined in relationship to outcomes on children's psychological health and function. It is accurate to say that both nature and nurture play a role in the development of psychopathology and substance use disorders. Multiple studies, including adoption studies, have found a link among familial alcoholism, dysfunctional parenting styles, and personality disorders in the parent to subsequent substance abuse and behavioral problems in children (Cadoret, Yates, Troughton, Woodworth, & Stewart, 1995; Kuperman,

Schlosser, Lidral, & Reich, 1999; Miles et al., 1998).

A complex set of factors place some older adults at high risk for substance problems. Changes at this phase of life often include major losses and role changes. Late life depression is not a normal part of aging. It is a serious illness and it is associated with a high risk for suicide, particularly in older adult men. Drinking can be a way to self-medicate in the face of overwhelming losses. The older adult is more susceptible to the effects of substances owing to the normal physiologic changes of aging.

Symptoms

The term **addiction** is used to describe a dependent pattern of behavior on drugs or alcohol in which the ability to moderate or stop use is repeatedly unsuccessful. There can be a sense of craving in the absence of the substance and an uncontrollable compulsion to use it again despite the knowledge of negative consequences. The loss of control over frequency or amount of use is a key indicator of addiction.

Tolerance is a pharmacologic property of some abused substances in which chronic use produces changes in the central nervous system so that more of the substance is needed to produce desired effects. With cessation or reduction of use, depending on the pharmacologic properties of the substance, a **withdrawal syndrome** may occur. Typically, the symptoms of withdrawal are the opposite of the effects of the substance. Addiction can be present even if a withdrawal syndrome does not occur. Tolerance and withdrawal can occur without addiction. Withdrawal syndromes are specific to the individual substance. All classes of substances, with the exception of caffeine and nicotine, may cause delirium and psychosis during intoxication as well as varying degrees of depression or anxiety with intoxication or after withdrawal (Schottenfeld & Pantalon, 1999).

Chemical dependency and **substance dependence** are often used interchangeably with the term *addiction*. Although

addiction and chemical dependency are not diagnostic labels in the *Diagnostic and Statistical Manual of Mental Disorders* (4th edition Text Revision) (*DSM-IV-TR*) (American Psychiatric Association [APA], 2000), they are terms commonly used (and misused) by health care professionals and the general public. **Substance abuse** and substance dependence are diagnostic terms with standard criteria that describe patterns of misuse and resulting adverse effects of mood-altering substances (Table 15–1).

Changes can be produced in alertness, coordination, attention, judgment, and thinking as well as in pulse, respiration, and blood pressure. Different substances can produce similar patterns of intoxication as in cocaine and amphetamine as stimulants, or alcohol and benzodiazepines as central nervous system (CNS) depressants.

Although it may be painfully clear to others that problems exist, the client with a substance-related disorder may offer little to no acknowledgment. The client may insist there are no problems and any expression of concern or suggestion to get help is viewed as unwelcome meddling. The client with a substance-related disorder may rationalize use of substances as a way to solve problems, fit in with a social group, expand creativity, enhance sexual drive, or cope with boredom, anxiety, or depression. And although some of those things may be true, serious consequences such as loss of job, school failure, disrupted interpersonal relationships, or health problems are routinely minimized, rationalized, or negated in the addict's view of reality.

Withdrawal symptoms appear about 6 to 8 hours after the last dose of heroin and peak in about 36 to 48 hours. Withdrawal resolves in approximately 4 to 5 days. Because of methadone's longer half-life, withdrawal symptoms are seen in about 2 to 3 days after the last dose and peak several days later. Complete symptom resolution can take up to 2 weeks (Olmedo & Hoffman, 2000).

Stimulant users will exhibit grandiosity, restlessness, pacing, talkativeness, hypervigilance, suspiciousness, anxiety, irritability, paranoia, and hallucinations.

Table 15–1 • *DSM-IV-TR* Diagnostic Criteria for Selected Substance-Related Disorders

Disorder	Criteria
Substance Abuse	A. A maladaptive pattern of substance use leading to clinically significant impairment or distress, as manifested by one (or more) of the following, within a twelve month period: 1. Recurrent substance use resulting in a failure to fulfill major role obligations at work, school, or home (e.g., repeated absences or poor work performance related to substance use; substance-related absences, suspensions, or expulsions from school; neglect of children or household). 2. Recurrent substance use in situations in which it is physically hazardous (e.g., driving an automobile or operating a machine when impaired by substance use). 3. Recurrent substance-related legal problems (e.g., arrests for substance-related disorderly conduct). 4. Continued substance use despite having persistent or recurrent social or interpersonal problems caused or exacerbated by the effects of the substance (e.g., arguments with spouse about consequences of intoxication, physical fights). B. The symptoms have never met the criteria for Substance Dependence for this class of substance.

Substance Dependence	A maladaptive pattern of substance use, leading to clinically significant impairment or distress, as manifested by three (or more) of the following, occurring at any time in the same twelve month period:
	
	1. Tolerance, as defined by either of the following:
	  a. A need for markedly increased amounts of the substance to achieve intoxication or desired effect
	  b. Markedly diminished effect with continued use of the same amount of the substance
	2. Withdrawal, as manifested by either of the following:
	  a. The characteristic withdrawal syndrome for the substance
	  b. The same (or closely related) substance is taken to relieve or avoid withdrawal symptoms
	3. The substance is often taken in larger amounts or over a longer period of time than was intended.
	4. There is a persistent desire or unsuccessful efforts to cut down or control substance use.
	5. A great deal of time is spent in activities necessary to obtain the substance (e.g., visiting multiple doctors or driving long distances), use the substance (e.g., chain smoking), or recover from its effects.
	6. Important social, occupational, or recreational activities are given up or reduced because of substance use.
	7. The substance use is continued despite knowledge of having a persistent or recurrent physical or psychological problem that is likely to have been caused or exacerbated by the substance (e.g., current cocaine use despite recognition of cocaine-induced depression, or continued drinking despite recognition that an ulcer was made worse by alcohol consumption).

(continues)

Table 15–1 *(continued)*

Disorder	Criteria
Substance Intoxication	1. The development of a reversible substance-specific syndrome due to recent ingestion (or exposure to) a substance.
	2. Clinically significant maladaptive behavioral or psychological changes that are due to the effect of the substance on the central nervous system (e.g., belligerence, mood lability, cognitive impairment, impaired judgment, impaired social or occupational functioning) and develop during or shortly after use of the substance.
	3. The symptoms are not due to a general medical condition and are not better accounted for by another medical disorder.
Substance Withdrawal	1. The development of a substance-specific syndrome due to the cessation of (or reduction in) substance use that has been heavy and prolonged.
	2. The substance-specific syndrome causes clinically significant distress or impairment in social, occupational, or other important areas of functioning.
	3. The symptoms are not due to a general medical condition and are not better accounted for by another medical disorder.

Note. From *Diagnostic and Statistical Manual of Mental Disorders* (4th edition Text Revision) (*DSM-IV-TR*), by American Psychiatric Association, 2000, Washington, DC: Author. Adapted with permission.

Appetite is suppressed sometimes to the point where users appear cachectic. Hyperpyrexia and seizures can occur. Cardiovascular effects include tachycardia, arrhythmias, elevated blood pressure, vasoconstriction, myocardial infarction, heart failure, and spinal cord and brain hemorrhages. Vasoconstriction can produce toxic renal complications.

Although acute intoxification effects from marijuana vary widely among individuals, common effects include an enhanced sense of well-being and euphoria. There can be a sense of time passing slowly, and perceptions can be distorted. Physical effects can include tachycardia, appetite stimulation, conjunctival injection, and dry mouth. Short-term memory is impaired. A sense of relaxation, drowsiness, or lethargy often follow the initial effects. Withdrawal from chronic high-dose use can include irritability and restlessness, which typically subside in a few days.

Intoxication effects from inhalants can include elated mood, slurred speech, slowed reflexes, ataxia, disorientation, hallucinations, and lethargy. There is

evidence of tolerance. Withdrawal is not common but discontinuation after chronic use can include sleep disturbance, irritability, nausea, and shakiness.

It is a myth to assume substance use disorders have no relevance to the older adult population (Table 15–2).

Key Fact

Compared to the 1970s and 1980s, rates of illicit substance abuse today are lower. SAMHSA (2000) reported that 14 million individuals had used an illicit substance in the month before the survey. The peak of illicit substance use was in 1979 with 25 million users. There was little difference among racial groups, with approximately 7 percent of whites, Hispanics, and blacks reporting illicit drug use. About 11 percent between ages 12 and 17 reported illicit drug use with marijuana—the major illicit substance used by almost 8 percent of this group.

Drug use among males is about twice that of females. Factors in the progression toward addiction and its consequences play out differently for men and women.

Table 15–2 • *DSM-IV-TR* and the Older Adult with Alcohol Problems

Criteria	Special Considerations for Older Adults
1. Tolerance	May have problems with even low intake due to increased sensitivity to alcohol and higher blood alcohol levels
2. Withdrawal	Many late onset alcoholics do not develop physiological dependence
3. Taking larger amounts or over a longer period than was intended	Increased cognitive impairment can interfere with self-monitoring; drinking can exacerbate cognitive impairment and monitoring
4. Unsuccessful efforts to cut down or control use	Same issues across life span
5. Spending much time to obtain and use alcohol and to recover from effects	Negative effects can occur with relatively low use
6. Giving up activities due to use	May have fewer activities, making detection of problems more difficult
7. Continuing use despite physical or psychological problem caused by use	May not know or understand that problems are related to use, even after medical advice

Note. From *Treatment Improvement Protocol Series 26 Substance Abuse Among Older Adults,* (DHHS Publication No. SMA 98-3179), by the Substance Abuse and Mental Health Services Administration Center for Substance Abuse Treatment, 1998, Rockville, MD: Department of Health and Human Services. Retrieved September, 2002 from http://www.samhsa.gov/centers/csat/csat2002/csat. Reprinted with permission; and *Diagnostic and Statistical Manual of Mental Disorders* (4th edition Text Revision) (*DSM-IV-TR*), by the American Psychiatric Association, 2000, Washington, DC: Author.

Drug abuse comes later for women and is often woven within the context of intimate relationships. Women become involved with cocaine often to develop or maintain an intimate relationship. Men's cocaine use is associated with friends and in relation to the drug trade. The onset of drug abuse occurs later for females, and a preexisting psychiatric disorder is often present. Histories of childhood sexual abuse and drug- or alcohol-dependent parents are more common for women.

According to the surgeon general (U.S. Public Health Service, 2000, June) tobacco use is most responsible for avoidable illness and death in millions of Americans. Approximately one third of all tobacco-dependent users will die prematurely. Tobacco contains nicotine, a psychoactive substance. Nicotine dependence is considered an addictive disorder.

TREATMENT

Medical and nursing interventions must be tailored to the features of the specific substance. As in the management of withdrawal syndromes, knowing the substance that has been used guides the plan of care in both degree and intensity of intervention (Table 15–3).

Detoxification refers to the process of systematically and safely managing withdrawal from a substance. Going through "detox" is often the first step of formal drug or alcohol treatment. Less-informed nurses assume a difficult drug or alcohol withdrawal ("let him go cold turkey") will motivate the individual to stop abusing substances. This is not accurate. The fear or discomfort of withdrawal can play a part in promoting continued compulsive

(continues)

Table 15–3 • **Selected Substances: Peak Time of Withdrawal Onset and Period of Detection**

Substance	Peak Time for Onset After Last Use	Detectable in Body
Alcohol	12–24 hours	6–10 hours
Benzodiazepines		1–6 weeks
Short acting	12–24 hours	
Long acting	5–8 days	
Barbiturates		2–10 days
Short acting	12–24 hours	
Long acting	5–8 days	
Nicotine	24 hours	1–2 days
Cocaine	4–6 hours	2–4 days
Crack cocaine	30–60 minutes	2–4 days
Amphetamines	12–24 hours	1–2 days
Heroin	10–12 hours	2–3 days
Methadone	24–96 hours	1 day–1 week
Marijuana		2 days–5 weeks
LSD		8 hours
PCP		2–8 days

LSD, lysergic acid diethylamide. PCP, phencyclidine.

TREATMENT *(continued)*

use, particularly if dependence is on alcohol or opiates.

Working with someone in denial is often a source of frustration for the nurse, especially when the client fails to take advantage of treatment resources or returns again and again to substance use. Facilitating a client's move out of denial requires patience, willingness to appropriately confront distorted thinking, and an acceptance that the individual is ultimately in charge of taking any steps toward **recovery**.

Increasingly, substance dependence is being understood as a chronic, relapsing disorder with similarities to other long-term chronic illnesses such as diabetes or chronic obstructive lung disease. **Abstinence**, avoiding all substances with abuse potential, is strongly encouraged as part of recovery. For the substance-

dependent individual, recovery is the process of experiencing life without the use of substances with abuse potential. Most in the addictions field define successful recovery in broader terms than just abstinence. This view of recovery includes an ongoing process of willingness to live a balanced lifestyle with a wellness focus within the context of healthy spiritual and interpersonal relationships. A **relapse** for the client implies the return to using substances in the characteristic dependent manner. As in most chronic diseases, relapses are part of the course of the illness. With the most diligent medical and personal management of chronic illness, relapses or exacerbations occur. In viewing addiction similarly, it is unproductive and possibly life threatening to "give up" on the chemically dependent. It is equally unreason-

(continues)

TREATMENT *(continued)*

able to judge treatment as having failed if relapse occurs. Treatment outcomes need to be viewed as effective on the basis of the decrease in substance use and the length of time that the person has been drug or alcohol free (Leshner, 1997).

The risks of drug interactions must be considered. A client taking a benzodiazepine for an anxiety disorder may be at risk for a lethal drug overdose if actively abusing alcohol. Suicide is greater in those with dual disorders, particularly substance use and depression (Berglund & Ojehagen, 1998).

As part of treatment, psychotherapy commonly uses psychodynamic principles. The therapist helps the individual or group develop self-awareness, interpersonal growth, and the resolution of current conflicts that may be rooted in the past (Frances, Frances, Franklin, & Borg, 1999).

Clients, particularly in early recovery, are urged to avoid their "drug hangouts" and the people with whom they used drugs because these can trigger the craving or the urge to use again.

If the family is to be an effective element in the treatment process, enabling behavior must be identified and addressed.

Culturally sensitive care requires identifying high-risk groups, reducing barriers to appropriate treatment, and assessing the role of families, communities, spirituality, and religion within the sociocultural context. The sociocultural context shapes the meaning of substances and affects treatment outcomes (Heath, 2001). Self-awareness, accurate diagnosing, and trust and family involvement are critical issues that must be addressed when working with the client with a substance-related disorder (Antai-Otong, 2002).

For prescription opioid dependence, a gradual decrease in dose over time can provide an effective and safe withdrawal. Opioids are cross-tolerant, which means drugs in the same class act in similar ways. Cross-tolerance allows methadone to be used for managing heroin withdrawal. Clonidine, though not an opioid, reduces sympathetic nervous system stimulation. Hypotension is the major adverse side effect, therefore, blood pressure must be monitored. Clonidine is not effective for muscle aches, restlessness, insomnia, or craving. Muscle relaxants, anxiolytics, and antiemetics are used to promote comfort and provide relief from cramping, anxiety, nausea, and vomiting.

Assessment for the use of substances should be a routine part of any health assessment. Physical complaints may have their basis in alcohol or drug abuse. The advanced-practice nurse should consider substance use disorders when making differential diagnoses.

Older adults are often taking a variety of medications that can produce adverse reactions in the presence of alcohol or other abused substances. A history of multiple falls or evidence of related trauma needs to be evaluated comprehensively, including medical conditions and substance use.

The role of the generalist nurse is based on basic nursing education that prepares the nurse to do a nursing assessment that includes taking vital signs, monitoring the client's response to treatment, and providing a safe and therapeutic healing environment. The generalist nurse's practice also includes 24-hour monitoring of the client's physical and medical status concerning withdrawal and intoxication from various substances. Assessing the client's safety requires close observation and continuous monitoring of her level of danger to self and others. Other responsibilities include psychoeducation; facilitating self-help groups; administering medications, monitoring the client's response, and reporting adverse reactions; and collaborating with the client, family, and other clinicians to provide holistic care.

The advanced-practice nurse's practice is based on advanced educational and

(continues)

TREATMENT *(continued)*

clinical expertise in managing complex client populations. Major responsibilities include collaborating with other clinicians to provide holistic care, prescribing psychotropic agents as allowed by the nurse's state regulation concerning prescriptive authority, and providing psychotherapy and health education. An in-depth discussion of the nurse's role in caring for the client with a substance-related disorder is forthcoming in this section.

Assessment of the client who is abusing substances is sometimes a difficult process because of the pervasiveness of denial. In addition to a variety of reasons why the client is reluctant to openly disclose substance use, other factors can hinder the process. How well informed the nurse is about addiction science and the nurse's own attitudes can influence the quality of the nurse's contribution to the assessment and treatment process. It is imperative for nurses to be aware of their attitudes toward those who abuse substances and to accept them as people in need of help managing a serious health problem.

Asking for information on current and past use of drugs and alcohol is part of a basic health history. Depending on the setting where health information is being gathered, it may be useful to begin asking about the use of less-threatening substances such as caffeine and nicotine. Clients may underestimate the quantity and frequency of use. To identify problematic use of mind-altering substances, not only do the type, amount, and frequency need to be assessed but also the consequences resulting from patterns of use. Information needed to perform a thorough assessment includes:

- Types of substances used
- Amounts typically used
- Time and amount of last use (critical in assessing for intoxication or withdrawal states)
- Duration and frequency of use

- Routes of use for those substances that are administered by various means
- Past history of any withdrawal states and characteristics of those states
- Occurrence and degree of adverse consequences
- Experience with any prior treatment modalities

The client should also be asked about any medical problems, past or current, that are often associated with substance use.

Numerous screening, assessment, treatment planning, and outcome evaluation tools are available. Selection is often based on the setting in which they are to be used and the intended objective for their use. One of the most commonly used assessment tools is the CAGE questionnaire. The individual is asked whether or not he has ever felt the need to Cut down on drinking, felt Annoyed by criticism or complaining by others about alcohol use, felt Guilty about drinking, or if an Eye opener in the morning has ever been needed to calm nerves or treat a hangover. Two or more affirmative answers indicate a clinically significant alcohol use disorder (Ewing, 1984). Other commonly used tools include the Michigan Alcohol Screening Test, the Alcohol Use Disorders Identification Test, and the Addiction Severity Index (NIAAA, 1998).

The level of preparation and setting may determine the degree and extent to which the nurse conducts a physical assessment. Basic components include:

1. Baseline vital signs
2. Mental status—level of consciousness, orientation, memory, mood, affect, reality testing, judgment, suicidal or homicidal ideation
3. Presence of any intoxication or withdrawal symptoms
4. Nutritional status
5. Assessment of skin integrity

Having a basic understanding of the expected effects of substances likely to be abused is helpful when assessing a client's behavior (Table 15–4).

Table 15–4 • Routes and Effects of Major Classes of Abused Substances

Drug and Routes	Effects	Overdose	Withdrawal Syndrome
Alcohol: Central nervous system depressant Route: Oral	Sedation, decreased inhibitions, relaxation, decreased coordination, impaired judgment; slowed reflexes; slurred speech; nausea; euphoria; depression; sexual dysfunction	Respiratory depression, stupor, circulatory collapse, cardiac arrest, coma, death Effects potentiated by combination with other central nervous system depressants	Tremors; increased temperature, pulse and respiration; psychomotor agitation; impaired attention and memory; illusions (misinterpretation of stimuli); auditory, visual, or tactile hallucinations; delusions; seizure, delirium tremens; circulatory collapse; death
Opiates: Central nervous system depressant Morphine Codeine Diacetylmorphine (heroin) Hydromorphone (Dilaudid) Dolophine (Methadone) Meperidine (Demerol) Hydrocodone (Vicodin) Propoxyphene (Darvon, Darvocet) Routes: Oral, inhalation, IM, IV, smoking	Analgesia; euphoria, calming sensation, sedation; clouding of consciousness; memory and concentration impairment; psychomotor retardation; constricted pupils; constipation; decreased libido	Respiratory depression, stupor; circulatory collapse; coma; death Effects potentiated by combination with other central nervous system depressants	Yawning; rhinorrhea; lacrimation; abdominal cramps; diaphoresis; irritability; restlessness; anxiety; agitation; sleep disturbance; body aches; muscle cramps; "gooseflesh"; sensations of hot and cold; nausea; diarrhea; anorexia; fever; dilated pupils; muscle twitching; increased blood pressure, pulse, respiration; dysphoria; craving
Sedative-Hypnotics and Anxiolytics: Central nervous system depressants *Barbiturates* Amobarbital (Amytal) Butabarbital (Butisol)	Relief of anxiety, euphoria; sedation; reduced libido; impaired judgment; dizziness; lack of coordination; impaired memory	Somnolence; hypotension; hypotonia; respiratory depression; coma; cardiac arrest; death	Tremor; nightmares; diaphoresis; blepharospasm; dilated pupils; agitation; ataxia; increased respiration and blood pressure;

(continues)

Table 15–4 *(continued)*

Drug and Routes	Effects	Overdose	Withdrawal Syndrome
Butalbital compound (Esgic, Fioricet) Pentobarbital (Nembutal) Phenobarbital (Luminal) Secobarbital (Seconal) *Barbiturate-like* Chloral hydrate (Noctec) Ethchlorvynol (Placidyl) *Benzodiazepines* Alprazolam (Xanax) Chlordiazepoxide (Librium) Clorazepate (Tranxene) Diazepam (Valium) Flurazepam (Dalmane) Lorazepam (Ativan) Oxazepam (Serax) Quazepam (Doral) Temazepam (Restoril) Triazolam (Halcion) Rohypnol ("date rape drug") *Other* Meprobamate (Equanil, Miltown) Glutethimide (Doriglute) Routes: Oral, IM, IV		Effects potentiated by combination with other central nervous system depressants	vomiting; hallucinations; delusions; apprehension; rebound anxiety or panic; clouded consciousness; muscle twitching; confusion; disorientation; memory impairment; seizures
Stimulants: Central nervous system stimulants Cocaine ("crack," "rock") Dextroamphetamine (Dexedrine)	Alertness; reduced fatigue; euphoria; initial CNS stimulation then depression when "coming down"; sleep disturbance; irritability; decreased appetite; paranoia;	Cardiac arrhythmias/ arrest; sudden cardiac death; elevated or lowered blood pressure; chest pain; vomiting; seizures; hallucinations; confusion;	Fatigue then insomnia; increased appetite; psychomotor retardation then agitation; severe dysphoria, anxiety; cravings; disturbed sleep; suicide

(continues)

Table 15-4 *(continued)*

Drug and Routes	Effects	Overdose	Withdrawal Syndrome
Methylphenidate (Ritalin) Pemoline (Cylert) Routes: Oral, buccal absorption, inhalation, smoking, IV	impaired judgment; hypertension; hyperpyrexia, slowing of cardiac conduction; aggression; dilated pupils; tremors; palpitations	dyskinesias; dystonias; weakness; lethargy; dysphoria; coma	
Cannabis santiva (marijuana, hashish) Routes: Usually inhalation by smoking; can be ingested orally ("Alice B. Toklas brownies")	Euphoria or dysphoria; relaxation; drowsiness; anxiety; panic attack; heightened perception of color, sound; loss of coordination; spatial perception and time distortion; unusual body sensations; dry mouth; conjunctival injection (blood shot eyes); food cravings; learning and memory impairment; increased heart rate	Unlikely	No recognized syndrome

Inhalants
Gases
Household:
  butane, propane, refrigerant gases, whipping cream aerosol
Propellants:
  aerosols—paint, hair spray, deodorants, air fresheners, fabric protectors, cooking oil spray
	Euphoria; giddiness; excitation; disinhibition; loss of consciousness; ataxia; nystagmus; dysarthria	Central nervous system depression; heart failure; coma; seizures; death	Similar to alcohol but milder, with anxiety, tremors, hallucinations, sleep disturbance

(continues)

Table 15–4 *(continued)*

Drug and Routes	Effects	Overdose	Withdrawal Syndrome
Medical anesthetics: nitrous oxide, halothane, chloroform, ether			
Solvents: Household: Cleaning agents— spot removers, dry cleaning fluid, degreasers, lighter fluid, acetone, spot removers, gasoline Adhesives: airplane glue, rubber cement			
Art/Office Supplies: Felt tip marker, correction fluid			
Nitrites: amyl, butyl, cyclohexyl			
Route: Inhalation ("huffing")			
Hallucinogenic Agent Phencyclidine (PCP) "Angel Dust" Routes: Oral, inhalation, smoking	Feelings of strength, power, invulnerability and a numbing effect on the mind; decreased awareness of and detachment from the environment; elevated pulse, respiration, blood pressure; flushing; disphoresis; ataxia; dysarthria; decreased pain perception; paranoid delusions; disordered thinking; catatonia; garbled and sparse speech	Decreased pulse respirations, blood pressure; extreme aggression; suicidality; nausea; vomiting; rapid eye movement; blurred vision; drooling; hallucinations; seizures; coma; death	None—supportive care with benzodiazepines or low dose neuroleptic agent for drug-induced psychosis

(continues)

Table 15–4 *(continued)*

Drug and Routes	Effects	Overdose	Withdrawal Syndrome
Caffeine Route: Oral	Stimulation; increased mental acuity; inexhaustability	Restlessness, nervousness; excitement; insomnia; flushing; GI distress; muscle twitching; rambling flow of thought and speech; tachycardia or cardiac arrhythmia; agitation	Headache; drowsiness; fatigue; craving; impaired psychomotor performance; difficulty concentrating; yawning; nausea
Nicotine Routes: Smoking, chewing	Stimulation; enhanced performance and alertness; appetite suppression	Anxiety	Mood changes; craving; anxiety; poor concentration; sleep disturbance; headaches; GI distress; increased appetite

ALCOHOLISM

The most commonly abused drug is alcohol. It is a staple of many social, cultural, and religious rituals and practices.

Causes

Although no known cause is apparent, alcoholism is viewed as a chronic, progressive disease that follows a predictable natural history (Figure 15–1). It progresses in predictable stages, with death as the eventual outcome barring some degree of intervention. There is widespread agreement at this time that addiction involves biological, psychological, and social factors (Figure 15–2).

Although alcohol and alcoholism have been studied most extensively, research is rapidly expanding our understanding of genetic factors associated with other substances of abuse. Studying twins born to parents with alcoholism, but raised in nonalcoholic homes, has provided strong evidence that the tendency to become alcoholic is inherited. Similar studies

Alcoholism is a primary, chronic disease with genetic, psychosocial, and environmental factors influencing its development and manifestations. The disease is often progressive and fatal. It is characterized by continuous or periodic: impaired control over drinking, preoccupation with the drug alcohol, use of alcohol despite adverse consequences, and distortions in thinking, most notably denial.

Figure 15–1 The American Society of Addiction Medicine definition of alcoholism. *(Note. From The American Society of Addiction Medicine, approved 1990. http://www.asam.org)*

examining abused drugs also support an increased vulnerability to addiction when a family history is present (Miller, Guttman, & Chawla, 1997). Family history of addiction does not guarantee the development of alcoholism or drug dependency but it makes an individual at higher risk.

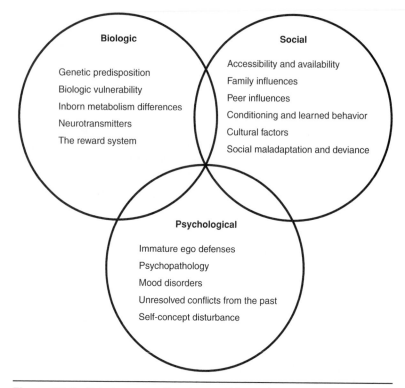

Figure 15–2 Substance use disorders and biopsychosocial influences

To cope with the greater responsibilities of adulthood and associated stressors, substance use may increase. Psychosocial stressors that are often cited as precipitants to chemical use include divorce, death of a spouse or child, and loss of job. The alcohol user may increase drinking to the point where blackouts begin to occur.

Symptoms

The classic physical appearance of an alcoholic includes a flushed face, spider angiomas, bulbous nose, abdominal fat accumulation, and a wasted appearance of the extremities. In chronic drinkers, inspection and palpation of the abdomen may reveal an enlarged liver, increased girth related to ascites,

and snake-like veins around the umbilicus (caput medusae related to the effects of portal vein obstruction). Bruising and other signs of traumatic injury are common.

Key Fact

Alcohol remains the most used and abused substance in all age groups. Of those age 12 and older, 105 million reported drinking alcohol in the month before being interviewed by SAMHSA (2000) researchers. Approximately 42 percent described patterns of **binge drinking** (five or more drinks on the same occasion in the past month) and 12 percent, **heavy drinking** (five or more drinks on the same occasion on each of five or more days in the past month) (SAMHSA, 2000).

TREATMENT

When individuals have a disease they *are not blamed* for having it; they are, however, held *responsible for participating in the management* of their disease for optimum health outcomes. Disease management in addiction involves a recovery process. Most addiction professionals view recovery as a lifelong process of abstinence, and physical, emotional, and spiritual healing. Some addiction professionals do not consider a spiritual component as necessary to managing addictive behavior. More emphasis is placed on correcting faulty cognitive processes. There is little disagreement that for the substance-dependent individual, abstinence is an essential element of the recovery process.

Medical complications of chronic alcohol dependence affect all body systems. Commonly seen medical problems are listed in Table 15-5. Alcohol use is also related to increased sexual risk taking such as risk for exposure to HIV infection and other sexually transmitted diseases. When working with older adults, evaluations for dementia must include a history of alcoholism. Chronic, excessive use results in the destruction and shrinkage of neurons, particularly in the frontal cortex of the brain (Dodd & Lewohl, 1998).

Table 15-5 • Medical Consequences of Alcoholism

Brain atrophy	Gastritis
Dementia	Peptic ulcers
Esophagitis	Acute and chronic
Esophageal varices	pancreatitis
Alcoholic cardiomyopathy	Testicular atrophy
	Alcoholic myopathy
Lowered resistance to infection	Coagulation deficits
	Anemia
Alcoholic hepatitis	Thiamine deficiency
Cirrhosis	Elevated lipids
Hypersplenism	Peripheral neuropathy

Tolerance and dependence occur in heavy alcohol use. Individuals with high tolerance can show little sign of intoxication at blood alcohol levels in which nontolerant individuals would be exhibiting significant impairment. Over time heavy drinking produces tolerance, whether the ethanol is delivered via very expensive bottles of Scotch whiskey or six packs of beer. This is a key point to emphasize when providing health education about alcohol use.

Withdrawal is associated with neuronal excitation in the face of abrupt cessation of the depressant action of alcohol. Its development is related to the amount of alcohol ingested on a daily basis. It is dose dependent in that heavier drinkers are more likely to develop withdrawal—the brain adapts to regular doses and cannot function sufficiently without the presence of alcohol. Withdrawal is mild in the majority of individuals who develop it, and it does not occur in every alcohol-dependent person. Early withdrawal can occur within hours of the last drink or with a decrease in the amount of drinking. The time the last drink was taken is an important assessment question.

Prompt identification of withdrawal risk can be more readily detected through an adequate nursing admission assessment regardless of setting. Repeated episodes of developing tolerance and experiencing withdrawal can increase the risk of seizure in subsequent withdrawal episodes. The client should be asked directly how many times she has gone through withdrawal (or detoxications) and whether or not DTs or seizures have occurred. Early management of withdrawal is preferable to managing DTs. Although no optimal treatment exists for withdrawal delirium, symptoms can be minimized and managed by appropriate pharmacotherapeutic agents.

Clients admitted to acute care hospital settings for medical or surgical reasons not directly related to alcoholism may

(continues)

TREATMENT *(continued)*

not disclose their heavy drinking even when queried on routine nursing admission assessment. The nurse discovers the client's alcoholism a few days after admission when the patient develops DTs. The importance of adequate assessment and early intervention cannot be overemphasized. The nurse may often be the one who discovers substance abuse issues not previously disclosed to the treating physician. Communicating this important piece of information is a nursing responsibility and should be documented in the medical record. Some physicians may not be familiar or comfortable with detoxification management and request assistance from psychiatric consultation liaison resources or physicians who specialize in addiction medicine.

Pharmacotherapy promotes prevention of serious withdrawal but it is not a guarantee. Benzodiazepines are the drugs of choice for managing alcohol withdrawal syndrome according to the American Society of Addiction Medicine's evidence-based practice guidelines (Mayo-Smith, 1997). Not only do they promote rest and are anxiolytic, they also decrease the risk for seizures and delirium (Mayo-Smith, 1997; Olmeda & Hoffman, 2000). They are cross-tolerant with alcohol in that each enhances GABA. GABA produces inhibitory effects in the central nervous system. Chlordiazepoxide (Librium), diazepam (Valium), or lorazepam (Ativan) are typical medications given in progressively decreasing doses over the course of several days to facilitate safe alcohol withdrawal. An objective withdrawal assessment scale, such as the Clinical Institute Withdrawal Assessment-Alcohol (CIWA-Ar) Tool (Table 15–6) is recommended to monitor the severity of symptoms and response to treatment. Dosing should be individualized based on severity of the withdrawal and half-life considerations. Benzodiazepine selection and dosing should also be guided by whether the client has a healthy liver, by potential drug interactions, and by the presence of any comorbid conditions that could create additional risks for respiratory depression, which can occur with benzodiazepine administration. When frank hallucinations or delusions occur, especially when severe agitation is present, antipsychotics, such as haloperidol, are indicated. Anticonvulsants are not routinely recommended for use in alcohol withdrawal. Reports are mixed regarding the benefit of adding anticonvulsants to routine benzodiazepine treatment. There are reports in the literature of anticonvulsant use in treating mild alcohol withdrawal. For persons with preexisting seizure disorders, the use of anticonvulsants appropriate to the type of seizure in addition to benzodiazepines is appropriate but routine use of anticonvulsants is not standard practice.

Vitamin therapy with parenteral thiamine 100 mg should also be given as soon as possible, followed by daily doses of 50 to 100 mg. Persons with alcoholism are at risk for thiamine deficiency owing to inadequate nutritional intake or poor gastrointestinal absorption. Thiamine administration is administered as treatment of choice to try to prevent **Wernicke's encephalopathy**, a reversible condition associated with thiamine deficiency. Symptoms include ataxia, delirium, and palsy of the sixth cranial nerve (abducens muscle of the eye). Thiamine administration may not prevent delirium in all clients.

Treatment for the adolescent ideally involves the entire family in an attempt to return the teen to normal growth and development. The earlier in life drinking behavior begins, the more likely alcohol use disorders will develop. Interventions aimed at postponing drinking until age 15 or 16 can avert substantial harm from drinking later in life (DeWit, Adlaf, Offord, & Ogborne, 2000). The most successful prevention approaches involve parents, schools, and the community, but parents have the greatest influence.

Table 15–6 • The Clinical Institute Withdrawal Assessment-Alcohol (CIWA-Ar) Tool

Patient: _____

Date: _____/_____/_____   Time: _____ : _____
     y   m   d   (24 hour clock, midnight = 00:00)

Pulse or heart rate, taken for one minute: Blood pressure: _____/_____

NAUSEA AND VOMITING—Ask "Do you feel sick to your stomach? Have you vomited?" Observation.

0 no nausea and no vomiting
1 mild nausea with no vomiting
2
3
4 intermittent nausea with dry heaves
5
6
7 constant nausea, frequent dry heaves and vomiting

TACTILE DISTURBANCES—Ask "Have you any itching, pins and needles sensations, any burning, any numbness, or do you feel bugs crawling on or under your skin?" Observation.

0 none
1 mild itching, pins and needles, burning, or numbness
2 mild itching, pins and needles, burning, or numbness
3 moderate itching, pins and needles, burning or numbness
4 moderately severe hallucinations
5 severe hallucinations
6 extremely severe hallucinations
7 continuous hallucinations

TREMOR—Arms extended and fingers spread apart. Observation.

0 no tremor
1 not visible, but can be felt fingertip to fingertip
2
3
4 moderate, with patient's arms extended
5
6
7 severe, even with arms not extended

AUDITORY DISTURBANCES—Ask "Are you more aware of sounds around you? Are they harsh? Do they frighten you? Are you hearing anything that is disturbing to you? Are you hearing things you know are not there?" Observation.

0 not present
1 very mild harshness or ability to frighten
2 mild harshness or ability to frighten
3 moderate harshness or ability to frighten
4 moderately severe hallucinations
5 severe hallucinations
6 extremely severe hallucinations
7 continuous hallucinations

PAROXYSMAL SWEATS—Observation.

0 no sweat visible
1 barely perceptible sweating, palms moist
2
3
4 beads of sweat obvious on forehead
5
6
7 drenching sweats

VISUAL DISTURBANCES—Ask "Does the light appear to be too bright? Is its color different? Does it hurt your eyes? Are you seeing anything that is disturbing to you? Are you seeing things you know are not there?" Observation.

0 not present
1 very mild sensitivity
2 mild sensitivity
3 moderate sensitivity
4 moderately severe hallucinations
5 severe hallucinations
6 extremely severe hallucinations
7 continuous hallucinations   *(continues)*

Table 15–6 *(continued)*

ANXIETY—Ask "Do you feel nervous?" Observation.

0 no anxiety, at ease
1 mildly anxious
2
3
4 moderately anxious, or guarded, so anxiety is inferred
5
6
7 equivalent to acute panic states as seen in severe delirium or acute schizophrenic reactions

HEADACHE, FULLNESS IN HEAD—Ask "Does your head feel different? Does it feel like there is a band around your head?" Do not rate for dizziness or lightheadedness. Otherwise, rate severity.

0 not present
1 very mild
2 mild
3 moderate
4 moderately severe
5 severe
6 very severe
7 extremely severe

AGITATION—Observation.

0 normal activity
1 somewhat more than normal activity
2
3
4 moderately fidgety and restless
5
6
7 paces back and forth during most of the interview, or constantly thrashes about

ORIENTATION AND CLOUDING OF SENSORIUM—Ask "What day is this? Where are you? Who am I?"

0 oriented and can do serial additions
1 cannot do serial additions or is uncertain about date
2 disoriented for date by no more than 2 calendar days
3 disoriented for date by more than 2 calendar days
4 disoriented for place and/or person

Total CIWA-A Score _____
Rater's Initials _____
Maximum Possible Score   67

This scale measures 10 symptoms associated with alcohol withdrawal. The scale can be administered by a nurse in about 5 minutes.

SCORING:

0–10	mild withdrawal
11–20	mild/moderate withdrawal
20–25	moderate withdrawal
> 25	severe withdrawal, possible impending delirium tremens (DT)

Scores 11–20   Indicate the use of medication is optional.

Scores 20–25   Require close monitoring either in an inpatient setting or outpatient setting where the patient can be reevaluated every hour until the score is below 20. Medication is required.

Scores > 25   Require inpatient detoxification until the patient is stable and the score is below 20. Medication is required.

Note: CIWA does not evaluate blood pressure (BP) or pulse. Neither BP nor pulse correlate with the severity of withdrawal. The indices measured by the CIWA are more reliable indicators of the severity of withdrawal. (Sullivan et al.)

The physician must, however, monitor vital signs as an integral part of detoxification, prescribing medication as necessary to control BP and/or tachycardia.

Elevated body temperature > 100°F, though not addressed in the CIWA or in CIWA studies, may signal incipient DT or early infection. The physician is advised to closely monitor any rise in body temperature over 100°F and to consider a hospital admission if DT is a possibility.

(continues)

Table 15–6 *(continued)*

Note. From "Assessment of Alcohol Withdrawal: The Revised Clnical Institute Withdrawal Assessment for Alcohol Scale," by J. T. Sullivan, K. Sakora, J. Schneiderman, C. A. Naranjo, and E. M. Sellers, 1989, *British Journal of Addictions, 84,* pp. 1353–1357. Adapted with permission.

RESOURCES

Please note that because Internet resources are of a time-sensitive nature and URL addresses may change or be deleted, searches should also be conducted by association or topic.

Internet Resources

http://www.alcoholics-anonymous.org
   Alcoholics Anonymous

http://www.adultchildren.org   Adult Children of Alcoholics World Service Organization

http://www.asam.org   American Society of Addiction Medicine

http://www.intnsa.org   International Nurses Society on Addictions

16 Violence Survivor Disorders

• Key Terms

Child Maltreatment: Refers to actions and behaviors that result in serious physical injury, neglect, sexual abuse, and serious mental injury to a child.

Elder Abuse: Abuse of a person over 60 years of age, which may include physical abuse but also sexual, emotional, or financial abuse and abandonment.

Intimate Partner Violence: Physical, sexual, or emotional and psychological abuse of men or women occurring in past or current intimate relationships, cohabiting or not, and including dating relationships.

Neglect: The failure to provide for the individual's basic needs for subsistence, including food, housing, clothing, education, medical care, and emotional care. At its most extreme, neglect results in death, especially in the older adults and in very young children.

Physical Abuse: Involves the intentional use of physical force against another person, including, but not limited to, pushing, slapping, biting, choking, punching, beating, and using a gun, knife, or other weapon.

Sexual Abuse: Abusive sexual contact, completed or attempted, against the will of the other, or in circumstances in which the other is unable to understand, refuse, or communicate unwillingness to engage in the sexual activity.

Violence is a leading worldwide public health problem (World Health Organization [WHO], 1996). Violence is also an inescapable public health problem, with an estimated 1.9 million women and

*3.2 million men being physically assaulted each year (Tjaden &
Toennes, 2000b). Prevalence of some types of violence varies based
on race or ethnicity, with some minority women and men reporting
more frequent and more violent victimization. Nurses and other
health care providers must guard against insensitivity when
working with survivors of violence.*

VIOLENCE SURVIVOR DISORDERS—GENERAL

The *Diagnostic and Statistical Manual
of Mental Disorders* (4th edition Text
Revision) (*DSM-IV-TR*) (American Psychiatric Association [APA], 2000), includes a
section categorizing severity of mistreatment (Table 16–1).

Causes

Many factors contribute to abuse and violence across the life span. Research shows
that survivors of abuse and violence are
also likely to become perpetrators. Similarly, inadequate family functioning contributes to neglect and child psychopathology (Moss, Lynch, Hardie, & Baron, 2002).

Table 16–1 • Problems Related to Abuse or Neglect as Defined by *DSM-IV-TR*

The focus of clinical attention is harsh
abuse of one person by another (e.g.,
physical and sexual abuse or child neglect).

Specify whether the client is a victim or
perpetrator.

The following categories apply:

1. Physical abuse of child
2. Sexual abuse of child
3. Neglect of child
4. Physical abuse of adult (e.g., intimate
   partner violence, elder abuse)
5. Sexual abuse of adult

Note. From *Diagnostic and Statistical Manual of Mental Disorders* (4th edition Text Revision) (*DSM-IV-TR*),
by American Psychiatric Association, 2000,
Washington, DC: Author. Adapted with permission.

Psychoanalytical theories suggest that
aggression is a basic instinct that is expressed or suppressed as a result of a wide
variety of interpersonal and intrapersonal
factors. When a basic need of the person
is not met, the person instinctively responds in an aggressive manner. This
instinctivist theory proposes that aggression is an innate drive and that humans
are fundamentally motivated by aggression (Ardrey, 1966; Lorenz, 1966.)

Studies on aggression or violence indicate dysregulation in neurochemical, neuroendocrine, and neuroanatomical structures and genetic-environmental factors.
Clients with an underlying brain disorder
are likely to exhibit aggressive, explosive,
and assaultive behaviors across the life
span (Coccaro, Kavoussi, Hauger, Coper,
& Ferris, 1998; Scarpa & Raine, 1997).
Biological theorists suggest that the limbic
system and neurotransmitters play a role
in the development of violent behavior.
The limbic system influences memory
storage, information interpreting and processing, and the autonomic functions of
the nervous system. Within the limbic
system's influence is the mediation of
the aggressive sexual and emotional
responses (Oquendo & Mann, 2000).
Interference with the processing of information through brain lesions, substance
use, head injury, malnutrition, and medical conditions such as epilepsy may contribute to the expression of aggression
(Bars, Heyrend, Simpson, & Munger,
2001; Coccaro et al., 1998).

Additionally, research has suggested
that exposure to trauma can evoke persistent biological abnormalities (Bars
et al., 2001; Coccaro et al., 1998). PTSD,
often diagnosed in survivors of sexual

and physical trauma, has been associated with a hyperadrenergic state, hypofunctioning of the hypothalamic-pituitary-adrenocortical system, and dysregulation of the endogenous opioid system (Widom, 1999; Yehuda, 1998; 2002).

Social learning theorists, such as Bandura (1973), postulated that behavior occurs as a result of cognitive and environmental factors and that aggression may be simulated and become a learned behavior. Children raised in abusive families are at risk of mimicking abuse or violent behaviors.

Sociological theories of violence address cultural attitudes toward aggression, societal structures that permit aggression, and social frustration and fragmentation. Violence as a cultural attitude is reflected in the glorification of violent behavior in movies and television, degradation of women, and in the acceptance of aggression or violence as part of daily living. In addition, social psychologists focus on the social learning that contributes to violence. When people grow up in a family context of violence, they learn that violence is a legitimate form of communication, often resulting in intergenerational transmission of violent behaviors (Fonagy & Target, 1995; Fonagy, Target, & Gergely, 2000).

Straus (1973) presented the following eight propositions to illustrate how general systems theory relates to family violence:

1. Violence among family members has many causes and roots. Normative structures, personality traits, frustrations, and conflicts are only some of them.
2. More family violence occurs than is reported.
3. Most family violence is either denied or ignored.
4. Stereotyped family violence imagery is learned in early childhood from parents, siblings, and other children.
5. Family violence stereotypes are continually reaffirmed for adults and children through ordinary social interactions and the mass media.
6. Violent acts by violent persons may generate positive feedback—that is, these acts may produce desired results.
7. Use of violence, when contrary to family norms, creates additional conflicts over ordinary violence. The conflict now becomes the use of violence, not the behavior, that elicited that response in the first place.
8. Persons who are labeled violent may be encouraged to play out a violent role, either to live up to others' expectations of them as violent or to fulfill their own concept of themselves as violent or dangerous.

Determining the proclivity for violence involves looking beyond pathology to maladaptive coping patterns. Role disturbance, power imbalance, and marital dissatisfaction all are correlates of abuse. Families with members who engage in maltreatment tend to exhibit a pattern of coping characterized by a low level of social exchange, low responsiveness to positive behaviors, and high responsiveness to negative behaviors. Failure to cope with or adapt to stress leads to low frustration tolerance, which, in turn, can escalate a situation to a crisis level. The resolution to the perceived crisis is often violence or abuse.

Alcohol abuse and substance abuse also play a role in abuse in the family. Maladaptive coping in the form of substance abuse can interfere with the person's ability to parent. Normally, family deficits in managing or coping with stress involve maltreatment and harsh and inconsistent interactions that result in transgenerational maladaptive coping patterns (Brook, Whiteman, Balka, & Cohen, 1995; Moss, Baron, Hardie, & Vanyukov, 2001; Moss et al., 2002).

Environmental stresses include financial problems, intergenerational transmission (i.e., parents usually raise their children the way they were brought up), or difficulties with family structures (i.e., single-parent families, large families, or blended families). These stressors can contribute to serious family dysfunction, resulting in child maltreatment.

Symptoms

Physiological changes include sympathetic hyperarousal, excessive startle reflex, abnormalities in sleep physiology, and traumatic nightmares.

Parents or guardians who abuse their children may present with issues of chronic low self-esteem, depression, dependency, immaturity, impulsiveness, suspiciousness, and lack of empathy.

TREATMENT

When working with families exhibiting maladaptive coping patterns, it is imperative for the nurse to assess their coping style, disciplining patterns, and cultural factors. Acting-out behaviors in the child or adolescent may indicate inadequate parenting or a mental or physical problem. When the nurse suspects child or elder abuse, the nurse must report it according to state laws governing abuse. Nursing interventions may include family crisis intervention, appropriate community referrals, or legal referrals.

The challenge for psychiatric nurses is grasping the scope of violence or abuse on the individual. It is also essential for nurses to understand the culture in which the survivor resides before assuming that abuse or violence exists. It is important for nurses to understand the differences between and within various cultural groups so that assessment can be structured to identify the unique needs of the clients from various cultural groups. Interventions also need to take into consideration the barriers that exist and limit access to culturally appropriate services (Yoshioka & Dang, 2000).

The specific type of intervention used with a family or individual experiencing abuse is determined by the family's or survivor's current situation, ability to verbalize feelings, and willingness to effect change.

Crisis intervention provides the family with immediate emotional support and facilitates adaptive coping responses and effective problem-solving skills. Initially, the child and parents or guardians may be seen separately and then together to assess family stressors, strengths, and coping patterns. It is important for the nurse to validate the survivor's feelings and provide safety.

Group therapy interventions provide unique opportunities for family members to work on issues of trust, differentiation, and responsibility. It enhances interpersonal communication and provides safe opportunities for social relationships. Group therapy reduces isolation by bringing parents together, and improve self-esteem by introducing parents to other families who are struggling.

Psychiatric assessment should be considered when clients are chronically depressed, suicidal, or express affective or thought disorders. Crisis situations require immediate management when the client is a danger to self and others. Short-term stabilization is usually the treatment of choice in these cases.

Pharmacologic interventions are useful in treating affective (mood) disorders, psychosis, acute anxiety reactions, and biological responses. A comprehensive physical and psychosocial assessment is necessary before beginning medication. These examinations provide information about differential diagnoses and the current health status.

Substance abuse therapy provides medical treatment, addictions treatment, and support services for nonabusers. Most communities have services for drug and alcohol abusers, including:

- Detoxification programs
- Inpatient hospital programs
- Outpatient programs
- Health services
- Parent education classes
- Employment training or retraining
- Self-help or support groups (e.g., Parents Anonymous, Narcotics and Alcoholics Anonymous, Al-Anon)
- Educational support (i.e., high school graduate equivalent degree [GED] courses)
- Legal referrals and resources

(continues)

TREATMENT *(continued)*

Certain competencies will help nurses to prepare for effective interventions with survivors, perpetrators, and witnesses of violence and abuse.

1. The nurse needs to recognize that interpersonal violence is a serious social problem worldwide that has persistent and severe physical and mental health consequences. Although violence and abuse are endemic, they are still not openly discussed in some families, communities, and cultures. The incidence is high and the consequences of some types of violence and abuse affect the remainder of the survivor's life.

2. The nurse needs to become familiar with the dynamics of abusive relationships and with the physical and mental health effects of ongoing and previous violence or abuse across the life span. In most states with legislation designed to protect survivors of violence, the nurse is expected to assess for and to report suspected abuse of children, women, and older adults, whether or not actual abuse can be documented (see Table 16–2, Child Abuse: How the Nurse Fits into the Reporting and Intervention Process). Ideally, the nurse's report activates a complex system, which not only furthers the assessment, but also, in the event of actual abuse, coordinates intervention activities from various agencies. These interventions are designed to provide safety for the individual being abused and, if possible, maintain the integrity of the family.

3. The nurse needs to be aware of the various resources in the community that can provide the supportive services needed by both survivors and perpetrators of violence. The nurse is less likely to blame the victim, avoid the problem, or use denial if she is aware of the resources available in the community to meet the needs of those involved in the violent situation.

Table 16–2 • Child Abuse: How the Nurse Fits into the Reporting and Intervention Process

Steps 1 through 3: The Nurse's Role

1. The nurse suspects reportable child abuse. A case conference is convened as indicated.

2. Reports are made to the state authority (child protective services or law enforcement) by telephone or in person.

3. A written report may be required. The content should include the following:
   a. Demographics of the child and the family
   b. Nature and content of injuries, in detail
   c. Caretaker information

Steps 4 through 7: The State's Role

4. The state agency initiates an investigation: High-risk assessments require response within 24 to 48 hours.

5. Family assessment takes place.

6. Case management ensues. If abuse is indicated, the child protective service worker may initiate any or all of the following:
   a. Treatment
   b. Referrals
   c. Court intervention

7. Closure of case is implemented.

---

4. The nurse must make a practice of assessing every client seen in any health care setting for experience with violence. The question must be asked directly, in a private setting, and in a manner that is comfortable for the nurse. Instruments developed by nurses can be incorporated into health history protocols to collect assessment data related to exposure to violence and abuse across the life span (Campbell, 1995; MacFarlane & Parker, 1994).

5. It is important for the nurse to recognize the effect that violence has had

(continues)

TREATMENT *(continued)*

on her own life. Because interpersonal violence is endemic, the nurse's life has also been affected by violence and abuse. The nurse's experience with violence will influence her attitude and response to experiences of violence of her clients. Introspection and processing of her own feelings regarding caring for survivors and perpetrators are important exercises for the nurse.

6. The nurse must identify a support network to assist in dealing with the feelings engendered by working with this truly vulnerable population. Sadness, rage, anger, fear, vulnerability, and frustration are just a few of the emotional consequences of working with survivors and perpetrators of violence and abuse. Self-care by the nurse will allow this important work to continue in the face of these stressful emotions.

The generalist nurse is integral to the mental health team that intervenes on behalf of the survivors and their families. The generalist nurse has the skill and expertise to provide client interventions at all junctures, and in all practice settings implements the nursing process to assist clients explore feelings related to the abuse. The generalist nurse acts as an advocate while helping clients negotiate the many systems (such as health care and protective services; schools; the workplace; community agencies' grassroot service organizations, food banks, day care centers, shelters, self-help or support groups; fraternal organizations; ethnic, cultural, and religious organizations; and social and recreational groups) that may affect them. The generalist nurse uses the nursing process to assess the clients' physical and mental health status, to determine the diagnoses and expected outcomes individual to the clients, to develop a plan of care and implement nursing interventions, and to evaluate client response and progress. In addition, the generalist nurse collaborates and coordinates the client care with other health professionals.

Advanced-practice psychiatric registered nurses conduct evaluations of children and families, provide treatment for survivors and perpetrators, and provide clinical consultation to other professionals. They may provide testimony in court, either as expert or as fact witnesses.

CHILD MALTREATMENT

Child maltreatment refers to actions and behaviors that result in serious physical injury, neglect, sexual abuse, and serious mental injury to a child.

Causes

Head trauma, which often results from shaking, accounted for the leading cause of death and disability among maltreated infants and children. The physical abuse of a child is any intentional injury inflicted by the child's caretaker. **Physical abuse** can be a single episode or repeated events and involves inflicting physical injury by punching, beating, kicking, shaking, or otherwise harming a child. Depending on the severity of the injury, the child's physical functioning is either permanently or temporarily impaired. The harm causes severe pain to the child and may be accompanied by a pattern of separate, unexplained injuries (see Table 16–3 for forms of child physical abuse).

The relationship between childhood maltreatment and mental disorders is well documented (Maxwell & Widom, 1996; Widom, 1998; 1999). Recent studies also implicate child maltreatment and neglect as markers for other factors that make an impact on the developing child and increase the risk of lifelong maladaptive behaviors. Examples of mental disorders associated with childhood maltreatment and abuse include post-traumatic stress disorder (PTSD) and other anxiety disorders, depression, and antisocial behaviors. Risk factors for emotional abuse and other forms of maltreatment include poverty, parental substance misuse, or inadequate social and family functioning

Table 16–3 • Forms of Child Physical Abuse

- Skin and soft tissue injury (i.e., bruises, hematomas, and abrasions)
- Internal injuries
- Dislocations and fractures
- Loss of teeth caused by shaking, slapping, punching, kicking, striking, and hitting
- Throwing of child or throwing objects against the child
- Branding or loop or restraint marks made by belt buckles, handprints, electric cords, ropes, or ligatures
- Hair loss caused by pulling the child by the hair
- Burns caused by spills, immersions, flames, and branding
- Wounds caused by gunshots, knives, razors, or other sharp objects

(Boney-McCoy & Finkelhor, 1996; Widom, 1999).

The psychosocial factors or characteristics of abusive families have also been identified. Starr (1988) and Widom (1999) have identified a set of risk factors or correlates for child abuse that includes the following:

- Isolation from family and friends
- High ratio of negative to positive interactions with various family members
- High level of expressed anger and impulsivity
- Inappropriate expectations of the child
- Relatively high rate of both actual and perceived stress

Symptoms

Nurses must always consider physical abuse when the child has bruises or other injuries that are difficult to explain or inconsistent with the given explanation. Oftentimes, these children are withdrawn, overly aggressive, or exhibit delay in developmental tasks. A child who has frequent visits to the hospital emergency room or other practice settings for the treatment of bizarre or strange complaints with overly doting parents or guardians may be a victim of Munchausen syndrome by proxy. Characteristics of this syndrome involve a parent or guardian asking or forcing the child to take substances that induce signs of physical illnesses (e.g., dehydration, diarrhea) and seeking medical attention to manage them (APA, 2000; Donald & Jureidini, 1996) (See Chapter 12 of the core text). Table 16–4 presents guidelines for assessing patterns of physical abuse of a child.

The CDC (2001) defines **neglect** as a failure to provide for the child's basic needs, including food, housing, clothing, education, medical care, and emotional care. See Table 16–5 for types of neglect and behaviors indicating neglect.

Emotional or psychological abuse refers to acts or behaviors or omissions by primary caregivers that result in or increase the risk of serious behavioral, cognitive, emotional, and mental disorders. This definition includes, but is not limited to, psychological, verbal, and mental injury.

Sexual abuse is defined as abusive sexual contact, completed or attempted, against the will of the other, or in circumstances in which the other is unable to understand, refuse, or communicate unwillingness to engage in the sexual activity. In addition, it refers to sexual contact with a person 5 or more years older than the child victim, whether by force or consent. The sexual contact includes a wide variety of sexual behaviors

Table 16–4 • Guidelines for Assessing Physical Abuse of a Child

- History of injury given by the parent or guardian does not match the injury observed
- Delay in seeking treatment for the child
- Past history of unexplained injuries
- Concealment of injuries by parents or guardian
- Recurrent injuries
- Failure to gain appropriate weight

Table 16–5 • Types of Neglect and Behaviors Indicating Neglect

Type of Neglect	Behavior Indicating Neglect
Failure to protect	Ingestion of poison, accidents (including falls, electric shocks, and burns), and disregard for the child's safety. Lack of appropriate supervision.
Physical neglect	Failure to provide food, clothing, and shelter. Failure to provide adequate heating, diet, and hygiene. Indicators include diaper dermatitis, lice, odors, scabies, dirty appearance, inappropriate clothing for the season, lack of adequate bedding, and a living environment infested with insects or rodents. Other signs include failure to immunize, poor dental hygiene, malnutrition, and failure to provide the child with hearing and seeing aids.
Medical neglect	Failure to provide for the medical needs of the child, including failure to seek timely intervention or failure to comply with prescribed medical treatment. Indicators include repeated urgent health care visits, delayed diagnosis, physical incapacity, and avoidable complications.
Emotional neglect and nonorganic failure to thrive	Failure to provide nurturing and psychological support. Indicators include delayed growth and development, depression, poor school performance, acute, psychiatric manifestations (withdrawal, phobias, hyperactivity, and acting out), and difficulties with relationships (inability to trust, attention-seeking behaviors, or suspiciousness).

such as touching and exposing of the child's sexual parts for the sexual gratification of the perpetrator; sexual intercourse, oral and anal penetration; rape; the prostitution of children; and the use of children in pornography. The sexual contact can also be observed contact (i.e., exposing the genitals to the child or having the child view sexually explicit activity). (Table 16–6 lists types of sexual abuse behaviors.)

Sexual abuse is differentiated from incest in that sexual abuse of children can involve a wide variety of perpetrators, not just blood relatives. Incest is a legal term describing a form of sexual abuse and is defined by each state's civil and criminal code. Incest is illegal in all states, but the behaviors that are considered incestuous may vary from state to state.

Disruptions in relationship can be observed in children through their interactions with their primary caregivers. Abused and neglected children may have difficulties in exploring and coping with the demands of new relationships and may demonstrate distortions in their relationships with their caregivers. These

Table 16–6 • Types of Sexual Abuse Behaviors

- Penile penetration of the anus and/or vagina
- Insertion of object into the anus and/or vagina (e.g., finger)
- Fellatio and cunnilingus
- Masturbation of the victim
- Masturbation of self in front of the victim
- Manipulation of the genitals (e.g., touching, caressing)
- Exposure of the perpetrator's genital to the victim
- Exposure of pornography to the victim (e.g., sexually explicit magazines, books, videos, or on the Internet)

distortions include a tendency to be passive with the abusing parent or guardian rather than being either difficult or compliant. Some abused children may exhibit excessive dependency, wariness, and an inability to form interpersonal relationships.

Key Fact

According to the Centers for Disease Control and Prevention's Injury Fact Book (2001–2002) (CDC, 2001) in 1998, nearly a million children in this country experienced or were at risk for child abuse, neglect, or both.

TREATMENT

The potential negative impact of emotional and other forms of maltreatment require nurses to recognize high-risk groups and clinical signs of maladaptive behaviors in both the child and caregiver. For instance, a child who appears overly anxious or frightened or a caregiver who fails to provide basic needs such as safety and nutrition may imply emotional abuse. Nurses must be careful and document observations and signs of maltreatment and report them according to state and federal laws. Health education is also pivotal in reducing child maltreatment and provides opportunities for nurses to teach parenting classes, anger management, and make appropriate community referrals to strengthen caregivers' coping skills.

Nurses are responsible for reporting suspected child maltreatment as mandated by these state reporting laws. All states and U.S. territories have laws and statutes requiring the reporting of child abuse and neglect to designated agencies or officials. Nurses who care for children and their families are in key positions to identify possible incidents of child abuse and neglect. Each state's reporting laws specify how to report, to whom, when, and the contents of the report. Most states have legal provisions to protect nurse reporters from civil lawsuits and criminal prosecution resulting from the reporting made in "good faith." Failure to report abuse by a designated mandated reporter, such as a nurse, could result in criminal penalties and loss of licensure. All nurses are urged to obtain copies of their state's reporting laws.

Nurses need to identify high-risk groups and maladaptive coping behaviors and initiate adaptive coping behaviors that enable the child to manage stress and feelings effectively. Teaching the family adaptive coping skills provides opportunities for the child to model healthy and appropriate behaviors.

Critical to an understanding of the effects of abuse on the child and adolescent is an appreciation of the components of the abuse. The nature of the act; the relationship of the perpetrator to the child; the response of other caregivers to the abuse; the frequency of the abuse; the duration and the severity of the abuse; and child-specific factors such as gender, coping and adaptation ability, and developmental level must be taken into account.

Children who are abused and neglected often present with varied acute symptoms. The nurse needs to consider the various defense mechanisms children may use to cope with the reality of the abuse. Common defense mechanisms used by children include denial, regression, projection, dissociation, and repression. Nurses also need to be aware of the immediate effects seen in children who are abused and neglected, some of which are delineated in Table 16–7. Nurses need to be very careful not to draw conclusions without a thorough assessment. Special educational preparation is necessary to perform a thorough assessment of a child who is suspected of being abused. Accurate documentation of social interactions with primary caregivers and the physical and mental status examinations is crucial to appropriate treatment planning.

The nursing interventions include interventions that facilitate healthy parenting skills, stress management, improve communication, foster positive parent-child interactions, and to help parents or guardians manage their conflicts. The nurse also needs to coordinate psychosocial services that link the family with necessary resources to reduce fragmented health care.

In families experiencing child maltreatment, couples therapy can be beneficial

(continues)

Table 16–7 • Immediate Effects of Abuse on the Child and Adolescent

Behavioral

- Acting out
- Aggression
- Hyperactivity
- Self-destructive acts
- Antisocial and delinquent behaviors (e.g., cruelty to animals, fire setting, and fecal smearing)
- Sexual acting out (promiscuity, prostitution, or sexualization)
- Somatic complaints and psychosomatic symptomatology

Emotional

- Depression
- Anxiety
- Anger
- Fears and phobias
- Psychotic processes
- Self-depreciating thoughts

Cognitive

- Distractability
- Concentration difficulties
- Memory impairment
- Poor judgment

Interpersonal

- Poor peer relationships
- Conflictual family relationships
- Disrespect and disregard for authority

TREATMENT *(continued)*

when parents or guardians realize that their anger toward and frustration with each other are being redirected onto the children. Couples can be taught direct styles of communication that encourage expression of their feelings, listening techniques, and effective verbalizations.

In families in which incest is occurring, the focus of couples therapy is on the effect of the incest on the dyad. Issues in therapy include the couple's capacity for intimacy, sexual relations, communication, respect, and an examination of roles and responsibilities.

Family therapy can also be a productive intervention if the family members are verbal, the children are old enough to participate, and the behavior related to anger in the family is controlled. The goal of intervention is to prevent further maltreatment. The following are examples of family therapy objectives:

- Confrontation of the abuse
- Identification of the pattern of abuse
- Setting of short- and long-term goals for the family in relation to the abuse
- Discussion of family roles and rules

Issues discussed with abusive families include the following:

- Impulse control
- Judgment errors (life choices)
- Conflicts with authority
- Manipulative behaviors, scapegoating, mixed or incongruent messages
- Tendency to act out rather than talk
- Blurred boundaries
- Role dysfunction
- Imbalance of power
- Communication skills
- Trust and intimacy

Art therapy allows children to express their feelings and thoughts rather than verbally expressing themselves. Art therapy is helpful as both a diagnostic and therapeutic tool.

Group therapy allows abused children to regain their status as children. The group provides peer interactions and age-appropriate tasks. If both sexes are in a group, the coleaders need to be a male and a female. Survivors are validated for their feelings and reinforced that they are not at fault. For example, if the child comments about being sad or upset, these feelings are accepted and validated by the group leader(s). Sometimes children from abusive families have been taught that expressing their feelings is not acceptable, and they begin to doubt their significance. By encouraging expressing

(continues)

TREATMENT *(continued)*

of feelings, the child begins to feel worthwhile and positive about self. Groups for sexually abused children can help correct the distortions in the parent-child relationship. Groups should be in a safe place for children to talk and play out their feelings. The group leaders are role models who help the children learn to relate to peers who have also been abused.

Individual therapy is suggested for children who can verbalize their feelings and needs. Therapy is directed toward their fears, conflicts, and the disclosure of the trauma associated with the abuse. Therapy helps the child process the abuse.

Play therapy is indicated for children too young to have the capacity for introspection and verbalization (toddler to 6 years old). Play therapy allows children to demonstrate their feelings through their actions. The abusive behaviors are observed in their play.

Special education programs for physically, developmentally, or emotionally disabled children should be considered by the nurse when these children present with maltreatment.

Self-neglect often manifests as an older adult's refusal or failure to provide self with basic needs (e.g., adequate food, water, clothing, shelter, and medication).

Survivors of elder abuse may present with unexplained physical injuries, such as fractures, bruises, abrasions, or hematomas, and may appear dehydrated, untidy, malnourished, or oversedated. The abused older adult may be in need of hearing, vision, and walking appliances, indicating that basic physical needs are not being met. Commonly, the psychological effects present in the abused older adult are withdrawal, passivity, hopelessness, and nonresponsiveness.

Key Fact

Each year an estimated 10 percent of adults 65 years and older are abused, and 4 percent experience moderate-to-severe abuse. By 2030, the U.S. population will comprise about 70 million people, thereby increasing the risk of elder abuse (Greenberg, 1996; Program Resources Department, American Association of Retired Persons [AARP] and Administration on Aging [ADA], U.S. Department of Health and Human Services, 1993).

ELDER ABUSE

Causes

Typically, the profile of the abused older adult is female, isolated socially and perhaps geographically, and economically and physically dependent on a family system, without skills to deal with longstanding intergenerational conflict. The perpetrator may be a close relative, highly stressed, and dependent on the abused older adult financially or psychologically, or both (Lachs, Williams, O'Brien, Pillemer, & Charlson, 1998; Steinmetz, 1993).

Symptoms

Elder abuse is abuse of a person over 60 years of age, which includes physical, sexual, financial, emotional, or psychological abuse; neglect; abandonment; material exploitation; and self-neglect.

INTIMATE PARTNER VIOLENCE

Intimate partner violence (IPV), or domestic violence, is the most common type of violence perpetrated toward women. Perpetrators of IPV include current or former spouse, boyfriend, or girlfriend (American Association of Colleges of Nursing [AACN], 2000). High-risk groups of IPV include young, childbearing women who are 16 to 24 years old (U.S. Department of Justice, 1998).

Causes

It is commonly accepted that men underreport their own assaults and may also tolerate a certain level of violence from their intimate partner as a result of traditional cultural norms. Survivors of IPV are likely to be faulted for their abuse and are less likely to seek professional guidance or mention the abuse than survivors assaulted by strangers.

Symptoms

Major types of IPV include actual or threatened physical abuse, sexual assault, emotional abuse, or verbal abuse. Physical abuse involves the intentional use of physical force against another person, including, but not limited to, pushing, slapping, biting, choking, punching, beating, and use of a gun, knife, or other weapon (CDC, 1997).

Acute biological responses include intense anxiety, hyperarousal, elevated heart rate and blood pressure, muscle tension, sleep and concentration disturbances, and panic reactions. Physical symptoms may include bruises; swellings; burns; lacerations; fractures; abdominal injuries (especially during pregnancy); unwanted pregnancies; miscarriage; sexually transmitted diseases (STDs), including HIV; and homicide. Survivors may also develop stress-related conditions such as headaches, asthma, pelvic pain, irritable bowel syndrome, or other gastrointestinal disturbances.

Psychological responses include feeling embarrassed or fearful to disclose the abuse or sometimes feeling fearful that the nurse will not believe these clients. They may feel the need to protect the perpetrator, may excuse the abusive behavior, or may cover for the perpetrator in an attempt to be viewed favorably by either the abuser or others. Additional psychological responses include intense fear, anxiety, sexual dysfunction, eating problems, sleep disorders, suicide, PTSD, depression, and alcohol and other drug abuse.

Many women who have experienced IPV develop a recognized pattern of psychological symptoms called *battered woman syndrome* (Walker, 1993). These symptoms are usually transient but are observed in a recognizable pattern in women who have been physically, sexually, or seriously psychologically abused by their partner. Components of battered woman syndrome are consistent with PTSD. For example, it is usual for abused women to experience flashbacks to the

violent incidents, and when the intrusive memories are too overwhelming, it is not uncommon for abused women to dissociate from the memories. Abused women experience avoidance of thoughts about the abuse, depression, and anxiety-based symptoms. See Table 16–8 for a summary of the general immediate and long-term effects of violence and abuse on the family.

Key Fact

A conservative estimate is that 1.3 million women and 835,000 men experience physical assault at the hands of an intimate partner each year (Tjaden & Theonnes, 2000b). Intimate partner violence is the foremost cause of injury to women, and as many as 45 percent of battered women report sexual abuse or rape in addition to repeated physical and psychological abuse (Campbell, Harris, & Lee, 1995; Liebshultz, Feinman, Sullivan, Stein, & Samet, 2000).

Table 16–8 • Effects of Abuse on the Family

Acute Effects

- Yelling, screaming, verbal outbursts
- Erratic discipline
- Corporal punishment
- Isolation of members
- Unrealistic expectations
- Disengagement or enmeshment
- Role disruption
- Power struggles

Chronic Effects

- Psychopathological/mental disturbances
- Separation or divorce
- Running away
- Court intervention
- Social service involvement
- Disturbances in school and work
- Health problems
- Drug or alcohol misuse
- Intrafamilial homicide

TREATMENT

Because the nurse is likely to be the first non-family member whom women encounter in emergency departments, battered women's shelters, college health clinics, primary care and office settings, or telephone crisis hotlines, she must be aware of symptoms that indicate acute stress reactions and provide immediate emotional support. The nurse also needs to screen for sexual, physical, and psychological abuse. Information about the survivor must be kept confidential, and discussions with the perpetrator concerning IPV should never be done in the presence of the survivor. Once IPV is discussed, the nurse needs to use a direct and calm approach and focus on the abuser's behavior rather than the survivor's (Ganley, 1998). Appropriate referrals to batterers intervention programs are important in dealing with IPV. Most states require participation in these programs as a stipulation of battering even when survivor objects or drops charges.

Initially, the client may be distant and untrusting, appear to be in a daze or state of shock, have problems answering questions spontaneously, and be emotionally distraught and tearful. Others may be overly compliant and exhibit very little emotion. Although the latter client appears less distraught than the former, the nurse must assess the emotional impact of this stressful situation. Nurses should also focus on the impact of the violence on the survivor's daily life, considering the social context and the degree to which the violence alienates the client from others. It is imperative for the nurse to assess the survivor's coping responses and offer help in resolving acute symptoms (Draucker & Madsen, 1999).

Warshaw (1998) delineates the following guiding principles when working with survivors of IPV:

- Providing safety of the survivors and their children must be a priority
- Respecting the woman's right and ability over her life choices
- Holding perpetrators responsible for the abuse and stopping it
- Advocating on behalf of survivors and their children
- Acknowledging the importance of making changes in the health care system to improve appropriate responses to violence

Nurses need to be aware of the reality that men are also survivors of intimate partner violence and that screening for exposure to violence must include all clients, not only women and girls presenting themselves for health care.

Overall, because survivors of IPV are less likely to disclose the abuse to nurses, it is important to create a supportive and empathetic environment that promotes expression of feelings. In addition, when the client reports IPV, the nurse needs to validate the client's feelings and grief and refrain from minimizing the emotional impact of violence. The nursing assessment of clients needs to include questions about abuse and violence, both as survivor and perpetrator. Issues concerning perpetrators of violence are crucial to the prevention of future violence. Inquiring about history of consequences of violence, such as legal issues, needs to be assessed along with appropriate referrals to batterers intervention programs. In addition, the client's spiritual needs must be assessed. By providing emotional support and spiritual care the nurse is likely to strengthen internal resources and coping patterns and buffer the client against distress and mental discomfort.

Implications for the nurse caring for the client in an abusive relationship must begin with understanding the emotional ties associated with the perpetrator. It is also important to understand that the survivor will leave the relationship when it feels safe. Acceptance and support of the client's decisions and feelings are critical elements of treatment planning and must be the foundation of the nurse-client relationship. Self-awareness about the client's decision enables the nurse to recognize the importance of client preferences and choices in dealing with abuse and violence.

(continues)

TREATMENT *(continued)*

Couples therapy is not advised in IPV until the abusive partner has demonstrated an ability to control the dangerous physically abusive behaviors.

RESOURCES

Please note that because Internet resources are of a time-sensitive nature and URL addresses may change or be deleted, searches should also be conducted by association or topic.

Internet Resources

http://www.famvi.com/   Domestic Violence, Family Violence, Child Abuse Page

http://www.sfms.org.org/domestic.html   Domestic Violence: A Practical Approach for Clinicians

http://www.mcadv.org/   National Coalition Against Domestic Violence (NCADV)

References

CHAPTER 1

American Psychiatric Association. (2000). *Diagnostic and statistical manual of mental disorders* (4th edition Text Revision) (*DSM-IV-TR*). Washington, DC: Author.

Antai-Otong, D. (2001). *Psychiatric emergencies*. Eau Claire, WI: Professional Educational Systems, Inc.

Beck, A. T., Brown, G., Berchick, R. J., Stewart, B. L., & Steer, R. A. (1990). Relationship between hopelessness and ultimate suicide: A replication with psychiatric outpatients. *American Journal of Psychiatry, 147,* 190–195.

Cheng, A. T. A., Chen, T. H. H., Chen, C. C. & Jenkins, R. (2000). Psychosocial and psychiatric risk factors for suicide. Case-control psychological autopsy study. *The British Journal of Psychiatry, 177,* 360–365.

Duberstein, P., & Conwell, Y. (1997). Personality disorders and completed suicide: A methological and conceptual review. *Clinical Psychology: Science and Practice, 4,* 359–376.

Gibbs, J. T. (1988). Conceptual, methodological, and sociological issues in black youth suicide: Implications for assessment and early intervention. *Suicide and Life-Threatening Behavior, 18,* 73–89.

Goldberg, J. F., Garno, J. L., Leon, A. C., Kocsis, J. H., & Portera, L. (1998). Association of recurrent suicidal ideations with nonremission from acute mixed mania. *American Journal of Psychiatry, 155,* 1753–1755.

Gunderson, J. G. (2001). *Borderline personality disorder: A clinical guide.* Washington, DC: American Psychiatric Publishing.

Harris, E. C., & Barraclough, B. (1998). Excess mortality of mental disorder. *The British Journal of Psychiatry, 173,* 11–53.

Helig, S. M., & Klugman, D. J. (1970). The social worker in suicide centers. In H. J. Parad (Ed.), *Crisis intervention: Selected readings* (5th ed., pp. 274–283). New York: Family Service Association of America.

Leon, A. C., Friedman, R. A., Sweeney, J. A., Brown, R. P., & Mann, J. J. (1990). Statistical issues in the identification of risk factors for suicidal behavior: The application of survival analysis. *Psychiatry Research, 31,* 99–108.

Mann, J. J. (1998). The neurobiology of suicide. *Nature Medicine, 4,* 25–30.

Mann, J. J., Waternaux, C., Haas, G. L., & Malone, K. M. (1999). Toward a clinical model of suicidal behavior in psychiatric patients. *American Journal of Psychiatry, 156,* 181–189.

McIntosh, J. L. (1995). Suicide prevention in the elderly (ages 65–99). *Suicide and Life Threatening Behavior, 25,* 180–192.

National Center for Health Statistics. (1991). *Vital statistics of the United States: Vol. 2, mortality—part A (for the years 1966–1988).* Washington, DC: US Government Printing Office.

Primeau, F., & Fontaine, R. (1987). Obsessive disorder with self-mutilation: A subgroup responsive to pharmacotherapy. *Canadian Journal of Psychiatry, 32,* 699–700.

Radomsky, E. D., Haas, G. L., Mann, J. J., & Sweeney, J. A. (1999). Suicidal behavior in patients with schizophrenia and other psychotic disorders. *American Journal of Psychiatry, 156,* 1590–1595.

Rauch, P. K., & Rappaport, N. (1994). Child psychiatric emergencies. In S. E. Hyman & G. E. Tesar (Eds.), *Manual of psychiatric emergencies* (3rd ed. pp. 53–59). Boston, MA: Little, Brown.

Rosenthal, P. A., & Rosenthal, S. (1984). Suicidal behavior by preschool children. *American Journal of Psychiatry, 141,* 520–525.

Roy, A. (1985). Suicide and psychiatric patients. *Psychiatric Clinics of North America, 8,* 181, 227–241.

Shaffer, D. (1988). The epidemiology of teen suicide: An examination of risk factors. *Journal of Clinical Psychiatry, 49,* 36–41.

Shneidman, E. S. (1985). *Definition of suicide.* New York: Wiley.

Smith, K. & Crawford, S. (1986). Suicidal behavior among "normal" high school students. *Suicide and Life-Threatening Behavior, 16,* 313–325.

Soloff, P. H., Lis, J. A., Kelly, T., Cornelius, J., & Ulrich, R. (1994). Risk factors for suicidal behavior in borderline personality disorder. *American Journal of Psychiatry, 151,* 1316–1323.

Strakowski, S. M., McElroy, S. L., Keck, P. E., Jr., & West, S. A. (1996). Suicidality among patients with mixed and manic bipolar disorder. *American Journal of Psychiatry, 153,* 672–676.

Waltzer, H. (1984). Suicide risk in the young schizophrenic. *General Hospital of Psychiatry, 6,* 219–225.

Winchel, R. M., & Stanley, M. (1992). Self-injurious behavior: A review of behavior and biology of self-mutilation. *American Journal of Psychiatry, 148,* 306–317.

Zayas, L. H., Kaplan, C., Turner, S., Romano, K., & Gonzalez-Ramos, G. (2000). Understanding suicide attempts by adolescent Hispanic females. *Social Work, 45,* 53–63.

CHAPTER 2

American Psychiatric Association (APA). (2000). *Diagnostic and statistical manual of mental disorders* (4th edition Text Revision) (*DSM-IV-TR*). Washington, DC: Author.

American Psychiatric Association Task Force on *DSM-IV*. (1991). *DSM-IV options book. Work in progress.* Washington, DC: Author.

Bleuler, E. (1950). *Dementia praecox or the group schizophrenias.* New York: International Universities Press.

Buckley, P. F. (2000). Treatment of schizophrenia: Improved therapies and evolving to higher standards of care. In *News Briefs, Special Issue.* Columbus: National Alliance for the Mentally Ill, Ohio.

Crespo-Facorro, B., Paradiso, S., Andreasen, N. C., O'Leary, D. S., Watkins, G. L., Ponto, L. L., et al. (2001). Neural mechanisms of anhedonia in schizophrenia: A PET study of response to unpleasant and pleasant odors. *Journal of the American Medical Association, 286,* 427–435.

Fox, J. C., & Kane, C. F. (1996). Information processing deficits in schizophrenia. In A. B. McBride & J. K. Austin (Eds.), *Psychiatric-mental health nursing* (pp. 321–347). Philadelphia: W.B. Saunders.

Freud, S. (1959). Inhibitions, symptoms, and anxiety. In J. Strachey (Trans. & Ed.), *The standard edition of the complete psychological works of Sigmund Freud* (Vol. 18, pp. 1–64). London: Hogarth Press.

Goldberg, R. J. (Ed.). (2001). Treating late-onset schizophrenia with newer antipsychotics. *Geriatric Psychopharmacology, 5*(6), 3–5.

Gottesman, I. I., & Moldin, S. O. (1997). Schizophrenia genetics at the millennium: Cautious optimism. *Clinical Genetics, 52,* 404–407.

Guyton, A, & Hall, J. (2000).1 *Textbook of medical physiology.* Philadelphia: W.B. Saunders.

Jerrell, J. M. (1999). Skill, symptom, and satisfaction changes in three service models for people with psychiatric disability. *Psychiatric Rehabilitation Journal, 22*(4), 342–348.

Lutz, W. J., & Warren, B. J. (2001). Symptomatology and medication monitoring for public mental health consumers: A cultural perspective. *Journal of the American Psychiatric Nurses Association, 7*(4), 115–124.

O'Connor, F. W. (1994). A vulnerability-stress framework for evaluating clinical interventions in schizophrenia. *Image: Journal of Nursing Scholarship, 158,* 163–175.

Owen, M. J. (2000). Molecular genetic studies of schizophrenia. *Brain Research and Brain Research Review, 31,* 179–186.

Perry, K., & Antai-Otong, D. (1995). The client with altered sensory perception: Schizophrenia and other psychotic disorders. In D. Antai-Otong (Ed.), *Psychiatric nursing: Biological and behavioral concepts* (pp. 223–229). Philadelphia: W.B. Saunders.

Raingruber, B. (2000). Settling into and moving in a climate of care: Styles and patterns of interaction between nurse psychotherapists and clients. *Perspectives in Psychiatric Care, 37*(1), 15–27.

Sadock, B. J., & Sadock, V. A. (Eds.). (1989). *Comprehensive textbook of psychiatry* (Vol. 1, 7th ed., pp. 134–142). Philadelphia: Lippincott Williams & Wilkins.

Srebnik, D. S., & La Fond, J. Q. (1999). Advance directives for mental health. *Psychiatric Services, 50*(7), 919–925.

U.S. Public Health Service, Department of Health and Human Services (DHHS). (1999). *Mental health: A report of the surgeon general.* Retrieved August 23, 2002, from http://www.surgeongeneral.gov/library/mentalhealth.html

Warren, B. J. (1999). Cultural competence in psychiatric nursing: An interlocking paradigm approach. In N. L. Keltner, L. Schwecke, & C. E. Bostrom (Eds.), *Psychiatric nursing* (3rd ed., pp. 199–218). St. Louis: Mosby.

Warren, B. J. (2000). Point of view: A best practice process for psychiatric-mental health nursing. *Journal of the American Psychiatric Nurses Association, 6*(4), 136–138.

Wuerker, A. K., Fu, V. K., Haas, G. L., & Bellack, A. S. (2002). Age expressed emotion and interpersonal controlling patterns in families of persons with schizophrenia. *Psychiatric Research, 109,* 161–170.

Wykes, T., Reeder, C., Corner, J., Williams, C., & Everitt, B. (1999). The effects of neurocognitive executive processing in patients with schizophrenia. *Schizophrenia Bulletin, 25*(2), 291–307.

CHAPTER 3

Albano, A. M., & Chorpita, B. F. (1995). Treatment of anxiety disorders of childhood. *Psychiatric Clinics of North America, 18,* 767–784.

American Academy of Child and Adolescent Psychiatry. (1998). Practice parameters for the assessment and treatment of children and adolescents with obsessive-compulsive disorder. *Journal of the American Academy of Child and Adolescent Psychiatry, 37,* 1110–1116.

American Psychiatric Association (1998). Practice guideline for the treatment of patients with panic disorder. *American Journal of Psychiatry, 155*(Suppl.), 1–34.

American Psychiatric Association. (2000). *Diagnostic and statistical manual of mental disorders* (4th edition Text Revision) *(DSM-IV-TR).* Washington, DC: Author.

Andrews, G., & Crino, R. (1991). Behavioral therapy of anxiety disorders. *Psychiatric Annals, 21,* 358–367.

Baldwin, D., Bobes, J., Stein, D. J., Scharwachter, I., & Faure, M. (1999). Paroxetine in social phobia/social anxiety disorder. *British Journal of Psychiatry, 175,* 120–126.

Ballenger, J. C., Wheadon, D. E., Steiner, M., Bushnell, W., & Gergel, I. P. (1998). Double-blind, fixed dose, placebo controlled study of paroxetine in the treatment of panic disorder. *American Journal of Psychiatry, 155,* 36–42.

Barlow, D. H. (1997). Cognitive-behavioral therapy for panic disorder: Current status. *Journal of Clinical Psychiatry, 58*(Suppl. 2), 32–36.

Barron, J., Curtis, M. A., & Grainger, R. D. (1998). Eye movement desensitization and reprocessing. *Journal of the American Psychiatric Nurses Association, 4,* 140–144.

Bauer, D. H. (1976). An exploratory study of developmental changes in children's fears. *Journal of Child Psychology and Psychiatry, 17,* 69–74.

Beck, A. T., Emery, G., & Greenberg, R. (1985). *Anxiety disorders and phobias: A cognitive perspective.* New York: Basic Books.

Beck, A. T., Skodol, L., Clark, D. A., Berchick, R., & Wright, F. (1992). A crossover study of focused cognitive therapy for panic disorders. *American Journal of Psychiatry, 149,* 778–783.

Bernstein, G. A., Borchardt, C. M., & Perwien, A. R. (1996). Anxiety disorders in children and adolescents: A review of the past 10 years. *Journal of American Academy of Child and Adolescent Psychiatry, 35,* 1110–1119.

Biederman, J., Hirsch-Becker, D. R., Rosenbaum, J. F., Herot, C., Friedman, D., Snidman, N., Kagan, J., & Faraone, S. V. (2001). Further evidence of association between behavioral inhibition and social anxiety in children. *American Journal of Psychiatry, 158,* 1673–1679.

Blazer, D., George, L. K., & Hughes, D. (1991). The epidemiology of anxiety disorders: An age comparison. In C. Salzman, & B. D. Lebowitz (Eds.), *Anxiety in the elderly* (pp. 17–30). New York: Springer.

Boney-McCoy, S., & Finkelhor, D. (1996). Is youth victimization related to trauma symptoms and depression after controlling for prior symptoms and family relationships: A longitudinal, prospective study. *Journal of Consulting Clinical Psychology, 64,* 1406–1416.

Bowlby, J. (1969). *Attachment and loss* (Vol. I). New York: Basic Books.

Cannon, W. B. (1914). The emergency functions of the adrenal medulla in pain and the major emotions. *American Journal of Physiology, 33,* 356–372.

Cloninger, C. R. (1986). A unified biosocial theory of personality and its role in the development of anxiety states. *Psychiatric Development, 5,* 167–226.

Connor, K. M., & Davidson, J. R. T. (1998). Generalized anxiety disorder: Neurobiological and pharmacotherapeutic perspectives. *Society of Biological Psychiatry, 44,* 1286–1294.

Coplan J. D., Papp, L. A., Martinez, J., Pine, D. S., Rosenblum, L. A., Cooper, T., et al. (1995). Persistence of blunted human growth hormone response to clonidine in panic disorder following fluoxetine treatment. *American Journal of Psychiatry, 152,* 619–622.

Dager, S. R., Friedman, S. D., Heide, A., Layton, M. E., Richards, T., Artru, A., et al. (1999). Two-dimensional proton echo-planar spectroscopic imaging or brain metabolic changes during lactate-induced panic. *Archives of General Psychiatry, 56,* 70–77.

Dager, S. R., Richards, T., Strauss, W. L., & Artru, A. (1997). Single-voxel H MRS investigation of brain metabolic changes during lactate-induced panic. *Psychiatry Research, 76,* 89–99.

DeVane, C. L., Grothe, D. R., & Smith, S. L. (2002). Pharmacology of antidepressants: Focus on Nefazodone. *Journal of Clinical Psychiatry, 63*(Suppl. 1), 10–17.

Eaton, W. W., Dryman, A., & Weissman, M. M. (1991). Panic and phobia. In L. N. Robins & D. A. Regier (Eds.), *Psychiatric disorder in America: The epidemiological catchment area study.* New York: Free Press.

Eysenck, H. J. (1981). *A model for personality.* New York: Springer-Verlag.

Eysenck, M. W. (1990). Anxiety and cognitive functioning. In G. D. Burrows, M. Roth, & R. Noyes (Eds.), *Handbook of anxiety: Vol. 2. The neurobiology of anxiety* (pp. 419–435). New York: Elsevier.

Feighner, J. P. (1999). Overview of antidepressants currently being used to treat anxiety disorders. *Journal of Clinical Psychiatry, 60*(Suppl. 22), 18–22.

Freud, S. (1936). *The problem of anxiety* (H. A. Bunker, Trans.). New York: Psychoanalytic Quarterly Press. (Original work published 1926)

Goenjian, A. K., Pynoos, R. S., Steinberg, A. M., Najarian, L. M., Asarnow, J. R., Karayan, I., et al. (1995). Psychiatric comorbidity in children after 1988 earthquake in Armenia. *Journal of the Academy of Child and Adolescent Psychiatry, 34,* 1174–1184.

Goldstein, G. D., Wampler, N. S., & Wise, P. H. (1997). War experiences and distress symptoms of Bosnian children. *Pediatrics, 100,* 873–878.

Gray, J. A. (1988). The neuropsychological basis of anxiety. In G. C. Last & M. Hersen (Eds.), *Handbook of anxiety disorder* (pp.10–40). New York: Pergamon Press.

Gurguis, G. N. M., Antai-Otong, D., Vo, S. P., Blakely, J. E., Orsulak, P. J., Petty, F., et al. (1999). Adrenergic receptors: G^1 protein coupling, effects of imipramine, and relationship to treatment outcome. *Neuropsychopharmacology, 20,* 162–176.

Hanna, G. L. (1995). Demographic and clinical features of obsessive-compulsive disorders in children and adolescents. *Journal of American Academy of Child and Adolescent Psychiatry, 34,* 19–27.

Kashani, J. J., & Orvaschel, H. (1990). A community study of anxiety disorders in children and adolescents. *American Journal of Psychiatry, 147,* 313–318.

Kendall, P. C. (1993). Cognitive behavioral therapies for youth: Guiding theory, current status, and emerging developments. *Journal of Consulting and Clinical Psychology, 61,* 235–247.

Kendler, K. S., Neale, M. C., Kessler, R. C., Heath, A. C., & Eaves, L. J. (1992a). Generalized anxiety disorder in women. *Archives of General Psychiatry, 49,* 267–272.

Kendler, K. S., Neale, M. C., Kessler, R. C., Heath, A. C., & Eaves, L. J. (1992b). The genetic epidemiology of

phobias in women: The interrelationship of agoraphobia, social phobia, situational phobia, and simple phobia. *Archives of General Psychiatry, 49,* 273–281.

Kirmayer, L. J., Young, A., & Hayton, B. C. (1995). The cultural context of anxiety disorders. *Psychiatric Clinics of North America, 18,* 503–521.

Lenane, M. C. (1991). Family therapy for children with obsessive-compulsive disorder. In M. S. Paton & J. Zohar (Eds.), *Current treatment of obsessive-compulsive disorder* (pp. 103–113). Washington, DC: American Psychiatric Press.

Leon, C. A., & Leon, A. (1990). Panic disorder and parental bonding. *Psychiatric Annals, 20,* 503–508.

Lindesay, J. (1991). Phobic disorders in the elderly. *British Journal of Psychiatry, 159,* 531–541.

Loerch, B., Graf-Morgenstern, M., Hautzinger, M., Schlegel, S., Hain, C., Sandmann, J., et al. (1999). Randomised placebo-controlled trial of moclobemide, cognitive-behavioral therapy and their combination in panic disorder with agoraphobia. *British Journal of Psychiatry, 174,* 205–212.

Longo, L. P. (1998). Anxiety: Neurobiologic underpinnings. *Psychiatric Annals, 28,* 130–138.

March, J. S., Mulle, K., & Herbel, B. (1994). Behavioral psychotherapy for children and adolescents with obsessive-compulsive disorder: An open trial of a new protocol-driven treatment package. *Journal of the Academy of Child Adolescent Psychiatry, 33,* 333–341.

Mataix-Cols, D., Rauch, S. L., Baer, L., Eisen, J. L., Shera, D. M., Goodman, W. K., Rasmussen, S. A., & Jenike, M. A. (2002). Symptom stability in adult obsessive-compulsive disorder: Data from a naturalistic two-year follow-up study. *American Journal of Psychiatry, 159,* 263–268.

Mavissakalian, M. R., Perel, J. M., Talbott-Green, M., & Sloan, C. (1998). Gauging the effectiveness of extended imipramine treatment for panic disorder with agoraphobia. *Society of Biological Psychiatry, 43,* 848–854.

May, R. (1977). *The meaning of anxiety* (2nd ed.). New York: W.W. Norton.

McNally, R. J. (2001). On the scientific status of cognitive appraisal models of anxiety disorders. *Behavioral Research Therapy, 39,* 513–521.

McNally, R. J., & Eke, M. (1996). Anxiety sensitivity, suffocation fear, and breath-holding duration as predictors of response to carbon dioxide challenge. *Journal of Abnormal Psychology, 105,* 146–149.

Mitchell, J. T., & Dyregov, A. (1993). Traumatic stress in disaster workers and emergency personnel: Prevention and intervention. In J. P. Wilson & B. Raphael (Eds), *International handbook of traumatic stress syndromes* (pp. 905–914). New York: Plenum.

Morgan, C. A., Hill, S., Fox, P., Kingham, P., & Southwick, S. M. (1999). Anniversary reactions in Gulf war veterans: A follow-up inquiry 6 years after the war. *American Journal of Psychiatry, 156,* 1075–1079.

Pavlov, I. P. (1927). *Conditioned reflexes: An investigation of the physiological activity of the cerebral cortex* (G. C. Andrep, Trans. and Ed.). London: Oxford University Press.

Price, L. H., Rasmussen, S. A., & Eisen, J. L. (1999). The natural history of obsessive-compulsive disorder. *Archives of General Psychiatry, 23,* 519–533.

Purcell, R., Maruff, P., Kyrios, M., & Pantelis, C. (1998). Neuropsychological deficits in obsessive-compulsive disorder: A comparison with unipolar depression, panic disorder, and normal controls. *Archives of General Psychiatry, 55,* 415–423.

Regier, D. A., Burke, J. D., & Burke, K. C. (1990). Comorbidity of affective and anxiety disorders in the NIMH Epidemiological Catchment Area Program. In J. D. Maser & C. R. Cloninger (Eds.), *Comorbidity of mood and anxiety disorders* (pp. 112–122). Washington, DC: American Psychiatric Press.

Regier, D. A., Narrow, W. E., Rae, D. S., Manderscheid, R. W., Locke, B. Z., &

Goodwin, F. K. (1993). The de facto U.S. mental and addictive disorders service system. Epidemiologic Catchment Area prospective 1-year prevalence rates of disorders and services. *Archives of General Psychiatry, 50,* 85–94.

Robinson, R. C., & Mitchell, J. T. (1993). Evaluation of psychological debriefings. *Journal of Traumatic Stress, 6,* 367–382.

Robinson, D., Wu, H., Munne, R. A., & Ashtari, M. (1995). Reduced caudate nucleus volume in obsessive-compulsive disorder. *Archives of General Psychiatry, 52,* 393–398.

Rosenbaum, B.O. (1997). A controlled study of eye movement sensitization and reprocessing in the treatment of post-traumatic stress disordered sexual assault victims. *Bulletin of Menninger Clinic, 61,* 317–334.

Rosenbaum, J. F., & Gelenberg, A. J. (1991). Anxiety. In G. Gelenberg, et al. (Eds.), *The practitioner's guide to psychoactive drugs* (3rd ed., pp. 179–218). New York: Plenum Press.

Schmidt, N. B., Lerew, D. R., & Jackson, R. J. (1999). Prospective evaluation of anxiety sensitivity in the pathogenesis of panic: Replication and extension. *Journal of Abnormal Psychiatry, 108,* 532–537.

Schmidt, N. B., Lerew, D. R., & Joiner, T. E., Jr. (2000). Prospective evaluation of the etiology of anxiety sensitivity: Test of a scar model. *Behavioral Research Therapy, 38,* 1083–1095.

Schneier, F. R., Goetz, D., Campeas, R., Fallon, B., Marshall, R., & Liebowitz, M. R. (1998). Placebo-controlled trial of moclobemide in social phobia. *British Journal of Psychiatry, 172,* 70–77.

Shapiro, F. (1995). *Eye movement desensitization and reprocessing: Basic principles, protocols, and procedures.* New York: Guilford Press.

Shaw, J. A., Applegate, B., & Schorr, C. (1996). Twenty-one-month follow-up study of school-age children exposed to hurricane Andrew. *Journal of American Academy of Child and Adolescent Psychiatry, 35,* 359–364.

Sheikh, J. I., King, R. J., & Taylor, C. B. (1991). Comparative phenomenology of early-onset versus late-onset panic attacks: A pilot survey. *American Journal of Psychiatry, 148*, 1231–1233.

Stein, M. B., Fyer, A. J., Davidson, J. R. T., Pollack, M. H., & Wiita, B. (1999). Fluvoxamine treatment of social phobia (social anxiety disorder): A double-blind, placebo-controlled study. *American Journal of Psychiatry, 156*, 756–760.

Stein, M. B., Liebowitz, M. R., Lydiard, R. B., Pitts, C. D., Bushnell, W., & Gergel, I. (1998). Paroxetine treatment of generalized social phobia (social anxiety disorder): A randomized controlled trial. *Journal of the American Medical Association, 280*, 708–713.

Sullivan, G. M., Coplan, J. D., & Gorman, J. M. (1998). Psychoneuroendocrinology of anxiety disorders. *The Psychiatric Clinics of North America, 21*, 397–412.

Swedo, S. E., Leonard, H. L., Garvey, M., Mittleman, B., Allen, A. J., Perlmutter, S., et al. (1998). Pediatric autoimmune neuropsychiatric disorders associated with streptococcal infections: Clinical description of the first 50 cases. *American Journal of Psychiatry, 155*, 264–271.

Taylor, S. (1995). Anxiety sensitivity: Theoretical perspectives and recent findings. *Behavioral Research Therapy, 33*, 243–258.

Taylor, S., & Cox, B. J. (1998). Anxiety sensitivity: Multiple dimensions and hierarchic structure. *Behavioral Research Therapy, 36*, 37–51.

Wang, S., Wilson, J. P., & Mason, J. W. (1996). Stages of decompensation in combat-related posttraumatic stress disorder: A new conceptual model. *Integration Physiology of Behavioral Science, 31*, 237–253.

Weissman, M. M., Bland, R. C., Canino, G. J., Faravelli, C., Greenwald, S., Hwu, H. G., et al. (1997). The cross-national epidemiology of panic disorder. *Archives of General Psychiatry, 54*, 305–309.

Widom, C. S. (1999). Posttraumatic stress disorder in abused and neglected children grown up. *American Journal of Psychiatry, 156*, 1223–1229.

Wolpe, J. (1961). The systematic desensitization treatment of neurosis. *Journal of Nervous and Mental Disease, 132*, 189–203.

Wolpe, J. (1973). *The practice of behavioral therapy*. New York: Pergamon Press.

Wolpe, J., & Lazarus, A. (1966). *Behavior therapy techniques: A guide to the treatment of neuroses*. London: Pergamon Press.

Yehuda, R. (1997). Sensitization of the hypothalamic-pituitary-adrenal axis in posttraumatic stress disorder. In R. Yehuda & A. C. McFarlane (Eds.), *Psychobiology of posttraumatic stress disorder* (pp. 57–75). New York: The New York Academy of Sciences.

Yehuda, R. (1998). Psychoneuroendocrinology of post-traumatic stress disorder. *The Psychiatric Clinics of North America, 21*, 359–379.

CHAPTER 4

American Psychiatric Association. (2000). *Diagnostic and statistical manual of mental disorders* (4th edition Text Revision) (*DSM-IV-TR*) Washington, DC: Author.

Barkley, R. A. (1997). *Attention deficit hyperactivity disorder and the nature of self-control*. New York: Guilford Press.

Bukstein, O. G., & Kolko, D. J. (1998). Effects of methylphenidate on aggressive urban children with attention deficit hyperactivity disorder. *Journal of Clinical Psychology, 27*, 340–351.

DuPaul, G. J., Barkley, R. A., & McMurray, M. B. (1994). Response of children with ADHD to methylphenidate: Interaction with internalizing symptoms. *Journal of the American Academy of Child and Adolescent Psychiatry, 33*, 894–903.

Feingold, B. F. (1974). *Why your child is hyperactive*. New York: Random House.

Ferguson, D. M., Horwood, L. J., & Lynskey, M. T. (1994). Structure of *DSM-III-R* criteria for disruptive childhood behavior: Confirmatory factors model. *Journal of the American Academy of Child and Adolescent Psychiatry, 33,* 1145–1155.

Gadow, K. D., & Spafkin, J. (1997). *ADHD symptom checklist-4 manual.* Stony Brook, NY: Checkmate Plus.

Gadow, K. D., & Spafkin, J. (1997). *Child symptom inventory-4 norms manual.* Stony Brook, NY: Checkmate Plus.

Goldstein, S., & Goldstein, M. (1999). *Managing attention deficit hyperactivity disorder in children: A guide for practitioners.* New York: Wiley.

Haenlin, M., & Caul, W. F. (1987). Attention deficit disorder with hyperactivity: A specific hypothesis of reward dysfunction. *Journal of the American Academy of Child and Adolescent Psychiatry, 26,* 356–362.

Kutcher, S. P. (1997). *Child and adolescent psychopharmacology.* Philadelphia: W.B. Saunders.

Nason, J. L., & Hiscock, M. (1990). Attention deficits in children exposed to alcohol prenatally. *Clinical and Experimental Research, 14*(5), 656–661.

North American Nursing Diagnosis Association (NANDA). (2001). *Nursing diagnosis, definitions and classification, 2001–2002.* Philadelphia: Author.

Steinhaus, H. C., Williams, J., & Spohr, H. L. (1993). Long term psychopathological and cognitive outcomes of children with fetal alcohol syndrome. *Journal of the American Academy of Child and Adolescent Psychiatry, 32,* 990–994.

Stewart, M. A., DuBlois, S., & Cummings, C. (1980). Psychiatric disorders in parents of hyperactive boys and those with conduct disorders. *Journal of Child Psychology and Psychiatry, 21,* 283–292.

Wilens, T. E., Biederman, J., Brown, S., Tanguay, S., Monuteaux, M. C., Blake, C., et al. (2002). Psychiatric comorbidity and functioning in clinically referred preschool children and school-aged youths with ADHD. *Journal of the American Academy of Child and Adolescent Psychiatry, 41,* 262–268.

Wyngarden, J. B. (1988). Adverse effects of low level lead exposure on infant development. *Journal of the American Medical Association, 259,* 2524.

CHAPTER 5

American Psychiatric Association. (2000). *Diagnostic and statistical manual of mental disorders* (4th edition Text Revision) *(DSM-IV-TR).* Washington, DC: Author.

American Psychiatric Association (2000). *Practice guidelines for the treatment of psychiatric disorders.* Washington, DC: Author.

Blanco, C., Lage, G., Olfson, M., Marcus, S. C., & Pincus, H. A. (2002). Trends in the treatment of bipolar disorder by outpatient psychiatrists. *American Journal of Psychiatry, 159,* 1005–1010.

Callahan, A. M., & Bauer, M. S. (1999). Psychosocial interventions for bipolar disorder. *Psychiatric Clinics of North America, 22*(3), 675–688.

Dasari, M., Friedman, L., Jesberger, J., Stuve, T. A., Findling, R. L., Swales, T. P., et al. (1999). A magnetic resonance imaging study of thalamic areas in adolescent patients with either schizophrenia or bipolar disorder as compared to health control. *Psychiatry Research: Neuroimaging, 91*(3), 155–162.

Ganong, W. F. (1999). *Review of medical physiology* (19th ed.). Stamford, CT: Appleton & Lange.

Goodwin, F. K., & Jamison, K. R. (1990). *Manic-depressive illness.* New York: Oxford University Press.

Lehne, R. A., Moore, L. A., Crosby, L. J., & Hamilton, D. B. (1998). *Pharmacology for nursing care* (3rd ed.) Philadelphia: W. B. Saunders.

Martinez-Aran, A., Vieta, E., Colom, F., Reinares, M., Benabarre, A., Gasto, C., et al. (2000). Cognitive dysfunction in bipolar disorder: Evidence of neuropsychological disturbances. *Psychotherapy & Psychosomatics, 69,* 2–18.

North American Nursing Diagnosis Association (NANDA). (2001). *Nursing Diagnosis: Definitions and classification, 2001–2002.* Philadelphia: Author.

Papolos, D., & Papolos, J. (1999). *The bipolar child.* New York: Broadway Books.

Pauls, D. L., Bailey, J. N., Carter, A. S., Allen, C. R., & Egeland, J. A. (1995). Complex segregation analyses of old order Amish families ascertained through bipolar I individuals. *American Journal of Medical Genetics, 60*(4), 290–297.

Robins, L., & Regier, D. (1991). *Psychiatric disorders in America: The epidemiologic catchment area study.* New York: Free Press.

Sachs, G. S., Printz, D. J., Kahn, D. A., Carpenter, D., & Docherty, J. P. (2000). The expert consensus guideline series. Medication treatment of bipolar disorder 2000. *Postgraduate medicine: A special report.* Minneapolis, MN: McGraw-Hill.

Torrey, E. F., Rawlings, R. R., Ennis, J. M., Merrill, D. D., & Flores, D. S. (1996). Birth seasonality in bipolar disorder, schizophrenia, schizoaffective disorder and stillbirths. *Schizophrenia Research, 21,* 141–149.

U.S. Department of Health and Human Services (U.S. DHHS). (1999). *Mental health: A report of the surgeon general.* Rockville, MD: U.S. Department of Health and Human Services Administration, Center for Mental Health Services, National Institutes of Health, National Institute of Mental Health.

Weissman, M. M., Bland, R. C., Camino, O. J., Faravelli, C., Greenwald, S., Hwu, H. G., et al. (1996). Cross-national epidemiology of major depression and bipolar disorder. *Journal of the American Medical Association,. 276,* 293–299.

Young, R. C., Biggs, J. T., Ziegler, W., & Meyer, D. A. (1978). A rating scale for mania: Reliability, validity, and sensitivity. *British Journal of Psychiatry, 133,* 429–435.

CHAPTER 6

American Psychiatric Association. (1987). *Diagnostic and statistical manual of mental disorders* (3rd ed.—Revised). Washington, DC: Author.

American Psychiatric Association. (1994). *Diagnostic and statistical manual of mental disorders* (4th ed.). Washington, DC: Author.

American Psychiatric Association. (2000). *Diagnostic and statistical manual of mental disorders* (4th edition Text Revision) *(DSM-IV-TR).* Washington, DC: Author.

Cummings, E., & Henry, W. E. (1961). *Growing old: The process of engagement.* New York: Basic Books.

Dawson, P., Kline, K., Wiancko, D., & Wells, D. (1986). Preventing excess disability in patients with Alzheimer's disease. *Geriatric Nursing, 1*(6), 298–330.

Erikson, E. H. (1963). *Childhood and society* (2nd ed.). New York: W.W. Norton.

Goetz, G. C. (1999). *Textbook of clinical neurology* (1st ed.). New York: W. B. Saunders.

Hall, G. R. (1991). Altered thought processes: SDAT. In M. Maas and K. Buckwalter (Eds.), *Nursing diagnoses and interventions in the elderly.* Menlo Park, CA: Addison-Wesley.

Hall, G. R., & Buckwalter, K. C. (1987). Progressively lowered stress threshold: A conceptual model for care of adults with Alzheimer's disease. *Archives of Psychiatric Nursing, 1*(6), 399–406.

Ham, R. J. (1992). Confusion, dementia, and delirium. In R. J. Ham & P. D. Sloane (Eds.), *Primary care geriatrics* (2nd ed., chap. 12). St. Louis: Mosby.

Havinghurst, R. J., & Albrecht, R. (1953). *Older people.* New York: Longmans.

Inouye, S. K., Rushing, J. T., Foreman, M. D., Palmer, R. M., & Pompei, P. (1998). Does delirium contribute to poor hospital outcomes: A three site epidemiologic study. *Journal of General Internal Medicine, 13,* 234–242.

Jarvik, L. F., Lavertsky, E. P., & Neshkes, R. E. (1992). Dementia and delirium in old age. In J. C. Brocklehurst, R. C. Tallis, & H. M. Fillit (Eds.), *Textbook of geriatric medicine and gerontology* (4th ed., pp. 326–348). Edinburgh, Scotland: Churchill-Livingstone.

Knopman, D. S. (1998). Current pharmacotherapies for Alzheimer's disease. *Geriatrics, 53*(Suppl. 1), S31–S34.

Levy-Lahad, E., Wasco, W., Pookaj, P., Ramano, D. M., Oshima, J., Pettingell, W. H., et al. (1995). Candidate gene for the chromosome 1 familial Alzheimer's disease locus. *Science, 269,* 973–977.

McKeith, I. G., Fairbairn, A. F., Perry, R. H., Jabeen, S., & Perry, E. K. (1992). Operational criteria for senile dementia of Lewy body type (SDLT). *Psychological Medicine, 22,* 911–922.

Mullan, M., Houlden, H., Windelspecht, M., Fidani, L., Lombardi, C., Diaz, P. L., et al. (1992). A locus for familial early-onset Alzheimer's disease on the long arm of chromosome 14, proximal to the alpha 1-antichymotrypsin gene. *Natural Genetics, 2*(4), 340–342.

Neugarten, B. (1968). *Middle age and aging.* Chicago: University of Chicago Press.

Rapp, C. G. (1998). *Research-based protocol: Acute confusion/delirium.* (Marita G. Titler, series editor). Iowa City, IA: The University of Iowa Gerontological Nursing Interventions Research Center.

Rasin, J. H. (1990). Confusion. *Nursing Clinics of North America, 25,* 909–919.

Reisburg, B., Ferris, S. H., DeLeon, M. J., & Crook, T. (1982). The global deterioration scale (GDS): An instrument for the assessment of primary degenerative dementia. *American Journal of Psychiatry, 139*(9), 1136–1139.

Salmon, E., Degueldre, C., Franco, G., & Franck, G. (1996). Frontal lobe dementia presenting as personality disorder. *Acta Neurologica Belgica,*

Schellenberg, G. D., Bird, T. D., Wijsman, E. M., Orr, H. T., Anderson, L., Nemens, E., et al. (1992). Genetic linkage evidence for a familial Alzheimer's disease locus on chromosome 14. *Science, 258*(5082), 668–671.

St. George-Hyslop, P., Haines, J., Rogaev, E., Mortilla, M., Vaula, G., Pericak-Vance, M., et al. (1992). Genetic evidence for a novel familial Alzheimer's disease locus on chromosome 14. *Natural Genetics, 2*(4), 330–334.

St. Pierre, M. N. (1996). Delirium in hospitalized elderly patients: Off track.

Critical Care Nursing Clinics of North America, 8(1), 53–55.

Stoehr, G.P. (1999). Pharmacology and older adults: The problem of polypharmacy. In M. Stanley & P. G. Beare (Eds.), *Gerontological nursing* (2nd ed., pp. 120–129). Philadelphia. F.A. Davis.

Strong, R. (1998). Neurochemical changes in the aging human brain: Implications for behavioral impairment and neurodegenerative disease. *Geriatrics, 53*(Suppl. 1), S9–S12.

U.S. Department of Health and Human Services. (1996). *Centers for Disease Control and Prevention: HIV/AIDS surveillance report.* Atlanta, 7(2), 15, 16–17.

Van Broeckhoven, C., Backhovens, H., Cruts, M., DeWinter, G., Bruyland, M., Crass, P. L., et al. (1992). Mapping of a gene predisposing to early-onset Alzheimer's disease to chromosome 14q24.3. *Natural Genetics, 2*(4), 335–339.

CHAPTER 7

Abraham, K. (1960). Notes on the psychoanalytic investigation and treatment of manic-depressive insanity and allied conditions. In *Selected papers on psychoanalysis* (pp. 137–156). New York: Basic Books. (Original work published 1911)

Abraham, K. (1960). A short study on the development of the libido. In *Selected papers on psychoanalysis* (pp. 418–501). New York: Basic Books. (Original work published 1924)

American Nurses Association, (2000). *Scope and standards of psychiatric-mental health nursing practice.* Washington, DC: American Nurses Publishing.

American Psychiatric Association Work Group. (2000). *Practice guideline for the treatment of patients with major depressive disorder* (Rev. ed.). Washington, DC: American Psychiatric Association.

American Psychiatric Association. (2000). *Diagnostic and statistical manual of* mental disorders (4th edition Text Revision) (*DSM-IV-TR*). Washington, DC: Author.

Antai-Otong, D. (2001). *Psychiatric emergencies*. Eau Claire, WI: PESI.

Antai-Otong, D. (2002). Culturally sensitive treatment of African Americans with substance-related disorders. *Journal of Psychosocial Nursing, 40*, 1–6

Beck, A. T. (1963). Thinking and depression, I: Idiosyncratic content and cognitive distortions. *Archives of General Psychiatry, 2*, 36–45.

Beck, A. T. (1964). Thinking and depression, II: Theory and therapy. *Archives of General Psychiatry, 10*, 561–571.

Beck, A. T. (1967). *Depression: Clinical, experimental, and theoretical aspects*. New York: Harper & Row.

Beck, A. T., Rush, A. J., Shaw, B. F., & Emery, G. (1979). *Cognitive theory of depression*. New York: Guilford.

Beekman, A. T. F., Copeland, J. R. M., & Prince, M. J. (1999). Review of community prevalence of depression in later life. *British Journal of Psychiatry, 174*, 301–311.

Belanoff, J. K., Kalehzan, M., Sund, B., Ficek, S. K. F., & Schatzberg, A. F. (2001). Cortisol activity and cognitive changes in psychotic major depression. *American Journal of Psychiatry, 158*, 1612–1616.

Berman, H. (1999). Stories of growing up amid violence by refugee children of war and children of battered women living in Canada. *Image: Journal of Nursing Scholarship, 31*, 57–63.

Biederman, J., Faraone, S. V., Hirschfeld-Becker, D. R., Friedman, D., Robin, J. A., & Rosenbaum, J. F. (2001). Patterns of psychopathology and dysfunction in high-risk children of parents with panic disorder and major depression. *American Journal of Psychiatry, 158*, 49–57.

Birmaher, B., Ryan, N. D., Williamson, D. E., & Brent, D. A. (1996). Childhood and adolescent depression: A review of the past 10 years. Part I. *Journal of the Academy of Child and Adolescent Psychiatry, 35*, 1427–1439.

Burnell, G. M., & Burnell, A. L. (1989). *Clinical management of bereavement:*

A handbook for healthcare professionals. New York: Human Sciences Press.

Charney, D. S. (1998). Monamine dysfunction and the pathophysiology of depression. *Journal of Clinical Psychiatry, 59*(Suppl. 14), 11–14.

Costello, E. J. (1989). Developments in child psychiatric epidemiology. *Journal of Child and Adolescent Psychiatry, 28*, 286–841.

Coyne, J. C. (1976). Toward an interactional description of depression. *Psychiatry, 39*, 28–40.

Faraone, S. V., & Biederman, J. (1997). Do attention deficit hyperactivity disorder and major depression share familial risk factors. *Journal Nervous and Mental Disorder, 185*, 533–541.

Fava, M., & Davidson, K. G. (1996). Definition and epidemiology of treatment-resistant depression. *Psychiatric Clinics of North America, 19*, 179–195.

Ganong, W. F. (1999). *Medical physiology* (19th ed.). Stamford: CT: Appleton & Lange.

Kendler, K. S., Kessler, R. C., Walters, E. E., MacLean, C., Neale, M. C., Heath, A. C., et al. (1995). Stressful life events, genetic liability, and onset of an episode of major depression in women. *American Journal of Psychiatry, 152*, 833–842.

Leonard, B. E. (1997). Noradrenaline in basic models of depression. *European Neuropsychopharmacology, 7*(Suppl.), S11–S16.

Lewinsohn, P. M (1974). A behavioral approach to depression. In R. Friedman & M. Katz (Eds.), *The psychology of depression: Contemporary theory and research* (pp. 157–185). New York: John Wiley & Sons.

Lewinsohn, P. M., Rohde, P., & Seely, J. R. (1998). Major depressive disorder in older adolescents: Prevalence, risk factors, and clinical implications. *Clinical Psychology Review, 18*, 765–794.

Lin, K.-M., & Cheung, F. (1999). Mental health issues for Asian Americans. *Psychiatric Services, 50*, 774–780.

Manson, S. M. (1997). Cultural considerations in the diagnosis of mood disorders. In *DSM-IV Sourcebook* (Vol. 3, pp. 909–923). Washington, DC: American Psychiatric Association.

Mavreas, V. G., Beis, A., Mouyias, A., Rigoni, F., & Lyketsos, G. C. (1986). Prevalence of psychiatric disorders in Athens. *Social Psychiatry, 21,* 172–181.

McDaniel, J. S., Musselman, D. L., & Porter, M. R. (1995). Depression in patients with cancer. *Archives of General Psychiatry, 52,* 89–99.

Murray, C. J., & Lopez, A. D. (1997a). Regional patterns of disability-free life expectancy and disability-adjusted life expectancy: Global burden of disease study. *Lancet, 349,* 1347–1352.

Murray, C. J., & Lopez, A. D. (1997b). Alternative projections of mortality and disability by cause 1990–2020: Global burden of disease study. *Lancet, 349,* 1498–1504.

Nelson, E. B., Sax, K. W., & Strakowski, S. M. (1998). Attentional performance in patients with psychotic and nonpsychotic major depression and schizophrenia. *American Journal of Psychiatry, 155,* 137–139.

Noyes, R., Jr., & Hoehn-Saric, R. (1998). *The anxiety disorders.* Cambridge, UK: Cambridge University Press.

Osterweis, M., Solomon, F., & Green, M. (1987). Bereavement reactions, consequences, and care. In S. Zisook (Ed.), *Biopsychosocial aspects of bereavement* (pp. 3–19). Washington, DC: American Psychiatric Press.

Pataki, C. S. (2000). Mood disorders and suicide in children and adolescents. In B. J. Sadock & V. A. Sadock (Eds.), *Kaplan & Sadock's comprehensive textbook of psychiatry* (7th ed., pp. 2740–2757). Philadelphia: Lippincott Williams & Wilkins.

Piccinelli, M., & Gomez-Homen, F. (1996). *Gender differences in the epidemiology of affective disorders and schizophrenia.* Geneva, Switzerland: World Health Organization.

Pincus, H. A., Zarin, D. A., Tanielian, T. L., Johnson, J. L., West, J. C., Pettit, A. R., et al. (1999). Psychiatric patients and treatment in 1997: Findings from the American Psychiatric Practice Research Project.

Archives of General Psychiatry, 56, 441–449.

Regier, D. A., Narrow, W. E., & Rae, D. S. (1990). The epidemiology of anxiety disorders: The Epidemiologic Catchment Area (ECA) experience. *Journal of Psychiatric Research, 24*(Suppl.), 3–14.

Rehm, L. P. (1990). Cognitive and behavioral theories. In B. B. Wolman & G. Stricker (Eds.), *Depressive disorders: Facts, theories, and treatment methods* (pp. 64–91). New York: John Wiley & Sons.

Sadovy, J. (2000). Psychosocial treatments: General principles. In B. J. Sadock & V. A. Sadock (Eds.), *Comprehensive textbook of psychiatry/VI* (Vol. 1, 7th ed., pp. 3112–3114). Philadelphia: Lippincott Williams & Wilkins.

Schatzberg, A. F. (1998). Noradrenergic versus serotonergic antidepressants: Predictors of treatment response. *Journal of Clinical Psychiatry* (Suppl 14), 15–18.

Stevenson, J. (1999). The treatment of long-term sequelae of child abuse. *Journal of Child Psychology, 40,* 89–111.

Terman, M., Terman, J. S., & Ross, D. C. (1998). A controlled trial of timed bright light and negative air ionization for the treatment of winter depression. *Archives of General Psychiatry, 55,* 875–882.

Uba, L. (1994). *Asian Americans: Personality patterns, identity, and mental health.* New York: Guilford Press.

Ustun, T. B. (2000). Cross national epidemiology of depression and gender. *Journal of Gender Specific Medicine, 3,* 54–58.

Wehr, T. A. (2000). Chronobiology. In B. J. Sadock & V. A. Sadock (Eds.), *Comprehensive textbook of psychiatry/VI* (Vol. 1, 7th ed., pp. 133–142). Philadelphia: Lippincott Williams & Wilkins.

Weiner, R. D. (1994). Treatment optimization with ECT. *Psychopharmacology Bulletin, 30,* 313–320.

Wells, K., Sturm, R., Sherbourn, C. D., & Meredith, L. S. (1996). *Caring for depression.* Cambridge, Mass: Harvard University Press.

Worden, J. W. (1991). *Grief counseling and grief therapy: A handbook for the mental health practitioner* (2nd ed.). New York: Springer.

CHAPTER 8

American Psychiatric Association. (2000). *Diagnostic and statistical manual of mental disorders* (4th edition Text Revision) (*DSM-IV-TR*). Washington, DC: Author.

Bernstein, E. M., & Putnam, F. W. (1986). Development, reliability, and validity of a dissociation scale. *Journal of Nervous and Mental Disease, 174*(12), 727–735.

Brunner, R., Parzer, P., Schuld, V., & Resch, F. (2000). Dissociative symptomatology and traumatogenic factors in adolescent psychiatric patients. *Journal of Nervous and Mental Disease, 188*(2), 71–77.

Casper, R. C. (1998). Serotonin, a major player in the regulation of feeding and affect [editorial]. *Biological Psychiatry, 44*(9), 795–797.

Chu, J. A., Frey, L. M., Ganzel, B. L., & Matthews, J. A. (1999). Memories of childhood abuse: Dissociation, amnesia, and corroboration. *American Journal of Psychiatry, 156*(5), 749–755.

Coons, P. M. (1998). The dissociative disorders: Rarely considered and underdiagnosed. *Psychiatric Clinics of North America, 21*(3), 637–648.

Coons, P. M. (2000). Dissociative fugue. In B. J. Sadock & V. A. Sadock (Eds.), *Comprehensive Textbook of Psychiatry* (Vol. I, pp. 1549–1552). Philadelphia: Lippincott Williams & Wilkins.

Draijer, N., & Langeland, W. (1999). Childhood trauma and perceived parental dysfunction in the etiology of dissociative symptoms in psychiatric inpatients. *American Journal of Psychiatry, 156*(3), 379–385.

Garcia, R., Vouimba, R. M., Baudry, M., & Thompson, R. F. (1999). The amygdala modulates the prefrontal cortex activity relative to conditioned fear. *Nature, 402,* 294–296.

Greyson, B. (2000). Dissociation in people who have near-death experiences: Out of their bodies or out of their minds? *Lancet, 355,* 460–463.

Herman, J. (1991). *Trauma and recovery.* New York: Basic Books.

Kirby, J. S., Chu, J. A., & Dill, D. L. (1993). Correlates of dissociative symptomatology in patients with physical and sexual abuse histories. *Comprehensive Psychiatry, 34,* 258–263.

McDowell, D. M., Levin, F. R., & Nunes, E. V. (1999). Dissociative identity disorder and substance abuse: The forgotten relationship. *Journal of Psychoactive Drugs, 31*(1), 71–83.

Meares, R. (1999). The contribution of Hughlings Jackson to an understanding of dissociation. *American Journal of Psychiatry, 156*(12), 1850–1855.

Peplau, H. (1952). *Interpersonal relations in nursing.* New York: G.F. Putnam & Sons.

Putnam, F. W. (1997). *Dissociation in children and adolescents. A developmental perspective.* New York: Guilford Press.

Rossini, E. D., Schwartz, D. R., & Braun, B. G. (1996). Intellectual functioning of inpatients with dissociative identity disorder and dissociative disorder not otherwise specified. Cognitive and neuropsychological aspects. *Journal of Nervous and Mental Disease, 184*(5), 289–294.

Silberg, J. L. (1998). Dissociative symptomatology in children and adolescents as displayed on psychological testing. *Journal of Personality Assessment, 71*(3), 421–439.

Spiegel, D. (1993). Multiple posttraumatic personality disorder. In R. P. Kluft & C. G. Fine (Eds.), *Clinical perspectives on multiple personality disorder* (pp. 87–99.). Washington, DC: American Psychiatric Press.

Spiegel, D., & Maldonado, J. R. (1999). Dissociative disorders. In R. E. Hales & S. C. Yudofsy (Eds.), *Essentials of clinical psychiatry* (3rd ed., pp. 453–469). Washington, DC: American Psychiatric Press.

Steinberg, M. (2000a). Dissociative amnesia. In B. J. Sadock & V. A. Sadock

(Eds.), *Comprehensive textbook of psychiatry* (Vol. I, pp. 1544–1549). Philadelphia: Lippincott Williams & Wilkins.

Steinberg, M. (2000b). Advances in the clinical assessment of dissociation: The SCID-D-R. *Bulletin of the Meninger Clinic, 64*(2), 146–163.

Sullivan, H. (1953). *The interpersonal theory of psychiatry.* New York: G. F. Putnam & Sons.

van der Kolk, B., & Saporta, J. (1991). The biological response to psychic trauma: Mechanisms and treatment of intrusion and numbing. *Anxiety Research, 4,* 199–212.

Whalen, P. J., Rauch, S. L., Etcoff, N. L., McInerney, S. C., Lee, M. B., & Jenike, M. A. (1998). Masked presentations of emotional facial expressions modulate amygdala activity without explicit knowledge. *Journal of Neuroscience, 18,* 411–418.

CHAPTER 9

Agras, W. S. (2001). The consequences and costs of the eating disorders. *Psychiatric Clinics of North America, 24,* 371–379.

American Psychiatric Association. (2000). *Diagnostic and statistical manual of mental disorders,* (4th edition Text Revision) (*DSM-IV-TR*). Washington, DC: Author.

American Psychiatric Association. (2000). *Practice guidelines for the treatment of patients with eating disorders* (2nd ed., Compendium 2000, pp. 627–697). Washington, DC: Author.

Anderson, A. (1984). Anorexia nervosa and bulimia in adolescent males. *Pediatric Annals, 13,* 901–907.

Benjamin-Coleman, R. (1998). Behavioral syndromes and disorders of adult personality. In C. Houseman (Ed). *Psychiatric certification review guide for the generalist and clinical specialist in adult, child, and adolescent psychiatric and mental health nursing* (2nd ed., pp. 358–408). Potomac, MD: Health Leadership Associates.

Bray, G. A. (1978). Definition, measurement, and classification of the syndromes of obesity. *International Journal of Obesity, 2,* 99–112.

Brewerton, T. D. (1995). Toward a unified theory of serotonin dysregulation in eating and related disorders. *Psychoendocrinology, 2016,* 561–590.

Brewerton, T. D. (1997, October). *Serotonin dysregulation in the eating disorder adolescent.* Paper presented at the meeting of Eating disorders at American Academy of Child and Adolescent Psychiatry (AACAP), Toronto, Ontario, Canada.

Bruch, H. (1982). Anorexia nervosa: Therapy and theory. *American Journal of Psychiatry, 139,* 1531–1538.

Colton, P. A., Rodin, G. M., Olmsted, M. P., & Daneman, D. (1999). Eating disorders in young women with type I diabetes mellitus: Mechanisms and consequences. *Psychiatric Annals, 29,* 213–218.

Cummings M. M., Waller D., Johnson C., Bradley K., Leatherwood D., & Guzzetta C. E. (2001). Developing and implementing a comprehensive program for children and adolescents with eating disorders. *Journal of Child and Adolescent Psychiatric Nursing 14*(4), 167–178

Dare, C., & Eisler, I. (1997). Family therapy for anorexia nervosa. In D. M. Carner & P. E. Garfinkel (Eds.). *Handbook of treatment of eating disorders* (pp. 307–324). New York: Guilford Press.

Fairburn, C. G., Cooper, Z., Doll, H. A., & Welch S. L. (1999). Risk factors for anorexia nervosa: Three integrated case-control comparisons. *Archives of General Psychiatry, 56,* 468–476.

Fairburn, C. G., Welch S. T., Doll H., Davies, B. A., & O'Connor, M. E. (1997). Risk factors for bulimia nervosa: A community based case-control study. *Archives of General Psychiatry, 54,* 509–517.

Fitzgibbon, M. L., & Stolley, M. R. (2001). *Dying to be thin: Minority women: The untold story.* Retrieved September, 2002, from http://www.pbs.org/wgbh/nova/thin/minorities.html

George, L. (1997). The psychological characteristics of patients suffering from anorexia nervosa and the nurses' role in creating a therapeutic relationship. *Journal of Advanced Nursing, 26*(5): 899–908.

Halmi, K. A. (1997, October). *Outpatient treatment of anorexia nervosa: Cognitive-behavioral and pharmacological therapies. Institute VI Adolescent Eating Disorders: A panorama.* Academy of Child & Adolescent Psychiatry Institute and Conference, Toronto, Ontario, Canada.

Hay, P. J., & Bacaltchuk, J. (2001). Psychotherapy for bulimia and binging. *Cochrane Database System Review, 3,* CD000562.

Herzog, D. B., Greenwood, D. N., Flores, A. T., Ekeblad, E. R., Richards, A., Blais, M. A., et al. (2000). Mortality in eating disorders: A descriptive study. *International Journal of Eating Disorders, 28,* 20–26.

Kaplan, H. I. S., & Sadock, B. J. (1998). *Synopsis of psychiatry* (8th ed.). Baltimore: Williams & Wilkins.

King, S. J., & deSales, T. (2000). Caring for adolescent females with anorexia nervosa: Registered nurses' perspective. *Journal of Advanced Nursing, 32*(1), 139–147.

Klump, K. L., Kaye, W. H., & Strober, M. (2001). The evolving genetic foundations of eating disorders. *Psychiatric Clinics of North America, 24,* 215–225.

Linehan, M. M. (1993). *Skills training manual for treating borderline personality disorder.* New York: Guilford Press.

Minuchin, S., Rosman, B., & Baker, L. (1978). *Psychosomatic families: Anorexia nervosa in context.* Cambridge, MA: Harvard University Press.

Nielsen, S. (2001). Epidemiology and mortality of eating disorders. *Psychiatric Clinics of North America, 24,* 201–214.

Roberto, L. G. (1986). Bulimia: The transgenerational view. *Journal of Marital and Family Therapy, 12,* 231–240.

Roberto, L. G. (1992). *Transgenerational family therapies.* New York: Guilford Press.

Rydall, A. C., Rodin, G. M., Olmsted, M. P., Devenyi, R. G., & Daneman, D. (1997). Disordered eating behavior and microvascular complications in young women with insulin-dependent diabetes mellitus. *New England Journal of Medicine, 336,* 1849–1854.

Safer, D. L., Telch, C. F., & Agras, W. S. (2001). Dialectical behavior therapy for bulimia nervosa. *American Journal of Psychiatry, 158,* 632–634.

Smolak, L., Murnen, S. K, & Ruble, A. E. (2000). Female athletes and eating disorders: A meta-analysis. *International Journal of Eating Disorders, 27,* 317–380.

Spitzer, R. L., Yanoski, S., Wadden, T., Wing, R., Marcus, M. D., Stunkard, A., et al. (1993). Binge eating disorder: Its further validation in a multisite study. *International Journal of Eating Disorders, 13,* 137–153.

Strober, M., Freeman, R., Lampert, C., et al (2000). Controlled family study of anorexia nervosa and bulimia nervosa: Shared liability and transmission of partial syndromes. *American Journal of Psychiatry, 157,* 393–401.

Swenson, C. R., Torrey, W. C., & Koerner, K. (2002). Implementing dialectical behavior therapy. *Psychiatric Services, 53,* 171–178.

Treasure, J., & Schmidt, U. (2001). *Anorexia nervosa in clinical evidence, 6,* 705–714. London: British Medical Journal Publishing Group.

U.S. Department of Health and Human Services (1999). *Mental Health: A Report of the Surgeon General—Executive Summary.* Rockville, MD: U.S. Department of Health and Human Services, Substance Abuse and Mental Health Services Administration, Center for Mental Health Services, National Institutes of Health, National Institute of Mental Health.

van Hoeken, D., Lucas, A. R., & Hoek, H. W. (1998). Epidemiology. In H. W. Hoek, J. L. Treasure, & M. A. Katzman (Eds.), *Neurobiology of eating disorders.*

(pp. 97–126). Chichester, UK: John Wiley & Sons.

Walsh, B. T., Agras, W. S., Devlin, M. J. (2000). Fluoxetine for bulimia nervosa following poor response to psychotherapy. *American Journal of Psychiatry, 157*, 1332–1334.

CHAPTER 10

American Psychiatric Association. (2000). *Diagnostic and statistical manual of mental disorders* (4th edition Text Revision) (*DSM-IV-TR*). Washington, DC: Author.

Black, D. W., Jr., (with Larson, C. L.). (1999). *Bad boys, bad men: Confronting antisocial personality disorder.* New York: Oxford University Press.

Brooner, R. F., Greenfield, L., Schmidt, C. W., & Bigelow, G. E. (1993). Antisocial personality disorder and HIV infection among intravenous drug abusers. *American Journal of Psychiatry, 150*(1), 53–58.

Cadoret, R. J., Yates, W. R., Troughton, E., Woodworth, G., & Stewart, M. A. (1995). Genetic-environmental interaction in the genesis of aggressivity and conduct disorders. *Archives of General Psychiatry, 52*, 916–924.

Comings, D. E., Gade-Andavolu, R., Gonzalez, N., Wu, S., Muhleman, D., Blake, H., et al. (2000). A multivariate analysis of 59 candidate genes in personality traits: The temperament and character inventory. *Journal of Clinical Genetics, 58*, 375–385.

Dadds, M. R., Barrett, P. M., Rapee, R. M., & Ryan, S. (1996). Family process and child anxiety and aggression: An observational analysis. *Journal of Abnormal Child Psychology, 24*, 715–734.

Egan, J. (1986). Etiology and treatment of borderline personality disorder in adolescents. *Hospital and Community Psychiatry, 37*(6), 613–618.

Erikson, E. (1963). *Childhood and society* (2nd ed.). New York: W. W. Norton.

Fletcher, K. E., Fischer, M., Barkley, R. A., & Smallish, L. (1996). A sequential analysis of the mother-adolescent interactions with ADHD, ADHD, and normal teenagers during neutral conflict discussions. *Journal of Abnormal Child Psychology, 24*, 271–297.

Fossati, A., Donati, D., Donini, M., Novella, L., Bagnata, M., & Maffei, C. (2001). Temperament, character, and attachment patterns in borderline personality disorder. *Journal of Personality Disorders, 15*, 390–402.

Freud, S. (1957). On narcissism: An introduction. In J. Strachey (Ed. and Trans.), *The standard edition of the complete psychological works of Sigmund Freud* (Vol. 19, pp. 69–102). London: Hogarth Press. (Original work published 1923)

Frosch, J. (1983). The psychosocial treatment of personality disorders. In J. Frosch (Ed.), *Current perspectives on personality disorders.* Washington, D.C.: American Psychiatric Press.

Gibb, B. E., Wheeler, R., Alloy, L. B., & Abramson, L. Y. (2001). Emotional, physical, and sexual mistreatment in childhood versus adolescence and personality dysfunction in young adulthood. *Journal of Personality Disorders, 15*, 505–511.

Gunderson, J. G. (1988). Personality disorders. In A. M. Nicholi (Ed.), *The new Harvard press guide to psychiatry* (pp. 337–357). Cambridge, MA: Harvard Press.

Hollander, E., Allen, A., Lopez, R. P., Bienstock, C., Grossman, R., Siever, L., et al. (2001). A preliminary double-blind, placebo-controlled trial of divalproex sodium in borderline personality disorder. *Journal of Clinical Psychiatry, 62*, 199–203.

Jang, K. L., Livesley, W. J., Vernon, P. A., & Jackson, D. N. (1996). Heritability of personality disorder traits: A twin study. *Acta Psychiatrica Scandinavica, 94*, 438–444.

Johnson, M., & Silver, S. (1988). Conflicts in the inpatient treatment of the borderline patient. *Archives of Psychiatric Nursing, 2*(5), 312–318.

Kalogerakis, M. G. (1992). Emergency evaluation of adolescents. *Hospital and Community Psychiatry, 43*, 617–621.

Kay, R. L., & Kay, J. (1986). Adolescent conduct disorders. In A. J. Frances &

R. E. Hales (Eds.), *Psychiatry update: American Psychiatric Association annual review* (Vol. 5, pp. 480–496). Washington, DC: American Psychiatric Press.

Keith, C. (1984). Individual psychotherapy and psychoanalysis with the aggressive adolescent: A historical review. In C. Keith (Ed.), *The aggressive adolescent: Clinical perspectives*. New York: Free Press.

Kernberg, O. (1984). *Severe personality disorders*. New Haven, CT: Yale University Press.

Khantzian, E. J., & Treece, C. (1965). *DSM-III* psychiatric diagnosis of narcotic addicts. *Archives of General Psychiatry, 42*, 1067–1071.

Links, P. S., Steiner, M., Boiago, I., & Irwin, D. (1990). Lithium therapy for borderline patients: Preliminary findings. *Journal of Personality Disorders, 4*, 173–181.

Livesley, W. J., Jang, K. L., & Vernon, P. A. (1998). Phenotype and genetic structure of traits delineating personality disorder. *Archives of General Psychiatry, 55*, 941–948.

Masterson, J. F. (2000). *Psychotherapy disorders: A new look at the developmental self and object relations approach*. Phoenix, AZ: Tucker.

Meares, R., Stevenson, J., & Gordon, E. (1999). A Jacksonian and biopsychosocial hypothesis concerning borderline and related phenomena. *Australian and New Zealand Journal of Psychiatry, 33*(6), 831–840.

Meissner, W. W. (1988). The psychotherapies: Individual, family and group. In A. Nicholi (Ed.), *The new Harvard guide to psychiatry* (pp. 449–480). Cambridge, MA: Belknap Press.

Mishne, J. M. (1986). *Clinical work with adolescents*. New York: Free Press.

Moss, H. B., Lynch, K. G., Hardie, T. L., & Baron, D. A. (2002). Family functioning and peer affiliation in children of fathers with antisocial personality disorder and substance dependence: Associations with problem behaviors. *American Journal of Psychiatry, 159*, 607–614.

Oquendo, M. A., & Mann, J. J. (2000). The biology of impulsivity and suicidality. *Psychiatric Clinics of North America, 23*, 11–25.

Parker, G. (1984). The measurement of pathogenic parental style and its relevance to psychiatric disorder. *Social Psychiatry, 19*, 75–81.

Perry, J. C., Banon, & Ianni, F. (1999). Effectiveness of psychotherapy for personality disorders. *American Journal of Psychiatry, 156*, 1312–1321.

Raine, A. (2002a). Annotation: The role of prefrontal deficits, low autonomic arousal, and early health factors in the development of antisocial and aggressive behavior in children. *Journal of Child Psychology & Psychiatry, 43*(4), 417–434.

Raine, A. (2002b). Bisocial studies of antisocial and violent behavior in children and adults. *Journal of Abnormal Child Psychology, 30*(4), 311–326.

Raine, A., Lencz, T., Bihrle, S., LaCasses, L., & Colletti, P. (2000). Reduced prefrontal gray matter volume and reduced autonomic activity in antisocial personality disorder. *Archives of General Psychiatry, 57*(2), 119–127.

Raine, A., Venables, P. H., & Williams, M. (1990). Relationships between central and autonomic measures of arousal at age 15 years and criminality at age 24. *Archives of General Psychiatry, 47*, 1003–1007.

Rinsley, D. B. (1982). *Borderline and other self-disorders*. New York: Jason Aronson.

Rounsaville, B. J., Weissman, M. M., Kleber, H., & Wilber, C. (1982). Heterogeneity of psychiatric diagnoses in the treatment of opiate addicts. *Archives of General Psychiatry, 39*, 161–166.

Salzman, C., Wolfson, A. N., Schatzberg, A., Looper, J., Henke, R., Albanese, M., et al. (1995). Effect of fluoxetine on anger in symptomatic volunteers with borderline personality disorder. *Journal of Clinical Psychopharmacology, 15*, 23–29.

Soloff, P. H. (2000). Psychopharmacology of borderline personality disorder. *Psychiatric Clinics of North America, 23*, 169–192.

Whiting, S. A. (1994). A delphi study of the defining characteristics of interdependence and dysfunctional independence. *Issues in Mental Health Nursing, 13*(1), 37–47.

Widom, C. S. (1999). Posttraumatic stress disorder in abused and neglected children grown up. *American Journal of Psychiatry, 156*, 1223–1229.

Zubieta, J. K., & Alessi, N. E. (1993). Is there a role of serotonin in the disruptive behavior disorders? A literature review. *Journal of Child and Adolescent Psychopharmacology, 3*, 11–35.

CHAPTER 11

American Nurses Association. (2000). *A statement on psychiatric-mental health nursing practices and standards of psychiatric-mental health practice.* Washington, DC: Author.

American Psychiatric Association. (2000). *Diagnostic and statistical manual of mental disorders* (4th edition Text Revision) (*DSM-IV-TR*). Washington, DC: Author.

Caine, D., & Caine, M. (1996). *When Benjamin wants to know: family conversations about the facts of life.* Chapel Hill, NC: Chapel Hill Press.

Crenshaw, T. L., & Goldberg, J. P. (1996). *Sexual pharmacology.* New York: W.W. Norton.

Dumas, L. S. (1996). *Talking with kids about tough issues.* Menlo Park, CA: Kaiser Family Foundation.

Fogel, C. I., & Lauver, D. (1990). *Sexual health promotion.* Philadelphia: W.B. Saunders.

Freud, S. (1962). *Three essays on the theory of sexuality.* New York: Avon.

Haffner, D. (1999). *From diapers to dating: A parents guide to raising sexually healthy children.* New York: New Market Press.

Hooper, A. (1992). *The ultimate sex book: A therapist's guide to sexual fulfillment.* New York: Dorling Kindersley Limited.

Hyde, J. S. (1986). *Understanding human sexuality* (3rd ed.). New York: McGraw-Hill.

Kaiser Family Foundation. (1999). *Talking with kids about tough issues.* Menlo Park, CA: Author.

Lehne, R. A., Moore, L. A., Crosby, L. J., & Hamilton, D. B. (1998). *Pharmacology in nursing* (3rd ed.). Philadelphia: W.B. Saunders.

Lubkin, I. M. (1986). *Chronic illness: Impact and interventions.* Boston: Jones & Bartlett.

Maslow, A. H. (Ed.), (1970). *Motivation and personality* (2nd ed.). New York: Harper & Row.

Masters, W. H., & Johnson, V. E. (1970). *Human sexual inadequacy.* Boston: Little, Brown.

North American Nursing Diagnoses Association (NANDA). (2001). *Nursing diagnosis: Definitions and classifications 2001–2002.* Philadelphia: Author.

Rogers, C. R. (1951). *Client-centered therapy: Its current practice, implications, and theory.* Boston: Houghton Mifflin.

Swaab, D., Jiang-Ning Z., Hofman, M., & Gooren, L. (1995). A sex difference in the human brain and its relation to transsexuality. *Letters to Nature, 378*, 68–70.

Williams, M. A. (1999, January). *FDA changes Viagra labeling.* Paper presented at the meeting of Contemporary Sexuality: The International Resource for Educators, Researchers and Therapists.

World Health Organization (WHO). (1975). *Education and treatment in human sexuality: The training of health professionals.* (Tech. Rep. No. 572). Geneva, Switzerland: Author.

CHAPTER 12

American Psychiatric Association. (2000). *Diagnostic and statistical manual of mental disorders* (4th edition Text Revision) (*DSM-IV-TR*). Washington, DC: Author.

Antai-Otong, D. (2000). The neurobiology of anxiety-disorders: Implications for psychiatric nursing practice. *Issues in Mental Health Nursing, 21,* 71–89.

Antai-Otong, D. (2001). Creative stress-management for self-renewal. *Dermatology Nursing, 13,* 31–32, 35–39.

Arnell, H., Hjalmas, M., Jagervall, G., Lackgren, G., Stenberg, A., Bengtsson, B., et al. (1997). The genetics of primary nocturnal enuresis: Inheritance and suggestion of a second major gene on chromosome 12q. *Journal of Medical Genetics, 34,* 360–365.

Bastien, C. H., & Morin, C. M. (2000). Familial incidence of insomnia. *Journal of Sleep Research, 9,* 49–54.

Benca, R. (1999). Sleep problems associated with mood and anxiety disorders. *Primary Psychiatry, 6,* 52–60.

Bexchlibynk-Butler, K. Z., & Jeffries, J. J. (2000). *Clinical handbook of psychotropic drugs.* Seattle, WA: Hogrefe & Huber.

Brown, D., (1999). Managing sleep disorders: Solutions in primary care. *Clinician Reviews, 9,* 51–71.

Currie, S. R., Wilson, K. G., Ponterfract, A. J. & deLaplante, L. (2000). Cognitive-behavioral treatment of insomnia secondary to chronic pain. *Journal of Clinical and Consulting Psychology, 68,* 407–416.

Dambro, M. (1998). *Griffith's five minute clinical consult.* Baltimore: Williams & Wilkins.

Elberg, H. (1998). Total genome scan analysis in a single extended family for primary nocturnal enuresis: Evidence for a new focus (ENUR 3) for primary nocturnal enuresis on chromosome 22q11. *European Urology, 33,* 34–36.

Folks, D. G., & Fuller, W. C. (1997). Anxiety disorders and insomnia in geriatric patients. *Psychiatric Clinics of North America, 20,* 137–164.

Freedman, N. S., Kotzer, N., & Schwab, R. J. (1999). Patient perception of sleep quality and etiology of sleep disturbances in the intensive care unit.

American Journal of Respiratory and Critical Care Medicine, 159(4, Pt. 10), 1155–1162.

Hauri, P. J. (1998). Insomnia. *Clinics of Chest Medicine, 19,* 157–168.

Hauri, P., Cleveland-Hauri, C. (1999). Diagnosing and treating insomnia. *Primary Psychiatry. 6,* 61–71.

Humphreys, J. C., Lee, K. A., Neylan, T. C., & Marmar, C. R. (1999). Sleep patterns of sheltered battered women. *Image: Journal of Nursing Scholarship, 31,* 139–143.

Kahn, D. M., Cook, T. E., Carlisle, C. C., Nelson, D. L., Kramer, N. R., & Millman, R. P. (1998). Identification and modification of environmental noises in an ICU setting. *Chest, 114,* 535–540.

Knill, R. J., Moote, C. A., Skinner, I., & Rose, E. A. (1990). Anesthesia with abdominal surgery leads to intense REM sleep during the first postoperative week. *Anesthesiology, 73,* 52–61.

Kupfer, D. J., & Reynolds, C. F. (1997). Management of insomnia: A meta-analysis of treatment efficacy. *New England Journal of Medicine, 336,* 341–346.

Kushida, C. (1999). Introductory clinical overview in sleep disorders. *Primary Psychiatry, 6,* 47–51.

Langer, S., Mendelson, W., & Richardson, G. (1999). Symptomatic treatment of insomnia. *Sleep, 22*(Suppl. 3), S437–S445.

Leger, D., Scheuermaier, K., Philip, P., Paillard, M., & Guilleminault, C. (2001). SF-36: Evaluation of quality of life in severe and mild insomniacs compared to good sleepers. *Psychosomatic Medicine, 63,* 49–55.

Leproult, R., Copinschi, G., Buxton, O., & Van Cauter, E. (1997). Sleep loss results in an elevation of cortisol levels next evening. *Sleep, 20,* 865–870.

McEvoy, G. K. (2001). *American hospital formulary service* (pp. 2311–2343). Bethesda, MD: American Society of Health-Systems Pharmacists.

Neubauer, D. N. (1999). Sleep problems in the elderly. *American Family Physician, 59,* 2551–2558.

Neylan, T. C., Reynolds, C. F., & Kupfer, D. F. (1999). In R. E. Hales, S. C. Yudofsky, & J. T. Talbott (Eds.), *American psychiatric press textbook of psychiatry*, (3rd ed., pp. 955–982). Washington, DC: American Psychiatric Press.

North American Nursing Diagnosis Association (NANDA). (2001). *Nursing diagnoses: Definitions & classification 2001–2002*. Philadelphia: Author.

Redwine, L., Hauger, R. L., Gillin, J. C., & Irwin, M. (2000). Effects of sleep and sleep deprivation on interleukin-6, growth hormone, cortisol, and melatonin levels in humans. *Journal of Clinical Endocrinology, 85,* 3597–3603.

Roth, T. (1999). Treating insomnia in the depressed patient: Practical considerations. *Hospital Medicine, 49,* 23–28.

Schultz, V., Hansel, R., & Tyler, V. E. (1998). *Restless and sleep disturbances. Rational Phytotherapy: A physician's guide to herbal medicine* (3rd ed., pp. 73–88). Berlin, Germany: Springer-Verlag.

Spitzer, R. L., Terman, M., Williams, J. B., Terman, J. S., Malt, U. F., Singer, F., et al. (1999). Jet lag: Clinical features, validation of a new syndrome-specific scale, and lack of responses to melatonin in a randomized, double-blind trial. *American Journal of Psychiatry, 156,* 1392–1396.

Vitiello, M. V. (1999). Effective treatments for age-related sleep disturbances. *Geriatrics, 54,* 47–52.

Walsh, J., & Unstun, T. B. (1999). Prevalence and health consequences of insomnia. *Sleep, 22*(Suppl. 3), S427–S436.

Yehuda, R. (1998). Psychoneuroendocrinology of post-traumatic stress disorder. *The Psychiatric Clinics of North America, 21,* 359–379.

CHAPTER 13

Abbruzzese, M., Bellodi, L., Lerri, S., & Scarone, S. (1995). Frontal-lobe dysfunction in schizophrenia and obsessive-compulsive disorder: A neuropsychology study. *Brain Cognition, 27,* 202–212.

American College of Rheumatology. (1990). *1990 criteria for the classification of fibromyalgia.* Retrieved June 28, 2002, from http://www.rheumatology.org/research/classification/fibro.html

American Psychiatric Association. (2000). *Diagnostic and statistical manual of mental disorders* (4th edition Text Revision) *(DSM-IV-TR).* Washington DC: Author.

Arnold, L. M., & Privitera, M. D. (1996). Psychopathology and trauma in epileptic and psychogenic seizure patients. *Psychosomatics, 37,* 438–443.

Arnold, L. M., Keck, P. E., & Welge, J. A. (2000). Antidepressant treatment of fibromyalgia: A meta-analysis and review. *Psychosomatics, 41,* 104–113.

Bass, C., & Murphy, M. (1995). Somatoform and personality disorders: Syndromal comorbidity overlapping developmental pathways. *Journal of Psychosomatic Research, 39,* 403–427.

Boisset-Pioro, M. H., Esdaile, J. M., & Fitzcharles, M. (1995). Sexual and physical abuse in women with fibromyalgia syndrome. *Arthritis and Rheumatology, 38,* 235–241.

Bowlby, J. (1973). *Attachment and loss: Volume 2. Separation.* New York: Basic Books.

Bowlby, J. (1977). The making and breaking of affectional bonds: Etiology and psychopathology in the light of attachment theory. *British Journal of Psychiatry, 130,* 201–210.

Bowlby, J. (1988). Developmental psychiatry comes of age. *American Journal of Psychiatry, 145,* 1–10.

Breuer, J., & Freud, S. (1893–1895). Studies in hysteria. In J. Strachey (Ed. & Trans.), *The standard edition of the complete psychological works of Sigmund Freud* (Vol. 2, pp. 1–311). London: Hogarth Press. (Original work published 1955)

Briquet, P. (1859). *Traite clinique et therapeutique y l'hysterie.* Paris: J.B. Balliere & Fils.

Demitrack, M. A., & Abbey, S. E. (1996). *Chronic fatigue syndrome: An integrative approach to evaluation and treatment.* New York: Guilford Press.

Dickens, C., Jayson, M., & Creed, F. (2001). Psychological correlates of pain behavior in patients with low back pain. *Psychosomatics, 43,* 42–48.

Escobar, J. I., Ribio-Stipec, M., Canino, G., & Karno, M. (1989). Somatic symptom index (SSI): A new and abridged somatization construct. *Journal of Nervous Mental Disorders, 177,* 140–146.

Fink, P., Rosendal, M., & Toft, T. (2002). Assessment and treatment of functional disorders in general practice: The extended reattribution and management mode—an advanced educational program for nonpsychiatric doctors. *Psychosomatics, 43,* 93–131.

Ford, C. V. (1986). The somatizing disorders. *Psychosomatics, 27,* 327–337.

Hanes, K. R. (1998). Neuropsychological performance in body dysmorphic disorder. *Journal of the International Neuropsychological Society, 4,* 167–171.

Hollander, E., Allen, A., Kwon, J., Aronowitz, C. Schmeidler, J., Wong, C., et al. (1999). Clomipramine versus desipramine: Crossover trial in body dysmorphic disorder. *Archives of General Psychiatry, 56*(11), 1033–1039.

Jorgensen, C. K., Fink, F., & Olesen, F. (2000). Psychological distress among patients with musculoskeletal illness in general practice. *Psychosomatics, 41,* 321–329.

Kaminsky, M. J., & Slavney, P. R. (1976). Methodology and personality in Briquet's syndrome: A reappraisal. *American Journal of Psychiatry, 133,* 85–88.

Kirmayer, L. J., & Young, A. (1998). Culture and somatization: Clinical, epidemiological, and ethonographic perspective. *Psychosomatic Medicine, 60*(4), 420–430.

Kirmayer, L. J., & Weiss, M. G. (1997). Cultural considerations on somatoform disorders. In T. A. Widiger, A. J. Frances, H. A. Pincus, R. Ross, M. B. First, & W. Davis (Eds.), *DSM-IV*

sourcebook (Vol. 3, pp. 933–941). Washington, DC: American Psychiatric Press.

Kroenke, K., & Swindle, R. (2000, July–August). Cognitive-behavioral therapy for somatization and symptom syndromes: A critical review of controlled clinical trials. *Psychotherapy-Psychosomatic Journal, 69*(4), 205–215.

Ladwig, K.-H., Marten-Mittag, B., Erazo, N., & Gundel, H. (2001). Identifying somatization disorder in a population-based health examination survey: Psychosocial burden and gender differences. *Psychosomatics, 42,* 511–518.

Lesser, R. P. (1996). Psychogenic seizures. *Neurology, 46,* 1499–1507.

Lilienfeld, S. (1992). The association between antisocial personality and somatization disorder: A review and integration of theoretical models. *Clinical Psychology Review, 12,* 641–662.

Lin, K.-M., Lau, J. K. C., Yamamoto, J., Zheng, Y. P., Kim, H. S., Cho, K. H., et al. (1992). Hwa-byung: A community study of Korean Americans. *Journal of Nervous and Mental Disorders, 180,* 386–391.

Macintyre, S., Hunt, K., & Sweeting, H. (1996). Gender differences in health: Are things really as simple as they seem? *Social Science Medicine, 42,* 617–624.

Maier, W., & Falkai, P. (1999). The epidemiology of comorbidity between depression, anxiety disorders and somatic diseases. *International Clinical Psychopharmacology, 14,* S1–S6.

Mumford, D. B. (1996). The "Dhat syndrome": A culturally determined form of depression? *Acta Psychiatrica Scandinavica, 94,* 163–167.

Ohaeri, J. U., & Odejide, O. A. (1994). Somatization symptoms among patients using primary health care facilities in a rural community in Nigeria. *American Journal of Psychiatry, 151,* 728–731.

Otto, M. W., Wilhelm, S., Cohen, L. S., & Harlow, B. L. (2001). Prevalence of body dysmorphic disorder in a community sample of women. *American Journal of Psychiatry, 158,* 2061–2063.

Perley, M., & Guze, S. B. (1962). Hysteria: The stability and usefulness of clinical criteria: A quantitative study based upon a 6–8 year follow-up of 39 patients. *New England Journal of Medicine, 266,* 421–426.

Phillips, K. A. (1996). Body dysmorphic disorder: Diagnosis and treatment of imagined ugliness. *Journal of Clinical Psychiatry, 57,* 61–65.

Phillips, K. A. (2000a). Quality of life for patients with body dysmorphic disorder. *Journal of Nervous Mental Disease, 88*(3), 170–175.

Phillips, K. A. (2000b). Pharmacologic treatment of body dysmorphic disorder: A review of empirical data and proposed treatment algorithm. *Psychiatric Clinics of North America, 7,* 59–82.

Phillips, K. A., Dwight, M. M., & McElroy, S. L. (1998). Efficacy and safety of fluvoxamine in body dysmorphic disorder. *Journal of Clinical Psychiatry, 59,* 156–171.

Phillips, A., Gunderson, C., Gophincth, M., & McElroy, S. L. (1998). A comparison study of body dysmorphic disorder and obsessive-compulsive disorder. *Journal of Clinical Psychiatry, 59*(11), 568.

Piccinelli, M., & Simon, G. (1997). Gender and cross-cultural differences in somatic symptoms associated with emotional distress: An international study in primary care. *Psychological Medicine, 27,* 433–444.

Purtell, J. J., Robins, E., & Cohen, M. E. (1951). Observations on clinical aspects of hysteria. *Journal of the American Medical Association, 146,* 902–909.

Ritsner, M., Ponizovsky, A., Kurs, R., & Modai, I. (2000). Somatization in an immigrant population in Israel: A community survey of prevalence, risk factors, and help-seeking behavior. *American Journal of Psychiatry, 157,* 385–392.

Stuart, S., & Noyes, R. (1999). Attachment and interpersonal communication in somatization. *Psychosomatics, 40,* 34–43.

Taylor, M. L., Trotter, D. R., & Csuka, M. E. (1995). The prevalence of sexual abuse in women with fibromyalgia syndrome. *Arthritis and Rheumatism, 38,* 229–234.

Tojek, T. M., Lumley, M., Barkley, G., Mahr, G., & Thomas, A. (2000). Stress and other psychosocial characteristics of patients with psychogenic non-epileptic seizures. *The Academy of Psychosomatic Medicine, 41,* 221–226.

von Knorring, L. (1994). Idiopathic pain and depression. *Quality of Life Research, 3,* S57–S68.

Walker, E. A., Keegan, D., Gardner, G., Sullivan, M., Bernstein, D., & Katon, W. J. (1997). Psychosocial factors in fibromyalgia compared with rheumatoid arthritis: I. Sexual, physical, and emotional abuse and neglect. *Psychosomatic Medicine, 59,* 572–577.

Wessely, S., Hotopf, M., & Sharpe, M. (1998). *Chronic fatigue and its syndromes.* London: Oxford University Press.

Wool, C. A., & Barsky, A. J. (1994). Do women somatize more than men? Gender differences in somatization. *Psychosomatics, 35,* 445–452.

Yazici, K. M., & Kostakoglu, L. (1998). Cerebral blood flow in patients with conversion disorder. *Psychiatry Research, 83,* 163–168.

CHAPTER 14

Alexander, F. (1950). *Psychosomatic medicine: Its principles and applications.* New York: W. W. Norton.

American Psychiatric Association. (2000). *Diagnostic and Statistical Manual of Mental Disorders* (4th edition Text Revision) (*DSM-IV-TR*). Washington, DC: Author.

Benson, H. (1975). *The relaxation response.* New York: William Morrow.

Biron, C. A., Nguyen, K. B., Pien, G. C., Cousens, L. P., & Salazar-Mather, T. P. (1999). Natural killer cells in antiviral defense: Function and regulation by innate cytokines. *Annual Review of Immunology, 17*, 189–220.

Cassileth, B. R., & Drossman, D. A. (1998). Psychosocial factors in gastrointestinal illness. In G. A. Fava & H. Freyberger (Eds.), *Handbook of psychosomatic medicine* (pp. 239–259). Madison, CT: International Universities Press.

Coelho, R., Ramos, E., Prata, J., Maciel M. J., & Barros, H. (1999). Acute myocardial infarction: Psychosocial and cardiovascular risk factors in men. *Journal of Cardiovascular Risk, 6*(3), 157–162.

Cohen, S., & Herbert, T. B. (1996). Health psychology: Psychological factors and physical disease from the perspective of human psychoneuro-immunology. *Annual Review of Psychology, 47*, 113–142.

Cottraux, J. (1998). Behavioral psychotherapy applications in the medically ill. In G.A. Fava & H. Freyberger, (Eds.), *Handbook of psychosomatic medicine* (pp. 519–539). Madison, CT: International Universities Press.

Drossman, D. A. (1998). Presidential address: Gastrointestinal illness and the biopsychosocial model. *Psychosomatic Medicine, 60*(3), 258–267.

Drossman, D. A. (1999). Do psychosocial factors define symptom severity and patient status in irritable bowel syndrome? *American Journal of Medicine, 107*(5A), 41S–50S.

Drossman, D. A., Whitehead W. E., Toner, B. B., Diamant, N., Hu, Y. J., Bangdiwala, S. I., et al. (2000). What determines severity among patients with painful functional bowel disorders? *American Journal of Gastroenterology, 95*(4), 974–980.

Emmelkamp, P. M. G., & Van Oppen, P. (1998). Cognitive interventions in behavioral medicine. In G. A. Fava & H. Freyberger (Eds.), *Handbook of psychosomatic medicine* (pp. 567–591). Madison, CT: International Universities Press.

Fletcher, M. A., Ironson, G., Goodkin K., Antoni, M. H., Schneiderman, N., & Klimas, N. G. (1998). Stress and immune function in HIV-1 disease. In J. R Hubbard & E. A. Workman (Eds.), *Handbook of stress medicine: An organ system approach* (pp. 229–242). New York: CRC Press.

Freud, S. (1958). On psycho-analysis. In J. Strackney (Ed. and Trans.), *The standard edition of the complete psychological works of Sigmund Freud* (Vol. 12, pp. 207–211). London: Hogarth Press. (Original work published 1911)

Friedman, M., & Rosenman, R. H. (1974). *Type A behavior and your heart.* New York: Knopf.

Fuller, G. D. (1977). *Biofeedback: Methods and procedures in clinical practice.* San Francisco: Biofeedback Press.

Garralda, M. E. (1992). A selective review of child psychiatric syndrome with a somatic presentation. *British Journal of Psychiatry, 161*, 759–773.

Greene, J. W., & Walker, L. S. (1997). Psychosomatic problems and stress in adolescence. *Pediatric Clinics of North America, 44*(6), 1557–1572.

Hendrix, W. H., & Hughes. R. L. (1997). Relationship of trait, type A behavior, and physical fitness variables to cardiovascular reactivity and coronary heart disease risk potential. *American Journal of Health Promotion, 11*(4), 264–271.

Hodges, W. B., & Workman, E. A. (1998). Pain and stress. In J. R. Hubbard & E. A. Workman (Eds.), *Handbook of stress medicine: An organ system approach* (pp. 251–271). New York: CRC Press.

Lanier, L. L. (2000). The origin and function of natural killer cells. *Clinical Immunology, 95*(1), S14–S18.

Littman, A. B. (1998). A review of psychosomatic aspects of cardiovascular disease. In G. A. Fava & H. Freyberger (Eds.), *Handbook of psychosomatic medicine* (pp. 261–293). Madison, CT: International Universities Press.

Menninger, K. (1963). *The vital balance.* New York: Viking Press.

Minuchin, S., Baker, L., Rosman, B. L., Liebman, R., Milman, L., & Todd, T. C. (1975). A conceptual model of psychosomatic illness in children. *Archives of General Psychiatry, 32*, 1031–1038.

O'Connor, T. M., O'Halloran, D. J., & Shanahan, F. (2000). The stress response and the hypothalamic-pituitary-adrenal axis: From molecule to melancholia. *Quarterly Journal of Medicine, 93*(6), 323–333.

Olff, M. (1999). Stress, depression, and immunity: The role of defense and coping styles. *Psychiatry Research, 85*(1), 7–15.

Selye, H. (1976). *Stress in health and disease.* New York: McGraw-Hill.

Smith, J. C. (1997). *Understanding stress and coping.* New York: Macmillan.

Weisberg, M. B., & Clavel, A. L. (1999). Why is chronic pain so difficult to treat? Psychological considerations from simple to complex care. *Post-graduate Medicine, 106*(6), 141–160.

CHAPTER 15

American Psychiatric Association. (2000). *Diagnostic and statistical manual of mental disorders* (4th edition Text Revision) (*DSM-IV-TR*). Washington, DC: Author.

American Society of Addiction Medicine. (1982). *Public policy of ASAM: State of recovery.* Retrieved September, 2002, from http://www.asam.org/asam

Antai-Otong, D. (2002). Culturally sensitive treatment of African Americans with substance-related disorders. *Journal of Psychosocial Nursing, 40,* 1–6

Berglund, M., & Ojehagen, A. (1998). The influence of alcohol drinking and alcohol use disorders on psychiatric disorders and suicidal behavior. *Alcohol, Clinical and Experimental Research, 22*(Suppl. 7), 333S–345S.

Cadoret, R. J., Yates, W. R., Troughton, E., Woodworth, G., & Stewart, M. A. (1995). Adoption study demonstrating two genetic pathways to drug abuse. *Archives of General Psychiatry, 52*(1), 42–52.

DeWit, D. J., Adlaf, E. M., Offord, D. R., & Ogborne, A. C. (2000). Age at first alcoholism: A risk factor for the development of alcohol disorders. *American Journal of Psychiatry, 157*(5), 745–750.

Dodd, P. R., & Lewohl, J. M. (1998). Cell death mediated by amino acid transmitter receptors in human alcoholic brain damage: Conflicts in the evidence. In S. F. Ali (Ed.). *Annals of the New York Academy of Sciences: The neurochemistry of drugs of abuse* (Vol. 844). New York: New York Academy of Sciences.

Ewing, J. A. (1984). Detecting alcoholism: The CAGE questionnaire. *Journal of the American Medical Association, 252,* 1905–1907.

Frances, R., Frances, J., Franklin, J., & Borg, L. (1999). Psychodynamics. In M. Galanter & H. D. Kleber (Eds.) *Textbook of substance abuse treatment* (2nd ed., pp. 309–322). Washington, D.C.: American Psychiatric Press.

Heath, D. B. (2001). Culture and substance abuse. *Psychiatric Clinics of North America, 24,* 479–496.

Hughes, J. R. (2000). Nicotine-related disorders. In B. Kaplan & V. Saddock (Eds.). *Comprehensive textbook of psychiatry* (7th ed., Vol. 1, pp. 1033–1038). Philadelphia: Lippincott Williams & Wilkins.

Jaffe, J. H. (2000a). Introduction and overview. In B. Kaplan & V. Saddock (Eds.). *Comprehensive textbook of psychiatry* (7th ed., Vol. 1, pp. 924–952). Philadelphia: Lippincott Williams & Wilkins.

Jaffe, J. H., & Jaffe, A. B. (2000b). Opioid-related disorders. In B. Kaplan & V. Saddock (Eds.). *Comprehensive textbook of psychiatry* (7th ed., Vol. 1, pp. 1038–1063). Philadelphia: Lippincott Williams & Wilkins.

Kuperman, S., Schlosser, S. S., Lidral, J., & Reich, W. (1999). Relationship of child psychopathology to parental alcoholism antisocial personality disorder. *Journal of the American Academy of Child and Adolescent Psychiatry, 38*(6), 686–692.

Leshner, A. I. (1997). Addiction is a brain disease, and it matters. *Science, 278*(3), 45–47.

Mayo-Smith, M. F. (1997). Pharmacological management of alcohol withdrawal: A meta-analysis and evidence-based practice guideline. *Journal of the American Medical Association, 278*(2), 144–151.

Miles, D. R., Stallings, M. C., Young, S. E., Hewitt, J. K., Crowley, T. J., & Fulker, D. W. (1998). *Drug and Alcohol Dependence, 49*(2), 105–114.

Miller, N. S., Guttman, J. C., & Chawla, S. (1997). Integration of generalized vulnerability to drug and alcohol addiction. *Journal of Addictive Disorders, 16*(4), 7–22.

National Institute on Alcohol Abuse and Alcoholism (NIAAA). (1998). *Alcoholism assessment and treatment instruments*. Bethesda, MD: Retreived September, 2002, from http://silk.nih.gov/silk/niaaa1/publication/aa13.htm

Olmeda, R., & Hoffman, R. S. (2000). Withdrawal syndromes. *Emergency Medicine Clinics of North America, 18*(2), 273–288.

Schottenfeld, R. S., & Pantalon, M. V. (1999). Assessment of the patient. In M. Galanter & H. D. Kleber (Eds.), *Textbook of substance abuse treatment*, (2nd ed., pp. 109–119). Washington, DC: American Psychiatric Press.

Substance Abuse and Mental Health Services Administration Center for Substance Abuse Treatment. (1998). *Treatment improvement protocol series 26 substance abuse among older adults* (DHHS Publication No. SMA 98-3179). Retrieved September, 2002, from http://www.samhsa.gov/centers/csat2002/csat

Substance Abuse and Mental Health Services Administration Center for Substance Abuse Treatment. (2000). *National treatment improvement evaluation study*. Rockville, MD: Author. Retrieved September, 2002, from http://www.health.org/govstudy/f027/index.htm

Sullivan, J. T., Sykora, K., Schneiderman, J., Naranjo, C. A., & Sellers, E. M. (1989). Assessment of alcohol withdrawal: The revised Clinical Institute Withdrawal Assessment for Alcohol scale (CIWA-AR). *British Journal of Addictions, 84*, 1353–1357.

United States Public Health Service. (2000, June). *Treating tobacco use and dependence*. Retrieved September, 2002, from http://www.surgeongeneral.gov/tobacco/smokesum.htm

CHAPTER 16

American Association of Colleges of Nursing. (2000). Position statement: Violence as a public health problem. *Journal of Professional Nursing, 16*(1), 63–69.

American Psychiatric Association. (2000). *Diagnostic and statistical manual of mental disorders* (4th edition Text Revision) (*DSM-IV-TR*). Washington, DC: Author.

Ardrey, R. (1966). *The territorial imperative*. New York: Antheneum.

Bandura, A. (1973). *Aggression: L A social learning analysis*. Englewood Cliffs, NJ: Prentice-Hall.

Bars, D. R., Heyrend, F. L. M., Simpson, C. D., & Munger, J. C. (2001). Use of visual evoked-potential studies and EEG data to classify aggressive, explosive behaviors of youths. *Psychiatric Services, 52*, 81–86.

Boney-McCoy, S., & Finkelhor, D. (1996). Is youth victimization related to trauma symptoms and depression after controlling for prior symptoms and family relationships? A longitudinal, prospective study. *Journal of Consulting and Clinical Psychology, 64*, 1406–1416.

Brook, J., Whiteman, M., Balka, E., & Cohen, P. (1995). Parent drug use, parent personality, and parenting. *Journal of Genetic Psychology, 156*, 137–151.

Campbell, J. (1995). *Assessing dangerousness*. Newbury Park, CA: Sage.

Campbell, J. C., Harris, M. J., & Lee, R. K. (1995). Violence research: An overview. *Scholarly Inquiry for Nursing Practice, 9*, 105–126.

Centers for Disease Control and Prevention (CDC). (1997). *Committee on violence definitions*. Atlanta, GA: Author.

Centers for Disease Control. National Center for Injury Prevention and

Control. (2001). Press Release: *Study finds school-associated violent deaths rare, fewer in events, but more deaths per event.* Retreived October, 2002, from http://www.cdc.gov/od/oc/media/pressrel/ro11204.htm

Coccaro, E. F., Kavoussi, R. J., Hauger, R. L, Coper, T. B., & Ferris, C. F. (1998). Cerebrospinal fluid vasopressor levels correlate with aggression and serotonin function in personality disordered subjects. *Archives in General Psychiatry, 55,* 708–714.

Dobash, R. P., & Dobash, R. E. (1992). *Women, violence, and social change.* New York: Routledge.

Donald, T., & Jureidini, J. (1996). Munchausen syndrome by proxy. Child abuse in the medicine system. *Archives of Pediatric Medicine, 150,* 753–758.

Draucker, C. B., & Madsen, C. (1999). Women dwelling with violence. *Image: Journal of Nursing Scholarship, 31,* 327–332.

Ferree, M. M. (1990). Beyond separate spheres: Feminism and family research. *Journal of Marriage and the Family, 52,* 866–884.

Fonagy, P., & Target, M. (1995). Understanding the violent patient. *International Journal of Psychoanalysis, 76,* 487–502.

Fonagy, P., Target, M., & Gergely, G. (2000). Attachment and borderline personality disorder. *Psychiatric Clinics of North America, 23,* 103–122.

Ganley, A. L. (1998). Health care responses to perpetrators of domestic violence. In C. Warshaw & A. Ganley (Eds.), *Improving the health care response to violence: A resource manual for health care providers* (2nd ed., pp. 89–106). San Francisco: Family Violence Fund.

Goldner, V., Penn, P., Sheinberg, M., & Walker, G. (1990). Love and violence: Gender paradoxes in volatile attachments. *Family Process, 29,* 343–364.

Greenberg, E. M. (1996). Violence and the older adult: The role of the acute care nurse practitioners. *Critical Care Nursing Quarterly, 19,* 76–84.

Lachs, M. S., Williams, C. S., O'Brien, S., Pillemer, K. A., & Charlson, M. E. (1998). The mortality of elder mistreatment. *Journal of the American Medical Association, 280,* 428–432.

Liebshultz, J. M., Feinman, G., Sullivan, L., Stein, M., & Samet, J. (2000). Physical and sexual abuse in women infected with the human immunodeficiency virus. *Archives in Internal Medicine, 160,* 1659–1664.

Lorenz, K. (1966). *On aggression.* New York: Harcourt, Brace, & World.

Maxwell, M. G., & Widom, C. S. (1996). The cycle of violence: Revisited six years later. *Archives of Pediatric and Adolescent Medicine, 150,* 390–395.

McFarlane, J., & Parker, B. (1994). Abuse during pregnancy: A protocol for prevention and intervention. In *March of Dimes Training Manual.* White Plains, NY: March of Dimes.

Moss, H. B., Baron, D. A., Hardie, T. L., & Vanyukov, M. M. (2001). Preadolescent children of substance-dependent fathers with antisocial personality disorder: Psychiatric disorders and problem behaviors. *American Journal of Addictions, 10,* 269–278.

Moss, H. B., Lynch, K. G., Hardie, T. L., & Baron, D. A. (2002). Family functioning and peer affiliation in children of fathers with antisocial personality disorder and substance dependence: Associations with problem behaviors. *American Journal of Psychiatry, 159,* 607–614.

Oquendo, M. A., & Mann, J. J. (2000). The biology of impulsivity and suicidality. *Psychiatric Clinics of North America, 23,* 11–25.

Paris, J. (2000). Childhood precursors of borderline personality disorder. *Psychiatric Clinics of North America, 23,* 77–88.

Program Resources Department, American Association of Retired Persons (AARP), and Administration on Aging (AOA), U.S. Department of Health and Human Services. (1993). *A profile of older Americans.* Washington, DC: American Association of Retired Persons.

Scarpa, A., & Raine, A. (1997). Psychophysiology of anger and violent behavior. *Psychiatric Clinics of North America, 20,* 375–394.

Schechter, S. (1982). *Women and male violence: The visions and struggles of the battered women's movement.* Boston: South End.

Starr, D. H. (1988). Physical abuse of children. In V. B. Val Hasselt, R. L. Morrison, A. S. Bellack, & M. Hersen (Eds.), *Handbook of family violence* (pp. 119–155). New York: Plenum.

Steinmetz, S. K. (1993). The abused elderly are dependent. In R. J. Gelles & D. R. Luseke (Eds.), *Current controversies on family violence* (pp. 222–236). Newbury Park, CA: Sage.

Straus, M. A. (1973). A general systems theory approach to a theory of violence between family members. *Social Science Information, 12,* 105–125.

Tjaden, P., & Thoennes, N. (2000). *Full report of the prevalence, incidence, and consequences of violence against women.* Washington, DC: National Institute of Justice and the Centers for Disease Control and Prevention.

U.S. Department of Justice. (1998). *Violence by intimates: Analysis of data on crimes by current or former spouses, boyfriends, and girlfriends* (NCJ Publication No. NCJ 167237). Washington, DC: Author.

Walker, L. (1993). The battered woman syndrome is a psychological consequence of abuse. In R. J. Gelles & D. R. Luseke (Eds.), *Current controversies on family violence* (pp. 133–153). Newbury Park, CA: Sage.

Warshaw, C. (1998). Identification, assessment, and intervention with victims of domestic violence. In C. Warshaw & A. Ganley (Eds.) *Improving the health care response to violence: A resource manual for health care providers* (2nd ed., pp. 49–86). San Francisco: Family Violence Fund.

Widom, C. S. (1998). Childhood victimization: Early adversity and subsequent psychopathology. In B. P. Dohrenwend (Ed.) *Adversity, stress, and psychopathology* (pp. 81–95). New York: Oxford Press.

Widom, C. S. (1999). Posttraumatic stress disorder in abused and neglected children grown up. *American Journal of Psychiatry, 156,* 1223–1226.

World Health Organization. (1996). Prevention of violence: A public health priority. *Handbook of Resolutions, 3,* 111.

Yehuda, R. (2002). Clinical relevance of biologic findings of PTSD. *Psychiatric Quarterly, 73,* 123–133.

Yoshioka, M. R., & Dang, Q. (2000). *Asian family violence report: A study of the Chinese, Cambodian, Korean, South Asian, and Vietnamese communities in Massachusetts.* Boston: Asian Task Force Against Domestic Violence, Inc.

Glossary

Abstinence: Refers to avoidance of all substances with abuse potential. It denotes cessation of addictive behaviors, such as substance abuse/dependence.

Abulia: Functional errors of omission; failing to perform activities to meet basic human needs; inability to make decisions; lack of will or willpower.

Acalculia: Inability to do simple arithmetic calculations.

Acting Out: Overt behavioral expression of a wish or conflict whereby the person avoids the conscious experience of unresolved developmental issues.

Active Listening: A dynamic process that requires using all senses to assess verbal and nonverbal messages.

Acute Confusion: Refers to the cognitive phenomenon of delirium (rapid onset of a disturbance in consciousness and cognition) before the actual diagnosis is made.

Adaptation: Sustaining homeostasis; the ability to mobilize resources and adjust to demands of internal and external environments.

Addiction: A pattern of out-of-control or compulsive use of psychoactive substances in which use continues despite negative consequences; often used interchangeably with the terms chemical dependency or substance dependence.

Advanced Sleep Phase Syndrome (ASPS): A circadian rhythm disorder common in the older adult, with early bedtime and related early rising time, inability to remain asleep during the night, and the perception of being "out of sync" with the rest of the population. Associated with napping, which worsens the problem.

Advocacy: Defending a cause or pleading a case in another's behalf (Bloom & Asher, 1982); putting the interest of the client before the interest of the nurse.

Affect: Emotional display or observable behaviors that are the expression of an experienced, subjective feeling. Examples of affect are appropriate, blunted, flat, inappropriate, labile, restricted, or constricted.

After Care: Involves that care occurring after a person's discharge from the hospital.

Aggressive: Physical or verbal behavior that is forceful, hostile, or enacted to intimidate others.

Akathisia: Subjective feelings of restlessness and an inability to sit still resulting from dopamine blockade by certain neuroleptics; part of the extrapyramidal side effects.

Akinesia: A condition characterized by the inability to make voluntary movements.

Al-Anon: A self-help group for spouses, parents, or significant others of alcoholics.

Alcoholics Anonymous: An international self-help organization whose purpose is to help alcoholics achieve and maintain sobriety.

Alexithymia: Refers to a lack of introceptive awareness, mistrust of self and others, cognitive dysfunction, and starvation-induced depression.

Alogia: Inability to speak owing to a mental condition or a symptom of dementia.

Altered Sensory Perception: Refers to the physical and psychological changes that affect brain functioning, behavior patterns, and the five senses.

Alters: A distinct identity with its own enduring pattern of perceiving, relating to, and thinking about the world and the self.

Alzheimer's Disease (AD): A condition characterized by progressive loss of memory, intellect, language, judgment, and impulse control. Neurofibrillary tangle and neuritic plaques are found in the cerebral cortex, particularly the hippocampus.

American Association of Sex Educators, Counselors and Therapists (AASECT): A multidisciplinary national organization of professionals dedicated to the study, education, and role of spokesperson for sexuality.

Amygdala: A nucleus in the limbic system or medial temporal lobe that affects neuroendocrine and behavioral functions. It also plays a role in behaviors, including eating, drinking, and sexuality, and the emotions linked to these behaviors. It plays a role in the emotional significance of events or memories and governs the level of hippocampal activity accordingly. Consequently, a traumatic or overwhelming event is permanently etched into the memory, whereas irrelevant events are immediately ignored.

Analytic Worldview: Worldview perspective that espouses and values specific detail to time, calculation, individuality, and acquiring material objects as being important in life. and its habitants in the context of peace and tranquility.

Anhedonia: The inability to experience pleasure from activities that usually produce pleasurable feelings.

Anima: The female aspect of the male personality.

Animus: The masculine aspect of the female personality.

Anomia: Inability to recall or recognize names of objects.

Anorexia Nervosa (AN): Self-induced starvation resulting from fear of fatness; not caused by true loss of appetite.

Anxiety: An affect or emotion arising from stress or change accompanied by biological arousal, behavioral responses, and elements of apprehension, impending doom, and tension.

Anxiolytic Agent: A drug used for the relief of anxiety; also called antianxiety agent or mild tranquilizer.

Anxiolytic: Drug used to reduce anxiety, and is synonymous to the term sedative. Examples include benzodiazepines such as diazepam, lorazepam, and clonazepam.

Aphasia: Loss of power of expression by speech, writing, or signs of loss of comprehension of spoken or written language owing to brain injury or pathology.

Apraxia: Loss of ability to carry out familiar, purposeful movements in the absence of paralysis or other motor or sensory impairments, especially the inability to make proper use of an object.

Apraxic Agraphia: Inability to express oneself in writing due to apraxia.

Archetypes: Primordial images that serve as the building blocks of collective unconscious.

Asimultanagnosia: Inability to visually integrate the components of an ordinarily complex scene into a coherent whole.

Assertive Community Treatment (ACT): Refers to a model of mental health care that provides the client and family with many case management functions, including ongoing assessments, treatment planning, and monitoring of mental, physical, and social functioning. The precise approach varies, but an individual is generally designated as the broker of care or treatment coordinator. ACT programs are available 24 hours a day.

Assertiveness: Clearly communicating one's needs, desires, or beliefs directly and tactfully with self-confidence.

Attachment System: A system that is instinctual or motivational and, like hunger and thirst, integrates the infant's memory processes, prompting the child to satisfy them by interacting with the caregiver.

Attachment: A classic term for the primary tie between a child and her caregiver and a process seen as evolving and biologically adaptive and critical to emotional and physiological development and survival.

Attachment Theory: Theory based on the classic works of Bowlby and Ainsworth that define attachment or bonding as an evolutionary and biological process of eliciting and maintaining physical closeness between a child and a parent or primary caregiver. This theory also infers that the infant's relationships with early caregivers are responsible for influencing future interactions and relationships.

Aural Comprehension: Understanding of stimuli perceived by the ear.

Autism: Denotes the presence of abnormal and impaired development in social and communication skills and severely restricted activity and interests.

Autonomy: The ability of individuals to make independent personal decisions and act in their own behalf, recognizing the inherent value of each individual.

Avoidant Behavior: Refers to constricted social interaction with unfamiliar people or situations that activate intense anxiety reactions, resulting in excessive social impairment and interactions with others.

Avolition: A marked decrease in motivation and inattention.

Behavior Management Plans: A plan designed to reinforce positive and reduce negative behaviors through the use of visual cues, charts, communication tools, and reward systems.

Behavioral/Cognitive Model: Combines behavioral and cognitive therapies. That is, the behavioral model focuses on behaviors that present in the here and now, identification of maladaptive behaviors that will become targets for change, motivation for the behaviors, and reinforcers of the behaviors.

Beneficence: Doing good and avoiding doing harm.

Binge Drinking: Five or more drinks on the same occasion at least once in the past month (SAMHSA, 2000).

Binge: A period of uncontrolled eating in which a large amount of food is consumed unrelated to physical hunger.

Bioethics: Ethics applied to health care.

Bipolar: The two extreme mood states of mania and depression illustrated in bipolar disorder.

Body Dysmorphic Disorder: A chronic and debilitating mental health condition characterized by a preoccupation with imagined defect in appearance (e.g., a "large" nose, "thinning" hair, or facial "scarring").

Body Image: One's physical perception, sense of identity, strengths, and limitations.

Body Image Disturbance: Refers to a distortion in the image of the body that is of near or actual delusional proportions; may include strong feelings of self-loathing projected onto the body, body parts, or perceived fat.

Body Language: Nonverbal communication or transmission of messages by way of physical gestures.

Body Mass Index (BMI): Refers to a mathematical formula that is highly correlated with body fat. It is weight in kilograms divided by height in meters squared (kg/m2). In the United States and in the United Kingdom, people with BMIs between 25 and 30 kg/m2 are considered overweight and those with BMIs of 30 kg/m2 are categorized as obese.

Boundary: Refers to rules defining who and how members participate in a subsystem or a relationship. The clearer the boundary, the healthier the relationship.

Brain Lesion: A condition in which an abnormality is noted in the brain such as a tumor or hematoma. A potentially reversible dementia.

Bulimia Nervosa (BN): Binge eating followed by self-inflicted vomiting, laxative or diuretic abuse, or starvation.

Case Management: A model of comprehensive and holistic health care delivery that concentrates the responsibility for all care given to a client in one person or agency.

Case Manager: A collaborative director with a consumer in the management of her holistic care.

Cataplexy: Sudden loss of motor control while awake, usually occurring with strong emotions, associated with narcolepsy.

Catecholamine: Any of the sympathomimetic amines such as epinephrine, dopamine, and norepinephrine. These biochemicals play critical roles in the stress response.

Catharsis: The healthy release of ideas that helps the client gain insight into conflicts and early developmental turmoil.

Character: Learned personality traits that influence behavioral patterns.

Chemical Dependency: A pattern of out-of-control or compulsive use of psychoactive substances in which use continues despite negative consequences; a popular term often used interchangeably with the terms addiction or substance dependence.

Child Maltreatment: Refers to actions and behaviors that result in serious physical injury, neglect, sexual abuse, and serious mental injury to a child.

Chorea: The ceaseless occurrence of a wide variety of rapid, jerky but well-coordinated movements performed involuntarily.

Choreiform: Resembling chorea.

Chronic Fatigue Syndrome: A chronic and debilitating disorder characterized by chronic fatigue, flulike symptoms, muscle pain, headaches, and malaise lasting more than 24 hours.

Chronic Insomnia: Refers to insomnia that lasts more than 3 weeks.

Chronobiology: Field of science and medicine that explores the many bodily changes governed by the hours and the seasons; includes studies of cellular rhythms all the way through those of populations and ecosystems.

Circadian Rhythm: The variation in sleep tendency over a slightly greater than 24-hour period, associated with core temperature control, neurotransmitter and hormone secretion, and light or dark exposure.

Circumstantiality: A thought and speech process in which an individual digresses into unnecessary details and inappropriate unrelated thoughts while trying to express a central idea.

Civil Commitment: The ability of the state to hospitalize a person without consent.

Clarifying Technique: Act of clearing or making a message understandable.

Classic Conditioning: A form of learning in which existing responses are attached to new stimuli by pairing those stimuli with those that naturally elicit the response; also referred to as respondent conditioning.

Client Advocate: A person who tries to ensure that the rights of all prospective research subjects and actual subjects are adequately protected.

Closed System: In system's theory, this refers to a limited exchange of energy and information about the environment. Boundaries are often rigid and impermeable.

Cognitive: The mental process involved in obtaining knowledge, including the aspects of perceiving, thinking, reasoning, and remembering.

Cognitive Disorders: Those conditions in which "the predominant disturbance is a clinically significant deficit in cognition or memory that represents a significant change from a previous level of functioning" (APA, 2000).

Cognitive Processes: Higher cortical mental processes, including perception, memory, abstraction, and reasoning, by which one acquires knowledge, solves problems, employs judgment, and makes plans.

Cogwheeling: Refers to rigidity or rhythmic contractions noted on passive stretching of muscles, as occurs in Parkinson's disease.

Communication: The act of transmitting feelings, attitudes, ideas, and behaviors from one person to another.

Communication/Systems Model: Communication theory applied to group therapy that considers both the content of messages of the group members and the method of transmission of these messages. The systems model aspect of this type of group considers subgroups, boundaries, and communication within and between these groups in relation to the whole group.

Community Mental Health: A treatment approach that provides various levels of mental health, wellness, and illness services to individuals living within various community settings.

Community Mental Health Centers: Treatment facilities located within the community that provide different specialized levels and varieties of mental health care as well as coordination of physical and mental health care to any person needing mental health treatment.

Community Support Systems (CSS): Integrative approaches to quality mental health care for consumers that combine various types of mental health at the primary, secondary, and tertiary levels of care.

Community Worldview: Worldview perspective that espouses and values the importance and needs of the community over the individual in the context of transcendence and meditation in life.

Comorbidity: Psychiatric or physical disorder that occurs with a primary psychiatric disorder.

Competency: The ability of a person to perform certain tasks; to be able to understand legal proceedings and assist in that process.

Complementary Therapies: Refer to unconventional therapies that encompass a spectrum of practices and beliefs, including herbs, visual imagery, acupuncture, and massage therapy.

Compulsion: Repetitive, ritualistic, unrealistic behaviors used to neutralize or prevent discomfort of stressful events, circumstances or recurring thoughts, images, or impulses such as obsessions.

Conflict: The opposition of mutually exclusive impulses, desires, or tendencies; controversy or disagreement.

Confrontation: The act of pointing out contradictions or incongruencies among feelings, thoughts, and behaviors, specifically pointing out parts of the assessment or treatment process that are contradictory or confusing.

Congruent Communication: Refers to messages that do not contradict each other. Normally, these messages promote clear and consistent boundaries and roles and effective problem solving.

Constructional Praxis: Inability to copy simple drawings or reproduce patterns of blocks or matchstick constructions.

Consultation: Rendering of an expert opinion in response to a request.

Consumerism: A movement seeking to protect the rights of those acquiring a service (in this instance, mental health care) by requiring standards of effectiveness and safety.

Containment: A term for safety, food, shelter, and medical care issues in milieu therapy.

Content Analysis: The evaluation of themes and specifics about what was said during the group therapy session. Examples of content themes are sadness, loneliness, leisure time activities, and relationship issues.

Continuous Quality Improvement: A method of ensuring the adequacy of care developed by Deming and adopted by health care systems.

Continuum of Mental Health Care: Refers to a model that is distinct from one area of treatment planning and encompasses a comprehensive or multisystem perspective mental health care delivery model.

Conversion Disorders: Refer to unexplained physical manifestations or deficits affecting voluntary motor or sensory function that suggest a neurological or other underlying medical condition.

Coping: An effort to reduce tension by minimizing, replacing, and resolving uncomfortable feelings such as anxiety, anger, frustration, and guilt.

Countertransference: Refers to intense emotional reactions to the client stemming from the therapist's early childhood experiences.

Creutzfeldt-Jakob Disease (CJD): A syndrome of motor, sensory, and mental disturbances. There is widespread degeneration and atrophy of the cerebral cortex, basal ganglia, and thalamus. Course of disease months to years.

Crisis: A turning point, or acute emotional turmoil, that stems from developmental, biological, situational, or psychosocial stressors that momentarily render the person's normal coping mechanisms inadequate.

Crisis Intervention: Short-term, here-and-now focus intervention that alleviates the impact of crisis-generated stress, enhances coping and problem-solving skills, and mobilizes resources of affected clients.

Critical Thinking: Systematic and purposeful process of reasoning.

Critiquer of Research Findings: A person who evaluates research findings and determines the usefulness of these findings to nursing practice.

Cues: Internal and external response signals that, if noticed, predict when, where, and what response will occur.

Cultural Competence: Refers to the synthesis and modification of knowledge concerning people and groups into distinct standards, practices, and attitudes.

Culturally Bound Factors: Health ideas and behaviors that a person exhibits in relationship to his environment and everyday life functioning.

Culture: A person, group, or community's internal and external daily expression of their beliefs, values, and norms.

Culture of Nursing: The nursing profession's body of values, knowledge, beliefs, and practices, which form the bases of how individual nurses delineate their nursing roles and functions within health care environments.

Cycle of Violence: A dynamic described by some survivors of intimate partner abuse. The cycle begins with low levels of abuse, which build to an acutely abusive incident involving levels of violence higher than that of the abuse experienced on a regular basis. Following the acute violence, the perpetrator engages in actions designed to keep the relationship from ending, creating an "ideal" dynamic to keep the survivor involved. If there is no change in the abusive behaviors, the tension building stage begins again, leading to another cycle of acute violence.

Cyclothymia: A condition in which numerous periods of abnormally elevated, expansive, or irritable moods are experienced interspersed with periods of depressed mood. Neither mood state reaches the height nor depth to qualify as bipolar disorder.

Data Collector: A person who gathers information for a research study, such as obtaining information from research subjects.

Decade of the Brain: Proclamation by the United States Congress that explains mental illness as a disease of the brain. It underscores the significance of technological advances in neurobiology and genetics and their impact on understanding mental illness.

Decerebrate: A sign characterized by adduction and extension of the arms, pronated wrists, and flexed fingers. The legs are stiffly extended, with plantar flexion of the feet. This sign indicates upper brain stem damage and usually heralds neurological deterioration.

Declaration of Sexual Rights: A document that identifies 11 human rights stating sexuality is an integral part of the personality of every human being.

Decompensation: The exacerbation of mental disorder symptomatology that affects a person's everyday functioning ability.

Decorticate: A sign characterized by adduction and flexion of the arms, with wrists and fingers flexed on the chest. The legs are extended and internally rotated with plantar flexion of the feet. Most often, it results from cerebrovascular accident or head injury. It is a sign of corticospinal damage and carries a more favorable prognosis than decerebrate posture.

Defense Mechanisms: Unconscious self-protective processes that seek to protect the ego from intense and overwhelming feelings of affect and impulses.

Deinstitutionalization: The release of clients from public state mental health hospitals into the general community settings (e.g., group homes, residential facilities, with their families).

Delayed Sleep Phase Syndrome (DSPS): A circadian rhythm disorder, common in adolescence, with late sleep onset, and resultant desire to oversleep.

Delirium: A medical syndrome characterized by acute onset and impairment in cognition, perception, and behavior. Also known as acute confusion.

Delirium Tremens (DTs): The most serious form of alcohol withdrawal that can be potentially fatal; characteristic symptoms include profound confusion, disorientation, and autonomic arousal; also known as alcohol withdrawal delirium.

Delusion: A fixed false belief unchanged by logic.

Dementia: A condition manifested in the insidious development of memory and intellectual deficits, disorientation, and decreased cognitive functioning.

Denial: An assertion that an allegation is false.

Depersonalization: A person's subjective sense of feeling unreal, strange, unfamiliar, or emotionally numb.

Depression: A mental disorder marked by sustained alteration in mood in which there is loss of interest and pleasure, altered weight, concentration, and sleep disturbance.

Derealization: A subjective sense that one's environment is unreal or unfamiliar.

Desensitization: A cognitive-behavioral therapy technique developed by Joseph Wolpe that involves three steps: relaxation training, gradual or hierarchy exposure (using visual imagery or real situations) to an anxiety-provoking or fearful situation or object, and desensitization to the stimulus. This technique is useful in the treatment of phobias.

Disaster: Refers to a sudden, unexpected, and calamitous event that leads to great loss, damage, or destruction.

Disengagement: Implies that family boundaries are rigid or impermeable and distant.

Disruptive: To throw into disorder or confusion; to disturb a balance.

Dissociation: The separation of thoughts, feelings, or experiences from the normal stream of consciousness and memory.

Dissociative Disorders: A continuum of disorders experienced by individuals exposed to trauma, including depersonalization disorder, dissociative amnesia, dissociative fugue, and dissociative identity disorder. These disorders involve a disturbance in the organization of identity, memory, perception, or consciousness.

Distractibility: The inability to maintain attention, shifting from one area or topic to another with minimal provocation, or attention being drawn too frequently to unimportant or irrelevant external stimuli.

Distributive Justice: The concept that resources should be distributed equitably across society or a collective group.

Dopaminergic Pathway: Nerve fibers in the mesocortical area that project to the cortex and hippocampus regions of the limbic system.

Double-Bind Messages: Refers to transactions that involve a binder and a victim.

Drive: Instinctual urges and impulses arising from biological and psychological needs.

Drug Polymorphism: Contextual chemical factors involved in individuals' genetic responses to pharmacologic agents.

Dual Diagnosis: The co-occurrence of a substance-related disorder(s) and psychiatric disorder(s).

Dyad: A two-person relationship, such as husband-wife and father-child.

Dysarthria: Imperfect articulation of speech caused by muscular weakness resulting from damage to the central or peripheral nervous system.

Dysphoria: A prevailing mood state of sadness and depression.

Dystonia: Slow sustained muscle spasms of the trunk, neck, or limb; the result of dopamine blockade from neuroleptic (antipsychotic) medications.

Eating Disorder (ED): A general term for abnormalities in behavior toward food, growing out of fear of fatness and pursuit of excessive thinness.

Echolalia: Stereotyped repetition of another person's words or phrases.

Eclecticism: Implies that the therapist uses two or more theories to develop an effective treatment to meet a client's needs.

Ecological Worldview: Worldview perspective that a person espouses, values, and accepts in his role of interconnectedness and responsibility for the world

Ego Dystonic: Discomfort in the presence of a disordered mental state.

Ego: The part of the mind that mediates between external reality and inner wishes and impulses.

Ego Function: Intrapsychic processes that enable people to mediate stress and adaptation using various defense mechanisms.

Ego Syntonic: Personal comfort with symptoms that create discomfort in others.

Elder Abuse: Abuse of a person over 60 years of age, which may include physical abuse but also sexual, emotional, or financial abuse and abandonment.

Electroconvulsive Therapy: Electric current induction of seizures, primarily for treatment of mental disorders; used most frequently in depression.

Embodied Language: Refers to a "meaning-making phenomenon" occurring simultaneously in the overlap of the physical (i.e., blood pressure) and linguistic descriptors related to spoken language concerning the meaning of a specific event.

Emotional Lability: An affective disturbance characterized by excessive and inappropriate emotional response.

Empathy: Refers to putting oneself into the psychological frame of reference of another. It conveys an understanding of the client's situation without becoming emerged or overwhelmed by the experience.

Enculturation: Process by which a person accepts and internalizes another person's or group's worldview into or in place of his existing worldview.

Enmeshment: Implies overinvolvement or lack of separateness of family members.

Entrepreneur: An individual who organizes, manages, and risks assumption of a business venture or enterprise.

Entropy: The tendency to increase randomness by the degradation of energy; the running-down of a system.

Enuresis: Bedwetting after having been toilet trained; generally resolves by school age.

Equifinality: The sameness of the end result starting from various points.

Equilibrium: Refers to the capacity of a system to use available resources to manage and reduce tension and stress.

Erogenous Zone: Part of the body that is a source of pleasure such as the lips, mouth, genitals, and anus.

Eros: The instinct or drive for love.

Ethnicity: Categorical determination of a group whose members have a common social and cultural heritage that is passed from generation to generation.

Ethnopsychopharmacology: The study of intensity and duration (e.g., absorption, distribution, metabolism, and elimination) of psychotropic medications for different racial groups of individuals.

Euphoria: An exaggerated feeling of well-being, or elation.

Evidence-Based Practice: Refers to interventions for which there is substantial empirical evidence that they improve client outcomes.

Evoked Potential: A short train of large slow waves recorded from the scalp to reflect dendritic activity and influenced by many variables—a useful indicator of brain activity in the processing of information.

Excitement Phase: First phase of the human sexual response cycle in which vasocongestion builds in the man and woman.

Executive Function: Ability to set a goal, make decisions, and implement appropriate activities toward meeting that goal.

Existential/Gestalt Model: Facilitates people's self-actualization processes by helping them become more aware of their full potential, their alternatives or choices, and their feelings and emotions. The primary goal in this model is to help individual members take responsibility for their emotions and behaviors through the process of support and feedback.

Exponential Kinetics: A pharmacokinetic model in which a constant fraction of a drug is eliminated in a set unit of time.

Extended Care: Involves long-term, more intensive care for someone who has been discharged from the hospital.

Extrapyramidal Side Effects (EPS): Involuntary motor movements; and muscle tone side effects that result primarily from dopamine blockade by neuroleptic medications.

Eye Movement Desensitization and Reprocessing (EMDR): Involves asking the client to imagine an anxiety-provoking or traumatic memory. This technique is used to treat post-traumatic stress disorder by processing a traumatic experience in a non-threatening manner.

Family: Refers to a dynamic system of people living together who are united by meaningful emotional bonds.

Family Roles: Expected patterns or specific behaviors within a social context.

Family Structure: The manner in which a family adapts and maintains itself.

Family Therapy: Also a specialized intervention that is used to treat clients within a social context, rather than individually.

Feedback Mechanism: A process that permits exchange of energy and matter across various boundaries.

Fetal Alcohol Syndrome (FAS): Specific pattern of malformation seen in the offspring of women who consume alcohol during pregnancy.

Fibromyalgia Syndrome: A nonspecific condition whose primary symptoms include diffuse musculoskeletal pain, fatigue, distress, and sleep disturbances.

Fidelity: Keeping promises and obligations.

Flight of Ideas: Overproductive speech characterized by rapid shifting from one topic to another and fragmented ideas.

Focal Neurological Signs: Specific signs of neurological impairment such as blurred vision, aphasia, and the like.

Focusing: The act of clarifying a perception or spotlighting a specific aspect of communication.

Foster Care: An alternative living arrangement for underage persons who legally cannot or choose not to live with their biological families or guardians.

Free Association: The client's spontaneous expression of thoughts.

Freebase Cocaine: A purer form of cocaine produced by removing the water-soluble base; commonly referred to as "crack" or "rock" cocaine.

Functional Family System: Refers to open systems composed of individuals, couples, children, and communities who are able to adapt to change or crisis.

Gender: A psychosocial construct that changes over time and is distinct from sex, which is an individual's biological state of maleness or femaleness.

Gender Dysphoria: An intense, persistent discomfort resulting from one's own perception of the inappropriateness of sex assignment made at birth.

Genetic Vulnerability: The relationship between genetic and enzymatic defects and vulnerability to mental illness. Genetic function is influenced by prenatal and environmental factors that activate intricate biochemical processes and affect behavior. A number of researchers have attempted to explore the relationship between genetic factors and mental disorders using twin, adoption, and family studies.

Genogram: A family assessment tool that maps pictorial illustration of family history (generations).

Genomics: The study of the human genome sequencing and its contributions to disease and treatment.

G-proteins: Part of the cell's second messenger system in the plasma involved in sending signals from regulatory chemicals such as hormones and neurotransmitters to target cells.

Grandiosity: An inflated appraisal of one's worth, power, knowledge, importance, or identity and may include delusional thinking.

Gratification: To be satisfied; receive pleasure from.

Grief: A normal profound response to loss.

Group Home Treatment: A structured living environment in which persons live with other individuals who are at various stages of their recovery process.

Group Therapy: In mental health, a modality of treatment for more than one person that provides therapeutic outcomes for each individual.

Hallucinations: Refer to a false sensory perception occurring in the absence of an external stimulus.

Hardiness: Refers to a personality trait that enables people to maintain health and cope with stressful events.

Heavy Drinking: Five or more drinks on the same occasion on each of 5 or more days in the past month (SAMHSA, 2000).

Hippocampus: Located in the medial temporal lobe, it is an important site for the formation and storage of immediate and recent memories, and it is influenced by the amygdala emotional rating of an event. This part of the brain is damaged by Alzheimer's disease.

Holding Environment: A descriptive term for a therapeutic milieu that incorporates traditional milieu therapy variables. The term healing environment is sometimes used interchangeably with holding environment.

Homeostasis: Refers to a state of adaptation or ability to effectively manage internal and external environmental demands.

Hopelessness: A state of despondency and absolute loss of hope.

Hospice: Refers to end-of-life health care for clients.

Human Genome: The entire genetic information present in a human cell.

Human Sexual Response Cycle: Encompasses four distinct stages in which the body responds to sexual arousal.

Hydrotherapy: Refers to the continuous baths and cold wet-sheet packs used to produce a calming effect to control emotional and mental disturbances.

Hyperactivity: Extra active; having too much energy to handle. An activity level that is out of proportion for the situation, setting, and person's developmental level.

Hyperphagia: Excessive amount of eating.

Hypersomnia: Excessive amount of sleep.

Hypochondriasis: Refers to persistent preoccupation with fears of having, or the idea that one has, a serious disease based on the person's misinterpretation or exaggeration of bodily functions.

Hypomania: A clinical syndrome that indicates an elated mood state similar but less severe than that described by the term mania or manic episode; it generally does not cause social or occupational impairment and has a duration of more than 4 days.

Hypothalamus: Combined with the pituitary gland, thyroid gland, adrenal glands, gonads, and the pancreas, the hypothalamus forms the major regulatory system and is involved in the biological aspects of behavior. The hypothalamus-pituitary-adrenal axis (HPA) is important in understanding certain mental disorders. The hypothalamus regulates autonomic, endocrine, and visceral integration and is surmised to be the foundation of the limbic system and the brain center for emotions and certain behaviors such as eating, drinking, aggression, and sexuality. Information in the hypothalamus is modulated by ascending sensory pathways, hormones, and descending pathways of the cerebral cortex.

Id: The sum total of biological instincts, including sexual and aggressive impulses.

Identified Client: Refers to the client whose symptoms are the focus and serve as the reasons for seeking treatment.

Illusion: Refers to a misinterpretation of an external stimulus such as a shadow for a person.

Impulsivity: The act of spontaneous actions without thinking about consequences.

Inattention: A failure to focus attention on those elements of the environment that are most relevant to the task at hand.

Incongruent Communication: Occurs when more than one message is sent and the messages contradict each other.

Inferiority Complex: An exaggeration of feelings of inadequacy and insecurity resulting in defensiveness and anxiety.

Infradian Rhythms: Biological variations with a frequency lower than circadian (rhythms that have longer, slower cycles than circadian rhythms).

Insight: Refers to the client's self-awareness and understanding of the meaning and reason for his behavior or motives.

Insight-Oriented or Process-Oriented Groups: For individuals with high levels of cognitive functioning. Insight-oriented groups focus on the development of intellectual awareness, thinking patterns, and emotional factors influencing behavior.

Insomnia: Inability to fall asleep, difficulty staying asleep, or early morning awakening.

Insulin-Shock Therapy: Refers to administering large doses of insulin to induce marked hypoglycemia, which produces a coma or seizure.

Intensive Case Management: A concept similar to ACT that has shown to be cost-effective and efficacious in the treatment of serious mental illnesses.

Intergenerational Transmission of Violence: Describes the phenomenon of violent behaviors being learned and repeated by subsequent generations of abusive families.

Internalized Relationships: Those relationships that are maintained as supportive or destructive to the psyche and which continue to affect the individual long after the experience.

Intimate Partner Violence: Physical, sexual, or emotional and psychological abuse of men or women occurring in past or current intimate relationships, cohabiting or not, and including dating relationships.

Intracultural Variations: Alterations in cultural ideation and psychological or physical characteristics between persons from different racial and ethnic groups.

Intrapreneur: An individual who expands the traditional role as direct health care provider to that of creator of quality of care products and services within an institution or organization.

Involvement: Includes the basic milieu therapy concept of the client's responsibility to participate actively in treatment and other decision making.

Justice: Treating all people fairly and equitably.

Kindling: The electrophysiological process that over time produces an action potential after repetitive subthreshold stimulation or progressive sensitization of a neuron. This concept is thought to play a role in recurrent mood disorders.

Korsakoff's Syndrome: A psychosis that is usually based on chronic alcoholism, and which is accompanied by disturbance of orientation, susceptibility to external stimulation and suggestion, falsification of memory, and hallucinations.

Language: A complex phenomenon and tool used to communicate.

Leadership: The ability to show others the way by going in advance; to act as a guide for others.

Learning Disability: A condition that makes it difficult for a person to learn information in a usual manner.

Lethality: Level of dangerousness or injury.

Lewy Body: Proteinaceous structures composed of a central core with radiating filaments, located in the substantia nigra in Parkinson's disease and in the cortex in diffuse Lewy body disease.

Liaison: The facilitation of the relationships between the client, the client's illness, the consultee, the health care team, and the environment.

Libidinal Object Constancy: The maintenance of the image of the primary caretaker in the growing infant's memory so that the figure remains in the mind even when the object is not immediately present and interactive.

Libido: Urge or desire for sexual activity.

Life Expectancy: Refers to the age at which an individual born into a particular cohort is expected to die.

Life Span: The maximum age that could be attained if an individual were able to avoid or be successfully treated for all illnesses and accidents.

Light Therapy: A biological intervention that increases exposure to artificial light, whose intensity is equivalent to outdoor levels, more than 2,000 lux. The aim of therapy is to suppress melatonin secretion and produce phase shifts of melatonin production.

Linear Kinetics: A pharmacokinetic model in which a constant amount of drug is eliminated in a set unit of time.

Loose Association: Manifests as a flow of thoughts or ideas unrelated to each other and shift from one subject to another. They are often seen in clients with schizophrenia and other major psychotic disorders.

Malpractice: Intentional professional misconduct that fails to comply with professional standards and results in injury.

Mania: A disorder characterized by exalted feelings, delusions of grandeur, elevated mood, psychomotor overactivity, and overproduction of ideas.

Marital Schism: A term used to describe intense marital conflict in which a parent attempts to enlist a child as an ally against the other parent.

Marital Skew: Severe marital discord arising from acceptance of maladaptive behaviors in one partner by the other partner.

Maturational Crisis: Refers to developmental stages marked by biological, psychosocial, and social transitions that generate predictable and characteristic disturbances in behavior and emotional responses.

Melatonin: A metabolite of serotonin produced by the pineal gland. It is produced during darkness and is involved in the feedback loop that is regulated according to the degree of environmental light. Melatonin is implicated in the regulation of seasonal and circadian variance and in the body's adjustment to time zones, and it is a biological marker for the effects of light therapy in SAD.

Memory: A complex brain function that involves storing and retrieving information that is later recalled to consciousness.

Mental Disorder or Illness: Any health condition that is identified by a change in thinking, mood, or behavior and one that creates distress or problems with everyday functioning.

Mental Health: A relative state of well-being that enables persons, couples, families, and communities to adaptively respond to external and internal stressors.

Mental Health Movement: A movement that began more than 25 years ago that focuses on humane treatment of the mentally ill, initially advocating their release from state institutions to community mental health centers.

Mental Health Team: An interdisciplinary group of mental health staff who collaborate to assess, intervene, and evaluate client responses to treatment.

Mental Illness: A mental disorder or condition manifested by disorganization and impairment of function that arises from various causes such as psychological, neurobiological, and genetic factors.

Mental Status Examination (MSE): Refers to the part of the clinical assessment that compiles nursing observations and impressions of the client during the interview. Data from this exam include general appearance, mood and affect, speech patterns, perception, thought content and processes, level of consciousness and cognition, impulsivity, ability to abstract, judgment and insight, and reliability.

Metabolic Pathways: Chemical sites (e.g., acetylation, debrisoquine-ds, mephenytoin) that are involved in the conversion of pharmacologic agents within a person's biological system.

Milieu: Environment, from French for middle space, or a safe place.

Milieu Therapy: A treatment modality that uses the total physical and social environment as a therapeutic agent to provide psychosocial rehabilitation for psychiatric clients. Traditionally, milieu therapy includes key variables or components that are also defined here. The term is sometimes used interchangeably with the term therapeutic milieu.

Mixed State: A behavioral condition displayed for a period of at least 1 week in which manic and major depressive mood states are exhibited every day. Symptoms are sufficiently severe to cause impairment in social and occupational functioning.

Modeling: A form of learning in which a person observes another person perform a desired response.

Mood: Refers to the client's sustained emotional state that reflects the client's perception of the world—depressed, sad, labile, elated, expansive, or anxious.

Moral Treatment: Humane treatment of the mentally ill; for example, releasing clients from mechanical restraints and improving physical care. Phillippe Pinel, a French physician, and Benjamin Rush, an American physician, were instrumental in promoting this movement.

Morgan Russel Scales: A widely used measure of outcome for anorexia nervosa that consists of two scores: an average outcome score and a general outcome score. The average outcome score is based on the outcome in five areas: nutritional status, menstrual function, mental state, sexual adjustment, and socioeconomic status.

Multi-infarct Dementia (MID): A probable irreversible dementia caused by many small strokes, or a large stroke.

Myoclonus: Shocklike contractions of a portion of a muscle, an entire muscle, or a group of muscles, restricted to one area of the body or appearing synchronously or asynchronously in several areas.

Narcolepsy: A rare disorder of chronic daytime sleepiness, cataplexy, and sleep paralysis. No amount of normal sleep ameliorates the disorder; individuals have disturbed nocturnal sleep, including vivid dreams, nightmares, or night terrors, or both.

National Institute of Mental Health: A federally funded agency whose goals include developing and helping various states to identify and use the most effective methods of prevention, diagnosis, and intervention of mental illnesses through research funding and staff development and education of mental health professionals to provide mental health treatment.

Negative Symptoms: Denote schizophrenic symptoms associated with structural brain abnormalities. Most negative symptoms include blunted affect, inability to experience pleasure, apathy, a lack of feeling, and impaired attention.

Negentropy: The counterforce to entropy; the evolving or more complete organization, complexity, and ability to convert resources.

Neglect: The failure to provide for the individual's basic needs for subsistence, including food, housing, clothing, education, medical care, and emotional care. At its most extreme, neglect results in death, especially in the older adults and in very young children.

Negligence: Unintentional injury that results from failure to act as a reasonable person would.

Neuritic Plaques: A patch or flat area of neurons.

Neurobiology: Biology of the nervous system, particularly the brain.

Neuroendocrinology: The study of how the neural and endocrine systems work together to maintain homeostasis. Communication between these systems is involved in biological and behavioral responses. Major organs of the neuroendocrine system are the hypothalamus, the pituitary, thyroid, and adrenal glands; the gonads; and the pancreas.

Neurofibrillary Tangles: Tangles of the neurofibril, the delicate threads running in every direction through the cytoplasm of the body of a nerve and extending into the axon and the dendrites of the cell.

Neuroleptic: Psychotropic medication; major tranquilizers; synonymous with antipsychotic or neuroleptic agent.

Neuroleptic Malignant Syndrome (NMS): A rare and potentially life-threatening syndrome primarily caused by antipsychotic medications and characterized by marked muscle rigidity, high fever, altered consciousness or delirium, tachycardia, hypoxia, hypertension, and diaphoresis.

Neuroscience: The science and study of the central nervous system.

Neurotransmitters: Biochemicals found in the central nervous system involved in the transmission of impulses across the synapses between neurons.

Neurovegetative: Refers to biological functions such as sleep pattern, eating pattern, energy level, sexual functioning, and bowel functioning.

Non-rapid Eye Movement (NREM) Sleep: Four stages of sleep occur: Stage I is light sleep; Stage II, eye movements are minimal or absent; Stages III and IV, slow EEG wave activity, with difficulty in arousal.

Non-Restorative Sleep: Associated with fatigue, difficulty awakening, poor concentration, and low productivity.

Nonverbal Communication: Refers to body language or transmission of messages without the use of words.

Normal Pressure Hydrocephalus (NPH): A condition in which the cerebral spinal fluid pressure reading is normal or high normal, but excessive fluid exists in the ventricles of the brain.

Nurse-Client Relationship: A dynamic, collaborative, therapeutic, interactive process between the nurse and the client.

Nursing Diagnosis: A statement of the client's nursing problem that includes both the adaptive or maladaptive health response and contributing stressors.

Nursing Informatics: The use of computers and information sciences to manage and process data, knowledge, and information in nursing practice and client care.

Nursing Process: An interactive, problem-solving process; a systematic and individualized problem-solving approach for administering nursing care that meets the client's needs comprehensively and effectively.

Object Relations: Internalized relationships recollected from early primary caregivers.

Obsession: Intrusive, recurrent, and persistent thoughts, impulses, or images.

Ocular Apraxia: Inability to voluntarily direct their gaze to a target of visual interest.

Open Communication: Active and honest sharing of feelings, thoughts, and information. Confidentiality is unit based and unhealthy secret keeping is discouraged, but privacy is respected.

Open System: In systems' theory, a term used to imply that members or parts are interrelated and responsive to each other's needs.

Operant Conditioning: A type of learning in which responses are modified by their consequences. Reinforcement increases the likelihood of future occurrences of the reinforced response; punishment and extinction decrease the likelihood of future occurrences of the responses they follow.

Optic Ataxia: The inability to benefit from visual guidance in reaching for an object.

Orgasm Phase: Third phase of the human sexual response cycle in which men and women experience rhythmic contractions followed by extreme pleasure.

Orientation: Refers to one's sense of time, person, or place.

Overarousal: To be excessively excited or stimulated.

Pain Disorder: Disorder whose major symptom is pain in one or more anatomical sites. It is the predominant focus of the clinical presentation and is of sufficient severity that necessitates clinical attention. It also produces significant distress that results in impaired occupational, interpersonal, and social performance.

Palliative Care: Combines the use of culturally competent, compassionate, therapeutic, and supportive therapies for persons who are diagnosed with a life-threatening disorder and for their families or significant others.

Paradoxical Reactions: A response to a drug that is opposite to what would be predicted by the drug's pharmacology.

Paraphasia: Speech defect characterized by disorderly arrangements of spoken words.

Parasomnias: Also called arousal disorders; include nightmares or night terrors, sleepwalking, and confusion with arousal.

Paresthesia: Unnatural tactile sensations manifested by tingling, tickling, or creeping sensations that have no physical basis. This sensation often results from activation of the hypothalamic-pituitary-adrenal axis.

Parkinson's Disease: The chronic condition marked by rigidity, tremor with intention. Pathology in the substantia nigra.

Partial Hospitalization/Day Treatment: A specific time-defined, outpatient, active psychiatric treatment program that is grounded in therapeutic communication and structured clinical services.

Patterns: A person's typical behavioral organization that resists change.

Pedophile: An adult who is sexually attracted to children and who abuses them sexually.

Perpetrator: A person who inflicts abuse or injury on another.

Persona: A disguised or masked attitude useful in interacting with one's environment but frequently at variance with one's true identity.

Personal Boundaries: A mental idea of how one experiences and maintains a line of separation between oneself and the world.

Personal Space: A subjective definition of comfortable space between one person and another.

Personality: Characteristic traits that are generally predictable in their influence on cognitive, affective, and behavioral patterns.

Pharmacodynamics: The study of biochemical and physiological actions and effects of drugs.

Pharmacokinetics: The study of a drug's absorption, distribution, metabolism, and excretion or elimination.

Pharmacology: The scientific study of chemical formulations (drugs), including their sources, properties, uses, actions, and effects.

Phase Advancing: A response to a light stimulus that is intentionally presented hours before the expected onset of solar or wavelength of environmental light.

Phase Delaying: Refers to a response elicited by a light stimulus presented hours later than expected.

Phase-Specific Community-Oriented Intervention: Those that target specific symptoms during various stages of treatment within an intensive case management model, specifically persons with first-episode psychosis.

Phobia: An exaggerated or irrational fear of an event or object, such as a presentation or spider, respectively.

Phonemic: Speech sounds that are the basic units of speech (e.g., "leviator" instead of "elevator," or grontologs" instead of "gerontology").

Physical Abuse: Involves the intentional use of physical force against another person, including, but not limited to pushing, slapping, biting, choking, punching, beating, and using a gun, knife, or other weapon.

Pick's Disease (PD): A rare, fatal degenerative disease of the nervous system, occurring mostly in middle-aged women. Characterized by signs of severe frontal or temporal lobe dysfunction. Overall symptomatology is very similar to Alzheimer's disease.

Plateau Phase: Second phase of the human sexual response cycle marked by vasocongestion and myotonia.

Play Therapy: An individualized intervention that offers children a symbolic way to express feelings, anxiety, aggressions, and self-doubt.

Positive Symptoms: Refer to schizophrenic symptoms with good premorbid functioning, acute onset, and positive response to typical and atypical antipsychotics. Common positive symptoms include hallucinations, delusions, disorganized thinking and speech, and gross behavioral disturbances. These symptoms are linked with dysregulation of biochemical processes.

Potentially Reversible Dementia: A condition characterized by an acute onset, causing neurological symptoms and changes in level of consciousness. If treated in time, the condition may be reversed. See delirium.

Praxis: The performance of an action; "doing."

Preoccupation: Refers to recurrent thoughts or centers on a particular idea or thought with an intense emotional component.

Pressured Speech: Disturbance in verbal expression of thought characterized by an overproduction of rapid speech that is frequently loud, unsolicited by social inter-action, and difficult to interrupt.

Primary Appraisal: Refers to initial responses to a stressor and the ultimate goal of pre-vailing over or effectively managing a given situation.

Primary Prevention: Includes those strategies and interventions that reduce a person's risk to develop mental illness.

Principal Investigator: A person who takes the major role in the development and conduct of a research study.

Probable Irreversible Dementia: Progressive loss of intellectual functioning caused by permanent brain damage.

Process: Refers to the manner in which clients talk about themselves and the way the group responds. Analysis of group process provides assessment of the therapy's effects on individual group members.

Progressive Relaxation: A form of relaxation training that involves visualizing and sequentially relaxing specific muscle groups, starting with the scalp to the tips of the toes. This technique involves teaching the client to tense and relax various muscle groups in an effort to reduce tension and stress.

Prosody: The variations in stress, pitch, and rhythms of speech that convey meanings.

Prosopagnosia: Inability to recognize faces.

Protein Kinase C (PKC): A group of enzymes that activate other enzymes.

Pseudoaddiction: A syndrome of behaviors resembling addiction that develops in chronic pain management; with adequate pain management, drug-seeking behaviors cease.

Pseudomutuality: A transaction that infers a sense of relatedness and emotional connectedness; in reality, it represents shallow and empty relationships.

Psyche Organizers: Repetitive developmental experiences that guide the person's experience and expectations resulting in the style of reaction that is typical of that person.

Psychoanalysis: A form of psychodynamic psychotherapy in which the therapist and client explore the client's conscious and unconscious conflicts and coping patterns.

Psychodynamic Model: A model of group therapy in which the problems of the members of a group are viewed as similar to the problems a person would present in individual therapy. That is, the problems of the people in the group are conceptualized to center on unconscious conflicts and basic love-hate instincts (constructive versus destructive forces). Freudian theory of psychoanalysis is the underlying foundation for psychodynamic therapy.

Psychoeducational Group: Group that offers information to a large number of people simultaneously, providing both information and emotional support. Persons who are motivated to learn about their illness or to develop self-awareness benefit from this type of group.

Psychological Abuse: Usually verbal abuse designed to control another through use of intimidation, degradation, or fear.

Psychological Autopsy: A standard procedure following a suicide that involves team members presenting and discussing the case with other staff with the intent of evaluating issues of quality of care and learning from the experience. It also offers an opportunity for staff to process their feelings and thoughts about the tragedy.

Psychomotor Retardation: A slowing of physical and emotional reactions, including speech, affect, and movement.

Psychoneuroimmunology: The study of the role of the immune system in health and illness in the face of biological and psycho-social stress. This field is a developing knowledge about the interconnectedness of the nervous system and the immune system.

Psychophysiologic Insomnia (PI): Refers to complaints of difficulty attaining or maintaining sleep during a normal sleep period.

Psychophysiological Disorder: Denotes emotional states producing or exacerbating physical problems.

Psychosis: A person's symptom state that refers to the presence of reality misinter-pretations, disorganized thinking, and lack of awareness regarding true and false reality.

Psychosocial Assessment: Refers to the data collection process that includes major elements such as psychosocial, biological, cultural, and spiritual data collections.

Psychosocial Rehabilitation: Refers to health services whose goal is to restore the client's ability to function in the community through social interaction, independent living, and vocational enhancement.

Psychostimulants: A class of medications that temporarily increases the functioning activity of the brain.

Psychosurgery: Surgical or chemical alteration involving severing brain fibers with the purpose of modifying behavioral disturbance, thoughts, or mood.

Psychotherapy: A global process in which people seek professional help to resolve problems, promote personal growth, and reduce or eliminate maladaptive responses.

Psychotropics: Various pharmacologic agents, such as antidepressants and antipsychotic, antimanic, and antianxiety agents used to affect behavior, mood, and feelings.

Purge: Self-induced vomiting or misuse of laxative, diuretics, or enemas.

Qualitative Research: Research that focuses on the meaning of the experiences to individuals rather than on the generalizability of study results.

Quantitative Research: Research that focuses on gathering numerical data, with the intent of generalizing the findings of the study.

Race: Taxonomy of a group's identity based on genetic factors that produce physical characteristics and distinguish the persons within that group from persons within another group.

Racing Thoughts: A rapid series of ideas that occur during manic episodes.

Rapid Cycling: A type of bipolar disorder characterized by at least four episodes of depression, mania, or mixed states each year.

Rapid Eye Movement (REM) Sleep: Associated with relative paralysis of skeletal muscles, rapid eye movement, penile erection, and dreaming.

Rapport: Refers to harmony or accord between people.

Reality Principle: A perception of the environment that fairly matches what others perceive and which fosters adaptive responses toward productivity, enjoyment of life, and maintenance of homeostasis.

Recovery: A state of physical and psychological health in which abstinence from dependency producing drugs is complete and comfortable (American Society of Addiction Medicine, 1982).

Reinforcement: In classical conditioning, the process following the conditioned stimuli with the unconditioned stimulus; in operant conditioning, the rewarding of desired responses.

Reinforcers: Personal, complex, learned, and biochemical rewards that are used to modify maladaptive behavior. Reinforcers can be positive, negative, or punishing, and are personally determined.

Relapse: Use of psychoactive substances after a maintained period of abstinence.

Relational Resilience: Refers to the family's ability to mobilize resources and confront psychosocial and biological stresses effectively using adaptive coping responses.

Relational Worldview: Worldview perspective that espouses and values the development of interactions, relationships, and spirituality as a contextual importance in life.

Repression: An unconscious process that removes anxiety-producing thoughts, desires, or memories from the conscious awareness.

Resolution Phase: Fourth phase of the human sexual response cycle in which the body returns to an unaroused state.

Restless Leg Syndrome (RLS)/Periodic Limb Movement Disorder (PLMD): Motor movement during sleep characterized during the day by akathesia, which is the inability to sit still, and a "deep uneasy" feeling in the legs, as well as aching, and "crazy legs," which is uncommon in the daytime, with an onset in the evening or at bedtime; associated with renal failure and iron deficiency anemia.

Restorative Sleep: Refers to sleep that restores normal brain activity and equilibrium in the central nervous system and bodily processes.

Ruminations: Repetitive or continuous thinking about a particular subject that then interferes with other thought processes.

Scapegoating: A form of displacement that involves blaming a member for the actions of others.

Schemata: Cognitive structures, or patterns, that consist of the person's beliefs, values, and assumptions.

Seasonal Affective Disorder: Recurrent depression that occurs during winter months and remits in the spring. Major symptoms include depressive mood, hypersomnia, tiredness, increased appetite, and cravings for carbohydrates.

Secondary Appraisal: Emerges with any form of perceived threat or harm if primary appraisals are ineffective or maladaptive. The rationale for secondary appraisal is to assess coping resources, options, and choices.

Secondary Gain: Attempting to earn the sympathy of others, receiving financial gain, or obtaining other benefits by suffering from a disorder.

Secondary Prevention: Refers to measures or interventions used to curtail disease processes.

Sedative: Drugs that are virtually synonymous to anxiolytics; used to calm nervousness, irritability, or excitement; these agents depress the central nervous system and tend to cause lassitude and reduced mental activity.

Self-Deprecatory Ideas: Negative thoughts about the self.

Self-Destructive Behavior: Behavior that tends to harm or destroy self.

Self-Disclosure: Exposing oneself to others; to make publicly known.

Self-efficacy: Refers to the expectation that one can effectively cope with and master situations, such as addictions, achieving desired outcomes through one's own personal efforts.

Self-Mutilation: The act of self-induced pain or tissue destruction void of the intent to kill oneself.

Semantic Paraphasia: Substituting a similar word for an object, e.g., "staple" for "paper clip."

Semantic Precision: Use of words appropriate or significant to the meaning of the intended communication, i.e., substituting "machine" for "automobile."

Separation Anxiety: Refers to a common childhood and adolescent anxiety disorder whose symptoms involve panic or intense fear of losing one's primary caregivers.

Serious Disabling Mental Disorders (SDMD): A term used to describe a person who has the diagnosis of schizophrenia, depressive disorders, and/or bipolar disorder.

Serotonin Syndrome: A condition characterized by serotonergic hyperstimulation that includes restlessness, hyperthermia, myoclonus, hypertension, hyperreflexia, diaphoresis, lethargy, confusion, and tremor and which may cause death.

Sexual Abuse: Abusive sexual contact, completed or attempted, against the will of the other, or in circumstances in which the other is unable to understand, refuse, or communicate unwillingness to engage in the sexual activity.

Sexual Attitude Reassessment (SAR): An intensive 2-day workshop to assist participants in reevaluation of sexual attitudes.

Sexual Desire: One's internal psychological state of pleasure governed by sexual pleasure centers in the brain.

Sexual Health: Integration of the somatic, emotional, intellectual, and social aspects of sexual being in ways that are positively enriching and that enhance personality, communication, and love (WHO, 1975).

Sexual Orientation: Sexual preference for erotic partners of the same, opposite, or either sex. An individual may be heterosexual, homosexual, lesbian, bisexual, or asexual.

Shadow: Carl Jung's term that refers to the unconscious.

Short-Term Hospitalization: A structured, inpatient treatment that provides clinical services, psychotherapy, counseling, and monitoring of physical, mental, and pharmacologic status.

Sick Role: Dependent, helpless, and ill behavior often associated with control and maintenance of maladaptive relationships.

Situational Crisis: Refers to unexpected crisis that arises from several sources, including environmental, physical or personal, or psychosocial.

Sleep Apnea: Various disorders arising from respiratory obstruction to cessation; associated with decreased oxygenation, fragmented sleep, and increased risk for injury, particularly with coexisting medical disorders such as chronic obstructive pulmonary disease (COPD), congestive heart failure (CHF), coronary artery disease (CAD), and myocardial infarction (MI). Characterized by snoring, gasping, or absence of breathing.

Sleep Cycles: Composed of cycles of REM and NREM sleep, with REM sleep occurring every 1 to 2 hours in normal situations.

Sleep Deprivation: Chronic lack of sleep, but may occur acutely, inability to get the needed 8.3 hours of sleep nightly.

Sleep Paralysis: Associated with narcolepsy, inability to move or speak just after or before awakening; breathing is not affected.

Sleepiness to Somnolence: Hypersomnia, common in shift workers, jet lag, and sleep disorders; individuals are likely to fall asleep if there is no stimulating or stressful activity occurring. Characterized by sleepiness, fatigue, poor concentration and memory lapses, depression, motor vehicle accidents (MVA), or on-the-job injuries.

Sleep-Wake Cycle: One of the body's biological rhythms normally determined by the day-night cycle.

Somatic Preoccupation: Excessively focused on one's own body functioning.

Somatization Disorder: Refers to a disorder whose primary symptoms are progressive, recurrent, and somatic complaints of pain, sexual, gastrointestinal (GI), and pseudo-neurological manifestations. These symptoms produce significant distress, and global disability.

Somatoform: Refers to a group of psychiatric disorders whose symptoms are severe enough to cause global impairment or functioning. Typically, these clients present with recurring, multiple, clinically significant somatic complaints. In addition, these complaints are colorful and exaggerated, but lack specific factual information to support the diagnosis.

Speech: The process of expressing ideas, thoughts, and feelings through language; use of words and language.

Spiritual Assessment: Process involving gathering data concerning the client's belief system, affirmation coping mechanisms, and psychosocial resources.

Spirituality: A dynamic phenomenon that enables a person to discover meaning and purpose in life, particularly during stressful life events.

Splitting: The internal mechanism wherein the person is unable to evaluate, synthesize, and accept imperfections in others so that a significant other is viewed as all good or all bad, and causing the phenomenon of setting persons up against each other.

Steady State: The state whereby the amount of drug eliminated from the body equals the amount being absorbed.

Stress Debriefing: A crisis intervention technique that relies on three therapeutic modalities: provide an opportunity to express one's feelings in the context of group support, facilitate normalization of reactions to an abnormal event, and learn about postdisaster reactions.

Stress: A stimulus or demand that has the potential to generate disruption in homeostasis or produce a reaction.

Substance Abuse: Repeated intentional use or misuse of a psychoactive substance; use is modified or discontinued with the occurrence of significant adverse consequences.

Substance Dependence: The accepted diagnostic term for a pattern of out-of-control or compulsive use of psychoactive substances in which use continues despite negative consequences; often used interchangeably with the terms addiction or chemical dependency.

Substance Intoxication: Substance-specific physical, psychological, and cognitive effects produced as a result of ingesting a psychoactive substance.

Subsystem: A smaller system within larger systems.

Suicidal Ideation: A thought or idea of suicide.

Suicidal Intent: Refers to the degree to which the person intends to act on his suicidal ideations.

Suicidal Threat: Verbalization of imminent self-destructive action, which, if carried out, has a high probability of leading to death.

Suicide: The act of killing oneself.

Superego: The part of the personality structure that evolves out of the ego and reflects early moral training and parental injunctions.

Switching: The process in which one alter is changed into another.

Synaptic Transmission: The process of nerve impulse transmission through the generation of action potentials from one neuron to another.

Tangentiality: A speech pattern that illustrates an inability to respond completely in a focused manner. Individuals may begin to respond appropriately but progress to related topics, never completing the originally desired response.

Tardive Dyskinesia: A complex range of involuntary movements associated with long-term and usually high-potency neuroleptic treatment. A chronic, progressive, and potentially fatal syndrome from prolonged dopamine blockade by neuroleptic medications. Major manifestations include choreiform movements of the face, tongue, upper and lower extremities, such as tongue movement or protrusion, lip sucking, chewing, and smacking; other symptoms include puffing of cheeks and pelvic thrusting.

T-cells: Viral- and tumor-fighting lymphocytes (all called natural killer cells) of the immune system. They are referred to as "T" cells because they are processed by the thymus gland.

Termination: The final phase of psychotherapy. This process involves exploring areas of accomplishment, goal attainment, and feelings generated by ending the relationship.

Tertiary Prevention: Refers to measures that minimize relapse and chronic disability, and restore the client to an optimal level of functioning.

Thanatos: The instinct toward death and self-destruction.

Theory: An organized and systematic set of statements related to significant questions in a discipline. Theories describe, explain, predict, or prescribe responses, events, situations, conditions, or relationships. Theories consist of concepts that are related to each other.

Therapeutic Alliance: Refers to a trusting relationship that helps the client explore interpersonal and intrapersonal conflicts and gain insight into maladaptive behaviors.

Therapeutic Communication: A healing or curative dialogue between people.

Therapeutic Factors: The standards for the conduct of group therapy. They include the following: imparting of information, instillation of hope, universality, altruism, corrective recapitulation of the primary family group member, development of socializing skills, imitative behavior, interpersonal learning, group cohesiveness, catharsis, and existential factors.

Therapeutic Use of Self: An intervention that involves self-awareness, empathy, acceptance, self-disclosure, and other means of facilitating a therapeutic relationship.

Thought Content: Refers to the content of the client's thoughts that may include

preoccupations, obsessions, compulsions, suicidal or homicidal ideations, and delusions.

Thought Process: Refers to the client's form of thinking or organization; examples include flights of ideas, phobias, tangentiality, circumstantiality, and racing thoughts.

Tolerance: A pharmacologic property of some abused substances in which increased amounts over time are required to achieve similar results as in earlier use.

Tort: Unintentional or intentional injury.

Traits: Personality structure that typifies a person's responses in various situations.

Transactional: Refers to a set of pattern interactions among family members.

Transference: Refers to unconscious displacement or reenactment of feelings and attitudes from the client to the psychotherapist.

Transgendered: Arching term that describes transsexuals, whose sense of themselves clashes with their original biological sex: cross-dressers, and others whose appearance is at odds with traditional gender expectations.

Transsexual: An individual who is profoundly unhappy in the sex assignment made at birth, and who seeks to change or has changed the body to be as much as possible like that of the opposite sex.

Trauma: An event that results in long-standing distress to the individual experiencing that event.

Triangulation: A term that describes a maladaptive triad transactional pattern.

Twin Studies: Researchers attempt to explore the relationship between genetic factors and mental disorders using these studies that usually include monozygotic or single ovum and dizygotic or two ova twins. Twin studies are helpful in isolating genetic and environmental influences and determining preventive and precipitating factors.

Type A Personality: A constellation of personality traits, such as highly driven, time-conscious, and competitive behavior, associated with high risk for coronary artery disease.

Type B Personality: A constellation of personality traits opposite from Type A and manifested by "easy-going, laid-back, and reposed" behavior.

Untradian Rhythms: Biological variations with a frequency higher (less than 24 hours) than circadian (rhythms that have shorter, faster cycles than circadian rhythms). Biological rhythms refer to cyclic variations in biological and biochemical function, activity, and emotional state.

Utilizer of Research Findings: A person who integrates research findings into clinical practice.

Validation: Affirmation of the client's individuality and right to be treated with respect and dignity.

Veracity: Telling the truth; honesty.

Verbal Memory: Ability to remember speech.

Visual Imagery: Refers to a stress or anxiety-reducing cognitive exercise that involves creating relaxing thoughts or visual images or place of serenity and calmness.

Visual Memory: Ability to remember what is seen.

Visuospatial Ability: Refers to time and space.

Vulnerability: The potential susceptibility of a person, family, or group to a health deviation.

Wernicke's Encephalopathy: A reversible delirium seen in alcoholics; it is associated with thiamine deficiency.

Wernicke-Korsakoff Syndrome: A complication of Wernicke's encephalopathy characterized by profound memory impairment and an inability to learn new material.

Withdrawal Syndrome: Substance-specific signs and symptoms precipitated by the abrupt cessation or reduction of a substance that produces tolerance and dependence after prolonged use.

World Association for Sexology (WAS): An international association of sexologists, researchers, and policy makers who develop international policies related to sex.

Worldview Perspective: A person's belief regarding what he considers to be true and valued.

Zeitgeber: A synchronizer or periodic environmental stimulus that is the dominant factor in determining a rhythm.

Index